2013
YEAR BOOK OF
ONCOLOGY®

The 2013 Year Book Series

Year Book of Critical Care Medicine®: Drs Dries, Zanotti-Cavazzoni, Latenser, Martinez, Rincon, and Zwank

Year Book of Emergency Medicine®: Drs Hamilton, Bruno, Handly, Minczak, Quintana, and Ramoska

Year Book of Endocrinology®: Drs Schott, Apovian, Clarke, Eugster, Meikle, Oetgen, Ovalle, Schteingart, and Toth

Year Book of Hand and Upper Limb Surgery®: Drs Yao, Adams, Isaacs, and Rizzo

Year Book of Medicine®: Drs Barker, Garrick, Gersh, Khardori, LeRoith, Panush, Talley, and Thigpen

Year Book of Neonatal and Perinatal Medicine®: Drs Fanaroff, Benitz, Donn, Neu, Papile, and Van Marter

Year Book of Neurology and Neurosurgery®: Drs Klimo, Minagar, Gandhi, Liu, Panagariya, Rezania, Riel-Romero, Riesenburger, Robottom, Schwendimann, Shafazand, and Yang

Year Book of Obstetrics, Gynecology, and Women's Health®: Drs Dungan and Shulman

Year Book of Oncology®: Drs Arceci, Chiorean, Lawton, Murphy, Thigpen, and Tsao

Year Book of Ophthalmology®: Drs Rapuano, Cohen, Flanders, Hammersmith, Milman, Myers, Nagra, Nelson, Penne, Pyfer, Sergott, Shields, Talekar, and Vander

Year Book of Orthopedics®: Drs Morrey, Huddleston, Rose, Swiontkowski, and Trigg

Year Book of Otolaryngology-Head and Neck Surgery®: Drs Sindwani, Balough, Franco, Gapany, and Mitchell

Year Book of Pathology and Laboratory Medicine®: Drs Raab and Bissell

Year Book of Pediatrics®: Dr Stockman

Year Book of Plastic and Aesthetic Surgery™: Drs Miller, Boehmler, Gosman, Gutowski, Ruberg, Salisbury, and Smith

Year Book of Psychiatry and Applied Mental Health®: Drs Talbott, Ballenger, Buckley, Frances, Krupnick, and Mack

Year Book of Pulmonary Disease®: Drs Barker, Jones, Maurer, Spradley, Tanoue, and Willsie

Year Book of Sports Medicine®: Drs Shephard, Cantu, Feldman, Galea, Jankowski, Janssen, Lebrun, and Nieman

2013

The Year Book of ONCOLOGY®

Editor-in-Chief

Robert J. Arceci, MD, PhD

Professor, Department of Child Health, University of Arizona, College of Medicine – Phoenix; Director, Children's Center for Cancer and Blood Disorders, Hematology/Oncology Co-Director of the Ron Matricaria Institute of Molecular Medicine at Phoenix Children's Hospital, University of Arizona, College of Medicine – Phoenix, Phoenix, Arizona

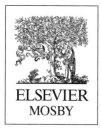

ELSEVIER
MOSBY

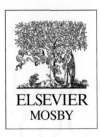

ELSEVIER
MOSBY

Vice President, Global Medical Reference: Mary Gatsch
Editor: Yonah Korngold
Production Supervisor, Electronic Year Books: Donna M. Skelton
Electronic Article Manager: Mike Rainey
Illustrations and Permissions Coordinator: Dawn Vohsen

Printed and bound by CPI Group (UK) Ltd, Croydon, CR0 4YY

Transferred to digital print 2012

Editorial Office:
Elsevier
Suite 1800
1600 John F. Kennedy Blvd.
Philadelphia, PA 19103-2899

International Standard Serial Number: 1040-1741
International Standard Book Number: 978-1-4557-7281-0

Editorial Board

Table of Contents

EDITORIAL BOARD   vii

JOURNALS REPRESENTED   xiii

1. Cancer Biology   1
2. Cancer Prevention.   7
3. Cancer Therapies   9
4. Chemotherapy: Mechanisms and Side Effects.   13
5. Breast Cancer   15
      General Issues in Breast Cancer   15
      Prevention   23
      Early Stage and Adjuvant Therapy.   26
      Diagnostic Imaging   29
      Sentinel Node Biopsy   47
      Surgical Treatment   50
      Tumor Biology   57
      Breast Conserving Therapy   62
      Hormonal Therapy   63
      Follow-up Care   67
      Prognostic Factors   69
      Economic, Legal, and Social Issues   71
6. Genitourinary   75
      Bladder.   75
      Prostate   76
7. Gynecology.   101
      Cervix   101
      Endometrial   107
      Ovarian   113
8. Gastrointestinal   123
      Colon: Advanced   123
      Colorectal Cancer   124
      Pancreas.   135
      Miscellaneous.   143

9. Hematologic Malignancies 145

    Leukemia and Myelodysplastic Syndrome 145

10. Thoracic Cancer 159

    Biology 159

    First Line Metastatic Non–Small-Cell Lung Cancer 167

    Second Line Metastatic Non–Small-Cell Lung Cancer 170

    Non–Small-Cell: Early Stage and Adjuvant Therapy 174

    Advanced Diseases 176

11. Head and Neck 179

12. Pediatric Cancer 199

    Hematologic Disorders 199

    Leukemia 202

    Neuro-Oncology 213

    Solid Tumors 215

    Miscellaneous 218

13. Sarcoma 221

14. Supportive Care 225

15. Miscellaneous 229

    ARTICLE INDEX 231

    AUTHOR INDEX 239

Journals Represented

Journals represented in this YEAR BOOK are listed below.

AJR American Journal of Roentgenology
American Journal of Obstetrics and Gynecology
Annals of Surgery
Annals of Surgical Oncology
Blood
Breast Journal
British Journal of Cancer
British Journal of Haematology
British Journal of Radiology
Cancer
Cancer Research
Cell
Gynecologic Oncology
Haematologica
Head and Neck
International Journal of Cancer
International Journal of Radiation Oncology *Biology* Physics
Journal of Clinical Oncology
Journal of the American College of Radiology
Journal of the American Medical Association
Journal of the American Medical Association Pediatrics
Journal of the National Cancer Institute
Journal of Thoracic Oncology
Journal of Urology
Lancet
Lancet Oncology
Nature
New England Journal of Medicine
Oral Oncology
Pain
Plastic and Reconstructive Surgery
Radiology
Seminars in Radiation Oncology
Science Translational Medicine
The American Journal of Managed Care

STANDARD ABBREVIATIONS

The following terms are abbreviated in this edition: acquired immunodeficiency syndrome (AIDS), cardiopulmonary resuscitation (CPR), central nervous system (CNS), cerebrospinal fluid (CSF), computed tomography (CT), deoxyribonucleic acid (DNA), electrocardiography (ECG), health maintenance organization (HMO), human immunodeficiency virus (HIV), intensive care unit (ICU), intramuscular (IM), intravenous (IV), magnetic resonance (MR) imaging (MRI), ribonucleic acid (RNA), ultrasound (US), and ultraviolet (UV).

NOTE

The YEAR BOOK OF ONCOLOGY is a literature survey service providing abstracts of articles published in the professional literature. Every effort is made to assure the accuracy of the information presented in these pages. Neither the editors nor the publisher of the YEAR BOOK OF ONCOLOGY can be responsible for errors in the original materials. The editors' comments are their own opinions. Mention of specific products within this publication does not constitute endorsement.

To facilitate the use of the YEAR BOOK OF ONCOLOGY as a reference tool, all illustrations and tables included in this publication are now identified as they appear in the original article. This change is meant to help the reader recognize that any illustration or table appearing in the YEAR BOOK OF ONCOLOGY may be only one of many in the original article. For this reason, figure and table numbers will often appear to be out of sequence within the YEAR BOOK OF ONCOLOGY.

1 Cancer Biology

Earlier Age of Onset of *BRCA* Mutation-Related Cancers in Subsequent Generations
Litton JK, Ready K, Chen H, et al (The Univ of Texas MD Anderson Cancer Ctr, Houston)
Cancer 118:321-325, 2012

Background.—Women who are diagnosed with a deleterious mutation in either breast cancer (*BRCA*) gene have a high risk of developing breast and ovarian cancers at young ages. In this study, the authors assessed age at diagnosis in 2 generations of families with known mutations to investigate for earlier onset in subsequent generations.

Methods.—Of the 132 *BRCA*-positive women with breast cancer who participated in a high-risk protocol at The University of Texas MD Anderson Cancer Center (Gen 2), 106 women could be paired with a family member in the previous generation (Gen 1) who was diagnosed with a *BRCA*-related cancer (either breast cancer or ovarian cancer). Age at diagnosis, location of the mutation, and year of birth were recorded. A previously published parametric anticipation model was applied in these genetically predisposed families.

Results.—The median age of cancer diagnosis was 42 years (range, 28-55 years) in Gen 2 and 48 years (range, 30-72 years) in Gen 1 ($P < .001$). In the parametric model, the estimated change in the expected age at onset for the entire cohort was 7.9 years ($P < .0001$). Statistically significant earlier ages at diagnosis also were observed within subgroups of *BRCA1* and *BRCA2* mutations, maternal inheritance, paternal inheritance, breast cancer only, and breast cancer-identified and ovarian cancer-identified families.

Conclusions.—Breast and ovarian cancers in *BRCA* mutation carriers appeared to be diagnosed at an earlier age in later generations. The authors concluded that patients who are younger at the onset of *BRCA*-related cancers should continue to be tracked to offer appropriate screening modalities at appropriate ages.

▶ Although *BRCA1* and *BRCA2* are known genetic abnormalities associated with an increase in breast and ovarian cancers, the timing of the risk for these malignancies in subsequent generations is not well understood. Given the autosome-dominant nature of the inheritance of these genes, it is important for subsequently affected generations to know when they are at increased cancer risk.

Oncologists tell their patients who have first-degree female relatives with breast and ovarian cancers to be screened approximately 10 years earlier than the first-degree relative was diagnosed. Yet data for *BRCA1* and *BRCA2* patients are lacking relative to this being the correct timing for screening.

These data certainly support the 10-year anticipation screening recommendation, but continued work is needed in this area as these data suggest an earlier and earlier age to diagnosis of these genetically associated tumors in subsequent generations.

C. Lawton, MD

Punctuated Evolution of Prostate Cancer Genomes

Baca SC, Prandi D, Lawrence MS, et al (Harvard Med School, Boston, MA; Univ of Trento, Povo, Italy; The Broad Inst of Harvard and MIT, Cambridge, MA; et al)

Cell 153:666-677, 2013

The analysis of exonic DNA from prostate cancers has identified recurrently mutated genes, but the spectrum of genome-wide alterations has not been profiled extensively in this disease. We sequenced the genomes of 57 prostate tumors and matched normal tissues to characterize somatic alterations and to study how they accumulate during oncogenesis and progression. By modeling the genesis of genomic rearrangements, we identified abundant DNA translocations and deletions that arise in a highly interdependent manner. This phenomenon, which we term "chromoplexy," frequently accounts for the dysregulation of prostate cancer genes and appears to disrupt multiple cancer genes coordinately. Our modeling suggests that chromoplexy may induce considerable genomic derangement over relatively few events in prostate cancer and other neoplasms, supporting a model of punctuated cancer evolution. By characterizing the clonal hierarchy of genomic lesions in prostate tumors, we charted a path of oncogenic events along which chromoplexy may drive prostate carcinogenesis.

▶ Whole genome sequencing of various cancers has provided important clues as to their etiology, molecular evolution, patient outcomes, and opportunities for potential new treatment approaches. A unique phenomenon, termed "chromothripsis" (shattering of chromosomes), has been described over the last several years and represents a yet unexplained disruption and reassembly of single chromosomes observed in some cancers. Baca et al describe what they term "chromoplexy" (weaving or stitching together chromosomes) that results in extensive interchromosomal rearrangements that, in turn, provides the possibility to generate multiple fusion gene products. Baca et al examined 57 prostate cancer samples and were able to classify them into 2 major groups, one characterized by TMPRSS2-ERG fusion and wild-type *CHD1* compared with those characterized by features of chromoplexy and negative for TMPRSS2-ERG fusion and having deletions of *CHD1*. That the rearrangements seen in the second group are most commonly associated with genes that are expressed strongly implies that there may be a transcriptional-mediated mechanism underlying this process. Both chromoplexy and chromothripsis suggest more cataclysmic evolutionary mechanisms for some cancers rather than the gradual acquisition of sequential mutations. Pondering how to therapeutically exploit such profound genome-wide alterations remains a major challenge.

R. J. Arceci, MD, PhD

Cytokine release syndrome after blinatumomab treatment related to abnormal macrophage activation and ameliorated with cytokine-directed therapy

Teachey DT, Rheingold SR, Maude SL, et al (Children's Hosp of Philadelphia, PA; et al)

Blood 121:5154-5157, 2013

Blinatumomab is a CD19/CD3-bispecific T-cell receptor-engaging (BiTE) antibody with efficacy in refractory B-precursor acute lymphoblastic leukemia. Some patients treated with blinatumomab and other T cell-activating therapies develop cytokine release syndrome (CRS). We hypothesized that patients with more severe toxicity may experience abnormal macrophage activation triggered by the release of cytokines by T-cell receptor-activated cytotoxic T cells engaged by BiTE antibodies and leading to hemophagocytic lymphohistiocytosis (HLH). We prospectively monitored a patient during blinatumomab treatment and observed that he developed HLH. He became ill 36 hours into the infusion with fever, respiratory failure, and circulatory collapse. He developed hyperferritinemia, cytopenias, hypofibrinogenemia, and a cytokine profile diagnostic for HLH. The HLH continued to progress after discontinuation of blinatumomab; however, he had rapid improvement after IL-6 receptor-directed therapy with tocilizumab. Patients treated with T cell-activating therapies, including blinatumomab, should be monitored for HLH, and cytokine-directed therapy may be considered in cases of life-threatening CRS. This trial was registered at www.clinicaltrials.gov as #NCT00103285.

▶ Activation or inhibition of the immune system often has dichotomous results. The recent clinical testing of chimeric antibody-modified cytotoxic T lymphocytes to treat patients with cancer is no exception. Teachey et al report the results of a single patient with acute lymphocytic leukemia treated with blinatumomab, a CD19/CD3-bispecific T cell receptor engager, who developed a life-threatening hypercytokinemia syndrome consistent with a hemophagocytic lymphohistiocytosis (HLH) or macrophage activation syndrome (MAS). Although the development of the hypercytokinemia would not seem to be completely unexpected, the response to anti–interleukin-6 receptor–directed therapy with tocilizumab, in light of it not being one of the most highly expressed cytokines, was dramatic. Although a fair bit of immunologic hand waving makes up the discussion as to why some cytokines might do this or that, the response to tocilizumab says the most...nothing like reality to straighten our thinking! In addition, it will now be important to determine how generalizable the response is to tocilizumab therapy in other patients with this type of reaction or in those with HLH/MAS from other causes.

R. J. Arceci, MD, PhD

Genomic and Epigenomic Landscapes of Adult De Novo Acute Myeloid Leukemia

The Cancer Genome Atlas Research Network (Genome Inst at Washington Univ and Siteman Cancer Ctr, St Louis; et al)
N Engl J Med 368:2059-2074, 2013

Background.—Many mutations that contribute to the pathogenesis of acute myeloid leukemia (AML) are undefined. The relationships between patterns of mutations and epigenetic phenotypes are not yet clear.

Methods.—We analyzed the genomes of 200 clinically annotated adult cases of de novo AML, using either whole-genome sequencing (50 cases) or whole-exome sequencing (150 cases), along with RNA and microRNA sequencing and DNA-methylation analysis.

Results.—AML genomes have fewer mutations than most other adult cancers, with an average of only 13 mutations found in genes. Of these, an average of 5 are in genes that are recurrently mutated in AML. A total of 23 genes were significantly mutated, and another 237 were mutated in two or more samples. Nearly all samples had at least 1 nonsynonymous mutation in one of nine categories of genes that are almost certainly relevant for pathogenesis, including transcription-factor fusions (18% of cases), the gene encoding nucleophosmin (*NPM1*) (27%), tumor-suppressor genes (16%), DNA-methylation—related genes (44%), signaling genes (59%), chromatin-modifying genes (30%), myeloid transcription-factor genes (22%), cohesin-complex genes (13%), and spliceosome-complex genes (14%). Patterns of cooperation and mutual exclusivity suggested strong biologic relationships among several of the genes and categories.

Conclusions.—We identified at least one potential driver mutation in nearly all AML samples and found that a complex interplay of genetic events contributes to AML pathogenesis in individual patients. The databases from this study are widely available to serve as a foundation for further investigations of AML pathogenesis, classification, and risk stratification. (Funded by the National Institutes of Health.)

▶ The molecular analysis of cancer has reached new heights with the evolution of high-throughput nucleic acid sequencing. Although to some critics of this type of science the effort has not generated a significantly increased number of new genes that are mutated, those on the other side of this fence have argued that only through extensive, detailed understanding of the entire molecular characteristics of cancer can we expect to understand and rationally treat patients with it. The Acute Myeloid Leukemia (AML) Cancer Genome Atlas Research Network paper moves the latter argument forward. Genomic (whole genome or exome) and RNA sequencing along with genomic methylation patterns are reported on 200 adult cases of de novo AML. Of interest, in spite of the complexity of AML, an average of only 13 mutations was found in individual cases. Recurrent mutations were less, and, overall, although about 2 dozen were more frequently mutated, about 240 were observed to be mutated in only a few individuals. The genes that were found mutated could, in turn, be partitioned into 9 biological function categories. Such data whet the appetite for an even more complete description of AML, including both protein and functional information, which will come in time. A key issue, of course, is how the key step to therapeutic application of molecular information will be used to more effectively treat patients, our ultimate goal.

R. J. Arceci, MD, PhD

Development of a Prognostic Model for Breast Cancer Survival in an Open Challenge Environment
Cheng WY, Ou Yang TH, Anastassiou D (Columbia Univ, NY)
Sci Transl Med 5:181ra50, 2013

The accuracy with which cancer phenotypes can be predicted by selecting and combining molecular features is compromised by the large number of potential features available. In an effort to design a robust prognostic model to predict breast cancer survival, we hypothesized that signatures consisting of genes that are coexpressed in multiple cancer types should correspond to molecular events that are prognostic in all cancers, including breast cancer. We previously identified several such signatures—called attractor metagenes—in an analysis of multiple tumor types. We then tested our attractor metagene hypothesis as participants in the Sage Bionetworks—DREAM Breast Cancer Prognosis Challenge. Using a rich training data set that included gene expression and clinical features for breast cancer patients, we developed a prognostic model that was independently validated in a newly generated patient data set. We describe our model, which was based on three attractor metagenes associated with mitotic chromosomal instability, mesenchymal transition, or lymphocyte-based immune recruitment.

▶ Although the complexity of a so-called simple organism such as a bacterium still eludes our ability to understand its biological responses but nevertheless seems solvable, the complexity of eukaryotic cells and, particularly, cancer, is almost impossible to understand with currently available methodologies. Despite these concerns, few truly innovative, analytical approaches have been applied to such biological systems. Instead, most scientists work in relative isolation with datasets that often are not open to a broader audience. Several efforts have been made over the last decade to change the way science is conducted. One approach is that of breaking down data silos and producing a system of sharing and open competition to solve major problems in biology and medicine. The so-called "crowd-sourcing" approach provides a means to exponentially expand the number of individuals and groups working on a particular problem through access to key, shared datasets. The report by Cheng et al represents an example of analytical model building though a crowd-sourcing initiative to develop criteria that would be prognostic in terms of the chance of surviving for women with breast cancer. Through multiple iterations, a single model was determined to outperform all other models, and this was validated on a second test set of data. Such approaches seem to validate that multiple heads are better than one. How such efforts can be translated into direct patient care decisions may provide the means to truly democratize medicine.

R. J. Arceci, MD, PhD

2 Cancer Prevention

Multivitamins in the prevention of cancer in men: the Physicians' Health Study II randomized controlled trial
Gaziano JM, Sesso HD, Christen WG, et al (Brigham and Women's Hosp and Harvard Med School, Boston, MA)
JAMA 308:1871-1880, 2012

Context.—Multivitamin preparations are the most common dietary supplement, taken by at least one-third of all US adults. Observational studies have not provided evidence regarding associations of multivitamin use with total and site-specific cancer incidence or mortality.

Objective.—To determine whether long-term multivitamin supplementation decreases the risk of total and site-specific cancer events among men.

Design, Setting, and Participants.—A large-scale, randomized, double-blind, placebo controlled trial (Physicians' Health Study II) of 14 641 male US physicians initially aged 50 years or older (mean [SD] age, 64.3 [9.2] years), including 1312 men with a history of cancer at randomization, enrolled in a common multivitamin study that began in 1997 with treatment and follow-up through June 1, 2011.

Intervention.—Daily multivitamin or placebo.

Main Outcome Measures.—Total cancer (excluding nonmelanoma skin cancer), with prostate, colorectal, and other site-specific cancers among the secondary end points.

Results.—During a median (interquartile range) follow-up of 11.2 (10.7-13.3) years, there were 2669 men with confirmed cancer, including 1373 cases of prostate cancer and 210 cases of colorectal cancer. Compared with placebo, men taking a daily multivitamin had a statistically significant reduction in the incidence of total cancer (multivitamin and placebo groups, 17.0 and 18.3 events, respectively, per 1000 person-years; hazard ratio [HR], 0.92; 95% CI, 0.86-0.998; $P = .04$). There was no significant effect of a daily multivitamin on prostate cancer (multivitamin and placebo groups, 9.1 and 9.2 events, respectively, per 1000 person-years; HR, 0.98; 95% CI, 0.88-1.09; $P = .76$), colorectal cancer (multivitamin and placebo groups, 1.2 and 1.4 events, respectively, per 1000 person-years; HR, 0.89; 95% CI, 0.68-1.17; $P = .39$), or other site-specific cancers. There was no significant difference in the risk of cancer mortality (multivitamin and placebo groups, 4.9 and 5.6 events, respectively, per 1000 person-years; HR, 0.88; 95% CI, 0.77-1.01; $P = .07$). Daily multivitamin use was associated with a reduction in total cancer among 1312 men with a baseline history of cancer (HR, 0.73; 95% CI, 0.56-0.96; $P = .02$), but this did not differ significantly from that among 13 329 men initially without cancer (HR, 0.94; 95% CI, 0.87-1.02; $P=.15$; P for interaction $= .07$).

Conclusion.—In this large prevention trial of male physicians, daily multivitamin supplementation modestly but significantly reduced the risk of total cancer.

Trial Registration.—clinicaltrials.gov Identifier: NCT00270647.

▶ The use of multivitamins to keep us healthy is a seemingly simple way to improve our health. But do we really know that multivitamins improve our health in terms of specific health outcomes? Particularly, can vitamin supplements help prevent heart disease and cancer, the 2 big killers in the United States of both men and women?

Data such as those presented in this study reported the correct way to answer these questions. This trial was randomized and double blinded, so truly the gold standard of level-1 type data. Yet the results showed that multivitamins, albeit significant in reducing total cancer risk, did not affect the incidence of prostate or colorectal cancer. In addition, they did not affect the risk of cancer mortality. Fortunately, the use of a daily multivitamin did decrease the risk of total cancer incidence in men, even those with a baseline history of cancer.

So what is the take-home message? Certainly we know that multivitamins can supplement nutritional losses or deficiencies, but these data tell us that they can also decrease the risk of developing cancer. Because cancer mortality was not statistically affected, we still need to look to other means, such as low-fat diets and exercise and likely other lifestyle changes, to continue to work toward a decrease in cancer incidence and mortality in adult men.

C. Lawton, MD

3 Cancer Therapies

Statin use and reduced cancer-related mortality

Nielsen SF, Nordestgaard BG, Bojesen SE, et al (Copenhagen Univ Hosp, Herlev, Denmark)

N Engl J Med 367:1792-1802, 2012

Background.—A reduction in the availability of cholesterol may limit the cellular proliferation required for cancer growth and metastasis. We tested the hypothesis that statin use begun before a cancer diagnosis is associated with reduced cancer-related mortality.

Methods.—We assessed mortality among patients from the entire Danish population who had received a diagnosis of cancer between 1995 and 2007, with follow-up until December 31, 2009. Among patients 40 years of age or older, 18,721 had used statins regularly before the cancer diagnosis and 277,204 had never used statins.

Results.—Multivariable-adjusted hazard ratios for statin users, as compared with patients who had never used statins, were 0.85 (95% confidence interval [CI], 0.83 to 0.87) for death from any cause and 0.85 (95% CI, 0.82 to 0.87) for death from cancer. Adjusted hazard ratios for death from any cause according to the defined daily statin dose (the assumed average maintenance dose per day) were 0.82 (95% CI, 0.81 to 0.85) for a dose of 0.01 to 0.75 defined daily dose per day, 0.87 (95% CI, 0.83 to 0.89) for 0.76 to 1.50 defined daily dose per day, and 0.87 (95% CI, 0.81 to 0.91) for higher than 1.50 defined daily dose per day; the corresponding hazard ratios for death from cancer were 0.83 (95% CI, 0.81 to 0.86), 0.87 (95% CI, 0.83 to 0.91), and 0.87 (95% CI, 0.81 to 0.92). The reduced cancer-related mortality among statin users as compared with those who had never used statins was observed for each of 13 cancer types.

Conclusions.—Statin use in patients with cancer is associated with reduced cancer-related mortality. This suggests a need for trials of statins in patients with cancer.

▶ Given the high incidence of many fatal cancers worldwide, is important that we constantly look for ways to decrease both cancer incidence and mortality. Many herbs and medicines have been thought to be helpful in decreasing the risk of cancer and decreasing its effect on mortality. The statin drugs have been in the literature of late because they help decrease cholesterol. Decreasing cholesterol can block protein prenylation and, therefore, could limit cell proliferation, which may result in decreased cancer growth and metastasis.

These data are an excellent example of the type of information that we need to evaluate the potential role of statin drugs on cancer progression and mortality. The Danish population, which is the basis for this work, has a health care system in which information on cancer diagnosis and medications prescribed are easily available. These results suggest a 15% reduction in cancer-related mortality for patients taking statin medications. These data are important in suggesting that a prospective trial be pursued for patients with cancer to establish the role of statin drugs in their long-term outcome.

C. Lawton, MD

Predictive Gene Signature in MAGE-A3 Antigen-Specific Cancer Immunotherapy

Ulloa-Montoya F, Louahed J, Dizier B, et al (GlaxoSmithKline Vaccines, Rixensart, Belgium; et al)
J Clin Oncol 31:2388-2395, 2013

Purpose.—To detect a pretreatment gene expression signature (GS) predictive of response to MAGE-A3 immunotherapeutic in patients with metastatic melanoma and to investigate its applicability in a different cancer setting (adjuvant therapy of resected early-stage non–small-cell lung cancer [NSCLC]).

Patients and Methods.—Patients were participants in two phase II studies of the recombinant MAGE-A3 antigen combined with an immunostimulant (AS15 or AS02$_B$). mRNA from melanoma biopsies was analyzed by microarray analysis and quantitative polymerase chain reaction. These results were used to identify and cross-validate the GS, which was then applied to the NSCLC data.

Results.—In the patients with melanoma, 84 genes were identified whose expression was potentially associated with clinical benefit. This effect was strongest when the immunostimulant AS15 was included in the immunotherapy (hazard ratio [HR] for overall survival, 0.37; 95% CI, 0.13 to 1.05; $P = .06$) and was less strong with the other immunostimulant AS02$_B$ (HR, 0.84; 95% CI, 0.36 to 1.97; $P = .70$). The same GS was then used to predict the outcome for patients with resected NSCLC treated with MAGE-A3 plus AS02$_B$; actively treated GS-positive patients showed a favorable disease-free interval compared with placebo-treated GS-positive patients (HR, 0.42; 95% CI, 0.17 to 1.03; $P = .06$), whereas among GS-negative patients, no such difference was found (HR, 1.17; 95% CI, 0.59 to 2.31; $P = .65$). The genes identified were mainly immune related, involving interferon gamma pathways and specific chemokines, suggesting that their pretreatment expression influences the tumor's immune microenvironment and the patient's clinical response.

Conclusion.—An 84-gene GS associated with clinical response for MAGE-A3 immunotherapeutic was identified in metastatic melanoma and confirmed in resected NSCLC.

▶ The hope of immunotherapies, and especially cancer vaccines, has had many high and low points, with accompanying excessive hype during the former periods and possibly excessive criticism in the latter periods. Ulloa-Montoya et al present an intriguing MAGE-A3 plus adjuvant vaccine study in patients with metastatic melanoma and non—small cell lung cancer. A twist of this study was to investigate, by microarray-based expression analysis of tumors, a gene signature that predicted response to vaccine plus adjuvant therapy. An 84-gene signature was observed that predicted a prolonged overall survival advantage to vaccine therapy. Of interest, this response prediction in part depended on the type of adjuvant utilized. So, there were 84 genes in the signature, which represents more than the number of patients with melanoma treated. It is also noted that the group that was positive for the predictive gene signature had more women and more patients with stage IV disease, which is interesting in that all patients with melanoma were stated in the abstract to have metastatic melanoma. More details within the report do state that patients with nonresectable stage III melanoma were included. Although the results are intriguing, they also raise questions that, in part because of the phenomenology of the therapeutic approach used, may not be easy to answer in terms of mechanistic explanations.

R. J. Arceci, MD, PhD

4 Chemotherapy: Mechanisms and Side Effects

Patients' Expectations about Effects of Chemotherapy for Advanced Cancer

Weeks JC, Catalano PJ, Cronin A, et al (Dana-Farber Cancer Inst, Boston, MA)

N Engl J Med 367:1616-1625, 2012

Background.—Chemotherapy for metastatic lung or colorectal cancer can prolong life by weeks or months and may provide palliation, but it is not curative.

Methods.—We studied 1193 patients participating in the Cancer Care Outcomes Research and Surveillance (CanCORS) study (a national, prospective, observational cohort study) who were alive 4 months after diagnosis and received chemotherapy for newly diagnosed metastatic (stage IV) lung or colorectal cancer. We sought to characterize the prevalence of the expectation that chemotherapy might be curative and to identify the clinical, sociodemographic, and health-system factors associated with this expectation. Data were obtained from a patient survey by professional interviewers in addition to a comprehensive review of medical records.

Results.—Overall, 69% of patients with lung cancer and 81% of those with colorectal cancer did not report understanding that chemotherapy was not at all likely to cure their cancer. In multivariable logistic regression, the risk of reporting inaccurate beliefs about chemotherapy was higher among patients with colorectal cancer, as compared with those with lung cancer (odds ratio, 1.75; 95% confidence interval [CI], 1.29 to 2.37); among nonwhite and Hispanic patients, as compared with non-Hispanic white patients (odds ratio for Hispanic patients, 2.82; 95% CI, 1.51 to 5.27; odds ratio for black patients, 2.93; 95% CI, 1.80 to 4.78); and among patients who rated their communication with their physician very favorably, as compared with less favorably (odds ratio for highest third vs. lowest third, 1.90; 95% CI, 1.33 to 2.72). Educational level, functional status, and the patient's role in decision making were not associated with such inaccurate beliefs about chemotherapy.

Conclusions.—Many patients receiving chemotherapy for incurable cancers may not understand that chemotherapy is unlikely to be curative, which could compromise their ability to make informed treatment decisions that are consonant with their preferences. Physicians may be able to improve patients' understanding, but this may come at the cost of patients' satisfaction with them. (Funded by the National Cancer Institute and others.)

▶ Metastatic lung and colon cancer are certainly treatable diseases, but long-term control (in other words cure) via any current medical/surgical modality is not possible short of a miracle. It is important, therefore, that all oncologists (surgical, medical, and radiation) are very clear with patients regarding the expectations of their modality with regard to both short-term and long-term outcomes.

With regard to both radiation and chemotherapy, both of which are often used in these metastatic patients, oncologists owe it to the patient to discuss the clinical endpoints that may or may not be achieved via their modality. We have all seen the metastatic patient referred for palliative radiation or chemotherapy who has not been told that their disease is incurable. Having that frank discussion is difficult at best but is vital for the patient in end-of-life planning and in trying to decide if they want to proceed with any form of oncologic treatment.

This study reinforces the need for all oncologists to be as clear as possible with their metastatic patients regarding the real risks and benefits of their modality. These data show that many patients with metastatic lung and colorectal cancer do not understand the noncurative role of chemotherapy in their case. Given the often limited benefit in terms of prolongation of life and effects on quality of life for chemotherapy in these patients, as oncologists we simply must make a concerted effort to help our patients better understand the reality of therapies. This empowers our patients to make the best decisions for their individual cases.

C. Lawton, MD

5 Breast Cancer

General Issues in Breast Cancer

Assessing the Impact of a Cooperative Group Trial on Breast Cancer Care in the Medicare Population

Soulos PR, Yu JB, Roberts KB, et al (Yale School of Medicine, New Haven, CT)
J Clin Oncol 30:1601-1607, 2012

Purpose.—The Cancer and Leukemia Group B (CALGB) C9343 trial found that adjuvant radiation therapy (RT) provided minimal benefits for older women with breast cancer. Although treatment guidelines were changed to indicate that some women could forego RT, the impact of the C9343 results on clinical practice is unclear.

Patients and Methods.—We used the Surveillance, Epidemiology, and End Results (SEER) —Medicare data set to assess the use of adjuvant RT in a sample of women ≥ 70 years old diagnosed with stage I breast cancer from 2001 to 2007 who fulfilled the C9343 inclusion criteria. We used log-binomial regression to estimate the relation between publication of C9343 and use of RT in the full sample and across strata of patient and health system characteristics.

Results.—Of the 12,925 Medicare beneficiaries in our sample (mean age, 77.7 years), 76.5% received RT. Approximately 79% of women received RT before study publication compared with 75% after (adjusted relative risk of receiving RT postpublication v prepublication: 0.97; 95% CI, 0.95 to 0.98). Although use of RT was lower after the trial within all strata of age and life expectancy, the magnitude of this decrease did not differ significantly by strata. For instance, among patients with life expectancy less than 5 years, RT use decreased by 3.7%, from 44.4% prepublication to 40.7% postpublication. Among patients with life expectancy ≥ 10 years, RT use decreased by 3.0%, from 92.0% to 89.0%.

Conclusion.—The C9343 trial had minimal impact on the use of RT among older women in the Medicare population, even among the oldest women and those with shorter life expectancies.

▶ In 2006, fresh out of residency training, I was eager to adhere to the new National Comprehensive Cancer Network guideline statement indicating that RT may be omitted for women with stage I estrogen receptor—positive breast cancer who underwent lumpectomy and endocrine therapy.[1] One of my first patients to meet these criteria was a woman in her late 70s with a 1.9-cm high-grade invasive ductal carcinoma with a close margin of less than 1 mm. She technically met all the criteria for endocrine therapy alone and opted for this approach. Two years later, when her mastectomy specimen was presented at our hospital's tumor board, I learned that she had a local recurrence. My second patient to elect observation was a woman in her early 80s with a T1c N0 intermediate-grade invasive ductal carcinoma who was fearful of RT side effects and opted for endocrine therapy. Approximately 4 weeks after our initial consultation, she was re-referred to my clinic after not tolerating endocrine therapy because of arthralgia. She then opted for whole-breast RT, completed a 4-week hypofractionated regimen, and did well, with minimal RT-related side effects and long-term local control.

These 2 anecdotes illustrate the challenge of trying to implement the omission of RT into clinical practice. Although the first patient technically satisfied all the criteria for the omission of RT, she clearly had a high risk of local failure and should have undergone at least re-excision, if not re-excision and RT. This scenario illustrates that the National Comprehensive Cancer Network guidelines, while well intentioned and evidence based, fail to provide sufficient granularity regarding tumor grade, margin status, and possibly other risk factors that are likely important for predicting the risk of local recurrence. The second scenario highlights the common clinical problem of endocrine therapy noncompliance. If a patient elects to omit RT but then subsequently fails to take endocrine therapy as prescribed, her adjuvant therapy is clearly suboptimal, and the risk of in-breast tumor recurrence is likely much higher than that quoted in the CALGB 9343 trial results.[2,3]

In this article, Soulos and colleagues suggested that financial incentives may have deterred the adoption of the CALGB 9343 trial results. While I agree that this is likely a contributing factor, more complex issues underlie the limited dissemination of this trial's findings into clinical practice. Without a more detailed understanding of the pathologic features that may or may not place patients at risk for recurrence with endocrine therapy alone, many radiation oncologists prefer to err on the side of treatment rather than no treatment. Furthermore, many patients may prefer a brief, 3- or 4-week course of hypofractionated whole-breast RT to a 5-year course of daily endocrine therapy, which often yields at least some impact on quality of life. Finally, at the time of radiation oncology consultation, it is impossible for either the patient or her physician to accurately predict the likelihood of long-term compliance with endocrine therapy. In the face of these issues, RT continues to be frequently recommended as a hedge against uncertainty.

B. D. Smith, MD

References

1. Carlson RW, Anderson BO, Burstein HJ, et al; National Comprehensive Cancer Network. Breast cancer. *J Natl Compr Canc Netw.* 2005;3:238-289.
2. Hughes KS, Schnaper LA, Berry D, et al; Cancer and Leukemia Group B; Radiation Therapy Oncology Group; Eastern Cooperative Oncology Group. Lumpectomy plus tamoxifen with or without irradiation in women 70 years of age or older with early breast cancer. *N Engl J Med.* 2004;351:971-977.

3. Lim M, Bellon JR, Gelman R, et al. A prospective study of conservative surgery without radiation therapy in select patients with stage I breast cancer. *Int J Radiat Oncol Biol Phys.* 2006;65:1149-1154.

Association Between Age at Diagnosis and Disease-Specific Mortality Among Postmenopausal Women With Hormone Receptor—Positive Breast Cancer

van de Water W, Markopoulos C, van de Velde CJH, et al (Leiden Univ Med Ctr, the Netherlands; Athens Univ Med School, Greece; et al)
JAMA 307:590-597, 2012

Context.—In addition to classic tumor-related prognostic factors, patient characteristics may be associated with breast cancer outcome.

Objective.—To assess the association between age at diagnosis and breast cancer outcome in postmenopausal women with hormone receptor—positive breast cancer.

Design, Setting, and Patients.—Study analysis of 9766 patients enrolled in the TEAM (Tamoxifen Exemestane Adjuvant Multinational) randomized clinical trial between January 2001 and January 2006. Age at diagnosis was categorized as younger than 65 years (n = 5349), 65 to 74 years (n = 3060), and 75 years or older (n = 1357).

Main Outcome Measures.—Primary end point was disease-specific mortality; secondary end points were other-cause mortality and breast cancer relapse.

Results.—During median follow-up of approximately 5.1 years, there were a total of 1043 deaths. Disease-specific mortality, as a proportion of all-cause mortality, decreased with categorical age group (78% [<65 years], 56% [65-74 years], and 36% [≥75 years]; $P < .001$). In multivariable analyses, compared with patients younger than 65 years, disease-specific mortality increased with age for patients aged 65 to 74 years (hazard ratio [HR], 1.25; 95% CI, 1.01-1.54); and patients aged 75 years or older (HR, 1.63; 95% CI, 1.23-2.16) ($P < .001$). Similarly, breast cancer relapse increased with age for patients aged 65-74 years (HR, 1.07; 95% CI, 0.91-1.25 and patients aged 75 years or older (HR, 1.29; 95% CI, 1.05-1.60) ($P = .06$). Other-cause mortality increased with age in patients aged 65 to 74 years (HR, 2.66; 95% CI, 1.96-3.63) and patients aged 75 years or older (HR, 7.30; 95% CI, 5.29-10.07) ($P < .001$).

Conclusion.—Among postmenopausal women with hormone receptor—positive breast cancer, increasing age was associated with a higher disease-specific mortality.

▶ It is well understood that age at diagnosis is a prognostic factor in breast cancer. Younger patients have a worse prognosis than older patients. This is also true regarding menopausal status, as patients with premenopausal breast cancer have a worse prognosis than postmenopausal breast cancer patients.

We know that hormone receptor status is also important, with hormone receptor–positive status a favorable prognostic factor. But within this more favorable group of breast cancer patients (ie, postmenopausal and hormone receptor–positive), how does age factor in?

These data on 9766 such patients, with follow-up of 5.1 years and 1043 deaths, help both patients and oncologists understand the age effect. Increasing age was associated with an increase in disease-specific mortality and supports the need for clinical trials targeting these patients so as to improve their outcome.

C. Lawton, MD

Pain Outcomes in Patients With Advanced Breast Cancer and Bone Metastases: Results From a Randomized, Double-Blind Study of Denosumab and Zoledronic Acid
Cleeland CS, Body J-J, Stopeck A, et al (Univ of Texas MD Anderson Cancer Ctr, Houston; Brugmann Univ Hosp, Brussels, Belgium; Univ of Arizona, Tucson; et al)
Cancer 119:832-838, 2013

Background.—In this study, the authors evaluated the effect of denosumab versus zoledronic acid (ZA) on pain in patients with advanced breast cancer and bone metastases.

Methods.—The prevention of pain, reduction in pain interference with daily life activities, and the proportion of patients requiring strong opioid analgesics were assessed in a randomized, double-blind, double-dummy phase 3 study comparing denosumab with ZA for preventing skeletal-related events in 2046 patients who had breast cancer and bone metastases. Patients completed the Brief Pain Inventory-Short Form at baseline and monthly thereafter.

Results.—Fewer patients who received denosumab reported a clinically meaningful worsening of pain severity ($\geq$2-point increase) from baseline compared with patients who received ZA, and a trend was observed toward delayed time to pain worsening with denosumab versus ZA (denosumab, 8.5 months; ZA, 7.4 months; $P = .08$). In patients who had no/mild pain at baseline, a 4-month delay in progression to moderate/severe pain was observed with denosumab compared with ZA (9.7 months vs 5.8 months; $P = .002$). Denosumab delayed the time to increased pain interference by approximately 1 month compared with ZA (denosumab, 16.0 months; ZA, 14.9 months; $P = .09$). The time to pain improvement ($P = .72$) and the time to decreased pain interference ($P = .92$) were similar between the groups. Fewer denosumab-treated patients reported increased analgesic use from no/low use at baseline to strong opioid use.

Conclusions.—Denosumab demonstrated improved pain prevention and comparable pain palliation compared with ZA. In addition, fewer denosumab-treated patients shifted to strong opioid analgesic use.

▶ Denosumab is a monoclonal antibody directed against the RANK ligand that is produced by osteoblasts in response to tumor growth in bone. The RANK ligand is thought to stimulate osteoclasts, which, in turn, cause bone resorption and weakening with resultant fractures or other skeletal-related events. Denosumab interrupts this cycle of growth and resorption and thus prevents skeletal-related events. In a pooled analysis of 3 large studies involving 5723 patients, denosumab showed a superior ability to prevent skeletal-related events in patients with bone metastases than was the case for zoledronic acid, a bisphosphonate. This superiority led to the approval of denosumab for the prevention of skeletal-related events associated with solid tumors that have metastasized to bone. This study provides further analysis of one of the 3 studies that made up the meta-analysis, a study of 2046 breast cancer patients. It looks at the ability of denosumab and zoledronic acid to prevent worsening of bone pain or to delay the time at which worsening occurred. The instrument used was the Brief Pain Inventory Short Form. Denosumab use resulted in fewer patients experiencing a meaningful worsening of pain than was the case with zoledronic acid, and denosumab significantly delayed the time to pain worsening. In short, denosumab is superior to zoledronic acid not only in preventing skeletal-related events but also in ameliorating and delaying pain associated with those metastases. Based on these data, one has to conclude that denosumab is the agent of choice in patients with bone metastases from solid tumors.

J. T. Thigpen, MD

Active Smoking and Breast Cancer Risk: Original Cohort Data and Meta-Analysis

Gaudet MM, Gapstur SM, Sun J, et al (American Cancer Society, Atlanta, GA)
J Natl Cancer Inst 105:515-525, 2013

Background.—The relationship between active cigarette smoking and breast cancer risk remains controversial because of unresolved issues of confounding and dose response.

Methods.—To investigate these issues further, we analyzed data from 73 388 women in the American Cancer Society's Cancer Prevention Study II (CPS-II) Nutrition Cohort. Analyses were based on 3721 invasive breast cancer case patients identified during a median follow-up of 13.8 years. Hazard ratios (HRs) and 95% confidence intervals (CIs) were estimated from multivariable-adjusted Cox proportional hazard regression models. *P* values were two-sided. We also conducted meta-analyses of our results with those published from 14 other cohort studies.

Results.—In CPS-II, incidence was higher in current (HR = 1.24, 95% CI = 1.07 to 1.42) and former smokers (HR = 1.13, 95% CI = 1.06 to 1.21) than in never smokers. Women who initiated smoking before menarche (HR = 1.61, 95% CI = 1.10 to 2.34) or after menarche but 11 or more years before first birth (HR = 1.45, 95% CI = 1.21 to 1.74) had higher risk (P_{trend} = .03). No relationships were observed with other smoking parameters. Alcohol consumption did not confound associations with smoking status, although neither current nor former smoking were associated with risk among never drinkers ($P_{interaction}$ = .11). In meta-analyses, current (HR = 1.12, 95% CI = 1.08 to 1.16) and former smoking (HR = 1.09, 95% CI = 1.04 to 1.15) were weakly associated with risk; a stronger association (HR = 1.21, 95% CI = 1.14 to 1.28) was observed in women who initiated smoking before first birth.

Conclusions.—These results support the hypothesis that active smoking is associated with increased breast cancer risk for women who initiate smoking before first birth and suggest that smoking might play a role in breast cancer initiation.

▶ Whether smoking is associated with an increased risk of breast cancer has been controversial. To attempt to settle this controversy, this article looked at 15 cohort studies, in particular the cohort of patients in the American Cancer Society Cancer Prevention Study II. The meta-analysis found a weak but statistically significant association between being a current or former smoker and the risk for breast cancer (hazard ratio [HR], 1.09—1.12). If one isolates those women who initiated smoking before first birth, a somewhat stronger association is noted (HR, 1.21), which was also statistically significant. There is biologic support for this observation because the terminal ductal-lobular units of the breast are not fully differentiated until the end of gestation and thus are more susceptible to exposure to potential carcinogens. There are several problems with declaring a firm association between smoking and breast cancer risk on the basis of these data. First, the association is weak. Second, there is no dose-response relationship such as that seen with other smoking-related cancers (ie, there is no relationship to overall duration of smoking, cigarettes smoked per day, or years since quitting). Third, in this analysis, the association between smoking and breast cancer was statistically significant only in current or former drinkers if one stratifies on alcohol consumption, a potential confounding factor. These problems leave the issue still open for debate. If there is a real association between smoking and breast cancer, it is a weak association at best, and there may well be no association at all.

J. T. Thigpen, MD

Effect of Three Decades of Screening Mammography on Breast-Cancer Incidence
Bleyer A, Welch HG (Oregon Health and Science Univ, Portland; Geisel School of Medicine at Dartmouth, Hanover, NH)
N Engl J Med 367:1998-2005, 2012

Background.—To reduce mortality, screening must detect life-threatening disease at an earlier, more curable stage. Effective cancer-screening programs therefore both increase the incidence of cancer detected at an early stage and decrease the incidence of cancer presenting at a late stage.

Methods.—We used Surveillance, Epidemiology, and End Results data to examine trends from 1976 through 2008 in the incidence of early-stage breast cancer (ductal carcinoma in situ and localized disease) and late-stage breast cancer (regional and distant disease) among women 40 years of age or older.

Results.—The introduction of screening mammography in the United States has been associated with a doubling in the number of cases of early-stage breast cancer that are detected each year, from 112 to 234 cases per 100,000 women—an absolute increase of 122 cases per 100,000 women. Concomitantly, the rate at which women present with late-stage cancer has decreased by 8%, from 102 to 94 cases per 100,000 women—an absolute decrease of 8 cases per 100,000 women. With the assumption of a constant underlying disease burden, only 8 of the 122 additional early-stage cancers diagnosed were expected to progress to advanced disease. After excluding the transient excess incidence associated with hormone-replacement therapy and adjusting for trends in the incidence of breast cancer among women younger than 40 years of age, we estimated that breast cancer was overdiagnosed (i.e., tumors were detected on screening that would never have led to clinical symptoms) in 1.3 million U.S. women in the past 30 years. We estimated that in 2008, breast cancer was overdiagnosed in more than 70,000 women; this accounted for 31% of all breast cancers diagnosed.

Conclusions.—Despite substantial increases in the number of cases of early-stage breast cancer detected, screening mammography has only marginally reduced the rate at which women present with advanced cancer. Although it is not certain which women have been affected, the imbalance suggests that there is substantial overdiagnosis, accounting for nearly a third of all newly diagnosed breast cancers, and that screening is having, at best, only a small effect on the rate of death from breast cancer.

▶ This article should be viewed with the other reviewed article reflecting the British experience with mammography. Approximately 3 decades ago, a series of 8 trials examined the role of mammography as a screening test for the early detection of breast cancer. All 8 studies showed a reduction in mortality caused by breast cancer on the order of 25% to 35% for women over the age of 50. A pooled analysis of the 8 trials also suggested no advantage for the use of mammography in women between the ages of 40 and 50 even though the guidelines over the years have included women in this decade of life in the recommendations for screening with mammography. Over the last decade, a number of studies have purported to show that mammography is not an effective screening tool for breast cancer. This article examining the US experience and the aforementioned article looking at the British experience both show that mammography results in substantial overdiagnosis as a price for the early detection of some breast cancers. This article concludes that "screening is having, at best, only a small effect on the rate of death from breast cancer." What, then, are we to conclude about the utility of mammography as a screening tool for breast cancer? First, we should note that, even though this study concluded that the effect was small, it still had to concede that there was reduction in mortality from breast cancer. Second, we must note that, in the era of widespread use of mammography, the absolute number of deaths from breast cancer has declined despite the discovery of more cases per year over time. Third, we must take into account the observation in the British study that a focus group of women, when given these observations, still concluded that mammographic screening was worthwhile. In short, mammography should remain a major screening test for breast cancer with our expectations for results tempered by the observations in this study.

J. T. Thigpen, MD

The benefits and harms of breast cancer screening: an independent review
Independent UK Panel on Breast Cancer Screening (UCL Dept of Epidemiology and Public Health, London, UK; Univ of Oxford, UK; Univ of Edinburgh, UK; et al)
Lancet 380:1778-1786, 2012

Whether breast cancer screening does more harm than good has been debated extensively. The main questions are how large the benefit of screening is in terms of reduced breast cancer mortality and how substantial the harm is in terms of overdiagnosis, which is defined as cancers detected at screening that would not have otherwise become clinically apparent in the woman's lifetime. An independent Panel was convened to reach conclusions about the benefits and harms of breast screening on the basis of a review of published work and oral and written evidence presented by experts in the subject. To provide estimates of the level of benefits and harms, the Panel relied mainly on findings from randomised trials of breast cancer screening that compared women invited to screening with controls not invited, but also reviewed evidence from observational studies. The Panel focused on the UK setting, where women aged 50–70 years are invited to screening every 3 years. In this Review, we provide a summary of the full report on the Panel's findings and conclusions. In a meta-analysis of 11 randomised trials, the relative risk of breast cancer mortality for women invited to screening compared with controls was $0 \cdot 80$ (95% CI $0 \cdot 73 – 0 \cdot 89$), which is a relative risk reduction of 20%. The Panel considered the internal biases in the trials and whether these trials, which were done a long time ago, were still relevant; they concluded that 20% was still a reasonable estimate of the relative risk reduction. The more reliable and recent observational studies generally produced larger estimates of benefit, but these studies might be biased. The best estimates of overdiagnosis are from three trials in which women in the control group were not invited to be screened at the end of the active trial period. In a meta-analysis, estimates of the excess incidence were 11% (95% CI 9–12) when expressed as a proportion of cancers diagnosed in the invited group in the long term, and 19% (15—23) when expressed as a proportion of the cancers diagnosed during the active screening period. Results from observational studies support the occurrence of overdiagnosis, but estimates of its magnitude are unreliable. The Panel concludes that screening reduces breast cancer mortality but that some overdiagnosis occurs. Since the estimates provided are from studies with many limitations and whose relevance to present-day screening programmes can be questioned, they have substantial uncertainty and should be regarded only as an approximate guide. If these figures are used directly, for every 10 000 UK women aged 50 years invited to screening for the next 20 years, 43 deaths from breast cancer would be prevented and 129 cases of breast cancer, invasive and non-invasive, would be overdiagnosed; that is one breast cancer death prevented for about every three overdiagnosed cases identified and treated. Of the roughly 307 000 women aged 50—52 years who are invited to begin screening every year, just over 1% would have an overdiagnosed cancer in the next 20 years. Evidence from a focus group organised by Cancer Research UK and attended by some members of the Panel showed that many women feel that accepting the offer of breast screening is worthwhile, which agrees with the results of previous similar studies. Information should be made available in a transparent and objective way to women invited to screening so that they can make informed decisions.

▶ This article provides the results of a meta-analysis of 11 randomized trials of screening for breast cancer. Some of these trials were conducted several years ago, and there was concern about the continued validity of the observations. These data were reviewed by an independent panel. The analysis produced several significant observations. First, the estimate of benefit is a 20% reduction in the mortality from breast cancer. Secondly, the trade-off was an estimated 3 overdiagnoses for every life saved by screening. For every 10000 patients screened over a 20-year period, 43 lives would be saved and 129 overdiagnoses would be encountered. These data thus tend to support the value of screening, as overdiagnosis seldom is fatal. A focus group convened by the panel agreed with the view that screening was worthwhile. Although this effort does not produce a definitive conclusion regarding the value of screening for breast cancer, it does lend support to the continued value of breast cancer screening.

J. T. Thigpen, MD

Prevention

Effect of three decades of screening mammography on breast-cancer incidence
Bleyer A, Welch HG (St. Charles Health System, Portland, OR)
N Engl J Med 367:1998-2005, 2012

Background.—To reduce mortality, screening must detect life-threatening disease at an earlier, more curable stage. Effective cancer-screening programs therefore both increase the incidence of cancer detected at an early stage and decrease the incidence of cancer presenting at a late stage.

Methods.—We used Surveillance, Epidemiology, and End Results data to examine trends from 1976 through 2008 in the incidence of early-stage breast cancer (ductal carcinoma in situ and localized disease) and late-stage breast cancer (regional and distant disease) among women 40 years of age or older.

Results.—The introduction of screening mammography in the United States has been associated with a doubling in the number of cases of early-stage breast cancer that are detected each year, from 112 to 234 cases per 100,000 women — an absolute increase of 122 cases per 100,000 women. Concomitantly, the rate at which women present with late-stage cancer has decreased by 8%, from 102 to 94 cases per 100,000 women — an absolute decrease of 8 cases per 100,000 women. With the assumption of a constant underlying disease burden, only 8 of the 122 additional early-stage cancers diagnosed were expected to progress to advanced disease. After excluding the transient excess incidence associated with hormone-replacement therapy and adjusting for trends in the incidence of breast cancer among women younger than 40 years of age, we estimated that breast cancer was overdiagnosed (i.e., tumors were detected on screening that would never have led to clinical symptoms) in 1.3 million U.S. women in the past 30 years. We estimated that in 2008, breast cancer was overdiagnosed in more than 70,000 women; this accounted for 31% of all breast cancers diagnosed.

Conclusions.—Despite substantial increases in the number of cases of early-stage breast cancer detected, screening mammography has only marginally reduced the rate at which women present with advanced cancer. Although it is not certain which women have been affected, the imbalance suggests that there is substantial overdiagnosis, accounting for nearly a third of all newly diagnosed breast cancers, and that screening is having, at best, only a small effect on the rate of death from breast cancer.

▶ The use of screening mammography has been a standard for adult women for decades in the United States. Its acceptance is so widespread among women in the US that when the US Preventative Task Force suggested that women less than 50 years of age need not be screened, there was a huge outcry of disagreement. Women in the US pushed for continued screening starting at age 40 so that insurers were essentially forced to continue to cover such screening. So now we have yet another dataset questioning the role of screening mammography for women older than 40 years of age. We know that for any screening test to be useful it has to diagnose significant cancers earlier so that treatment can result in a decrease in mortality from the disease. Screening mammography based on the data presented here clearly diagnoses breast cancer earlier. But the challenge is that there appears to be a real issue of overdiagnosis of cancers not likely to impact a woman's survival. Thus, the concern of overtreatment is raised.

These data add to the growing literature questioning the role of screening mammography. It will be very interesting to watch the response of adult women across the US who, at least to date, have not accepted any of this type of data. Women in the US want to be screened and will likely continue to push for this until we truly see a risk to doing so. Overdiagnosis and overtreatment of some mammographically detected breast cancers, as shown in this article, may not be enough to convince women in the US to change their minds regarding the benefits of screening mammography in detecting breast cancer early.

C. Lawton, MD

Estrogen Plus Progestin and Breast Cancer Incidence and Mortality in the Women's Health Initiative Observational Study
Chlebowski RT, Manson JE, Anderson GL, et al (Los Angeles Biomedical Res Inst at Harbor-UCLA Med Ctr, Torrance, CA; Harvard Med School, Boston, MA; Fred Hutchinson Cancer Res Ctr, Seattle, WA; et al)
J Natl Cancer Inst 105:526-535, 2013

Background.—In the Women's Health Initiative (WHI) randomized trial, estrogen plus progestin increased both breast cancer incidence and mortality. In contrast, most observational studies associate estrogen plus progestin with favorable prognosis breast cancers. To address differences, a cohort of WHI observational study participants with characteristics similar to the WHI clinical trial was studied.

Methods.—We identified 41 449 postmenopausal women with no prior hysterectomy and mammogram negative within 2 years who were either not hormone users (n = 25 328) or estrogen and progestin users (n = 16 121). Multivariable-adjusted Cox proportional hazard regression was used to calculate hazard ratios (HRs) with 95% confidence intervals (CI). All statistical tests were two-sided.

Results.—After a mean of 11.3 (SD = 3.1) years, with 2236 breast cancers, incidence was higher in estrogen plus progestin users than in nonusers (0.60% vs 0.42%, annualized rate, respectively; HR = 1.55, 95% CI = 1.41 to 1.70, P < .001). Women initiating hormone therapy closer to menopause had higher breast cancer risk with linear diminishing influence as time from menopause increased (P < .001). Survival after breast cancer, measured from diagnosis, was similar in combined hormone therapy users and nonusers (HR = 1.03, 95% CI = 0.79 to 1.35). On a population basis, there were somewhat more deaths from breast cancer, measured from cohort entry (HR = 1.32, 95% CI = 0.90 to 1.93, P = .15), and more all-cause deaths after breast cancer (HR = 1.65, 95% CI = 1.29 to 2.12, P < .001) in estrogen plus progestin users than in nonusers.

Conclusions.—Consistent with WHI randomized trial findings, estrogen plus progestin use is associated with increased breast cancer incidence. Because prognosis after diagnosis on combined hormone therapy is similar to that of nonusers, increased breast cancer mortality can be expected.

▶ The Women's Health Initiative study evaluated the impact of postmeno-pausal hormone replacement therapy on women's health and found an increase in risk of breast cancer in women taking estrogen/progesterone combinations. This study examines 41 449 women, 16 121 of whom used estrogen/progesterone combinations. The data show that, after a mean of 11.3 years of follow-up, breast cancer incidence was higher in those who used estrogen/progesterone than in those who did not use hormone replacement therapy (hazard ratio = 1.55). The highest breast cancer risk was seen in women who initiated hormone therapy closer to the menopause. Because the survival rate in patients with breast cancer in both groups was similar, these data strongly suggest that an increased breast cancer mortality rate in those using hormone replacement therapy can be expected. From a practice standpoint, this is an issue that needs to be thoroughly discussed with women who are contemplating the use of hormone replacement therapy. It does not constitute an absolute contraindication to hormone use, as there are potential beneficial effects as well.

J. T. Thigpen, MD

Early Stage and Adjuvant Therapy

Exemestane Versus Anastrozole in Postmenopausal Women With Early Breast Cancer: NCIC CTG MA.27—A Randomized Controlled Phase III Trial
Goss PE, Ingle JN, Pritchard KI, et al (Massachusetts General Hosp, Boston; Mayo Clinic, Rochester, MN; Sunnybrook Odette Cancer Centre, Toronto, Canada; et al)
J Clin Oncol 31:1398-1404, 2013

Purpose.—In patients with hormone-dependent postmenopausal breast cancer, standard adjuvant therapy involves 5 years of the nonsteroidal aromatase inhibitors anastrozole and letrozole. The steroidal inhibitor exemestane is partially non–cross-resistant with nonsteroidal aromatase inhibitors and is a mild androgen and could prove superior to anastrozole regarding efficacy and toxicity, specifically with less bone loss.

Patients and Methods.—We designed an open-label, randomized, phase III trial of 5 years of exemestane versus anastrozole with a two-sided test of superiority to detect a 2.4% improvement with exemestane in 5-year event-free survival (EFS). Secondary objectives included assessment of overall survival, distant disease–free survival, incidence of contralateral new primary breast cancer, and safety.

Results.—In the study, 7,576 women (median age, 64.1 years) were enrolled. At median follow-up of 4.1 years, 4-year EFS was 91% for exemestane and 91.2% for anastrozole (stratified hazard ratio, 1.02; 95% CI, 0.87 to 1.18; $P = .85$). Overall, distant disease–free survival and disease-specific survival were also similar. In all, 31.6% of patients discontinued treatment as a result of adverse effects, concomitant disease, or study refusal. Osteoporosis/osteopenia, hypertriglyceridemia, vaginal bleeding, and hypercholesterolemia were less frequent on exemestane, whereas mild liver function abnormalities and rare episodes of atrial fibrillation were less frequent on anastrozole. Vasomotor and musculoskeletal symptoms were similar between arms.

Conclusion.—This first comparison of steroidal and nonsteroidal classes of aromatase inhibitors showed neither to be superior in terms of breast cancer outcomes as 5-year initial adjuvant therapy for postmenopausal breast cancer by two-way test. Less toxicity on bone is compatible with one hypothesis behind MA.27 but requires confirmation. Exemestane should be considered another option as up-front adjuvant therapy for postmenopausal hormone receptor-positive breast cancer.

▶ There are 4 agents that function as inhibitors of aromatase and that are approved for the treatment of patients with breast carcinoma. One of these, fulvestrant, is a parenteral medication given monthly. The other 3 are given orally and are used more commonly because of the route of administration. Of these, 2 (anastrozole and letrozole) are nonsteroidal aromatase inhibitors and one (exemestane) is a steroidal aromatase inhibitor. The 2 nonsteroidal agents are by far the most commonly prescribed aromatase inhibitors. Exemestane, however, does have some potential advantages over anastrozole and letrozole in that it is partially non—cross resistant with anastrozole and letrozole and also has mild androgenic effects. Because of these differences, it is conceivable that exemestane may offer some advantages. This article reports a phase III trial directly comparing anastrozole with exemestane. The study design randomly assigned 7576 patients to 5 years of therapy with one or the other of the 2 agents with a primary endpoint of event-free survival (seeking a difference of 2.4% at 5 years). The data show an essentially identical event-free, distant disease-free, and disease-specific survival. Toxicity differences included fewer bone effects, hypertriglyceridemia, vaginal bleeding, and hypercholesterolemia in patients on exemestane but more mild liver test abnormalities and atrial fibrillation (rare with both). Vasomotor and musculoskeletal effects were similar. These data support exemestane as another valid option with essentially identical efficacy for aromatase inhibitor therapy.

J. T. Thigpen, MD

Long-term effects of continuing adjuvant tamoxifen to 10 years versus stopping at 5 years after diagnosis of oestrogen receptor-positive breast cancer: ATLAS, a randomised trial

Davies C, for the Adjuvant Tamoxifen: Longer Against Shorter (ATLAS) Collaborative Group (Univ of Oxford, UK; et al)
Lancet 381:805-816, 2013

Background.—For women with oestrogen receptor (ER)-positive early breast cancer, treatment with tamoxifen for 5 years substantially reduces the breast cancer mortality rate throughout the first 15 years after diagnosis. We aimed to assess the further effects of continuing tamoxifen to 10 years instead of stopping at 5 years.

Methods.—In the worldwide Adjuvant Tamoxifen: Longer Against Shorter (ATLAS) trial, 12 894 women with early breast cancer who had completed 5 years of treatment with tamoxifen were randomly allocated to continue tamoxifen to 10 years or stop at 5 years (open control). Allocation (1:1) was by central computer, using minimisation. After entry (between 1996 and 2005), yearly follow-up forms recorded any recurrence, second cancer, hospital admission, or death. We report effects on breast cancer outcomes among the 6846 women with ER-positive disease, and side-effects among all women (with positive, negative, or unknown ER status). Long-term follow-up still continues. This study is registered, number ISRCTN19652633.

Findings.—Among women with ER-positive disease, allocation to continue tamoxifen reduced the risk of breast cancer recurrence (617 recurrences in 3428 women allocated to continue *vs* 711 in 3418 controls, $p=0.002$), reduced breast cancer mortality (331 deaths *vs* 397 deaths, $p=0.01$), and reduced overall mortality (639 deaths *vs* 722 deaths, $p=0.01$). The reductions in adverse breast cancer outcomes appeared to be less extreme before than after year 10 (recurrence rate ratio [RR] 0.90 [95% CI 0.79−1.02] during years 5−9 and 0.75 [0.62-0.90] in later years; breast cancer mortality RR 0.97 [0.79-1.18] during years 5-9 and 0.71 [0.58-0.88] in later years). The cumulative risk of recurrence during years 5−14 was 21.4% for women allocated to continue versus 25.1% for controls; breast cancer mortality during years 5−14 was 12.2% for women allocated to continue versus 15.0% for controls (absolute mortality reduction 2.8%). Treatment allocation seemed to have no effect on breast cancer outcome among 1248 women with ER-negative disease, and an intermediate effect among 4800 women with unknown ER status. Among all 12 894 women, mortality without recurrence from causes other than breast cancer was little affected (691 deaths without recurrence in 6454 women allocated to continue versus 679 deaths in 6440 controls; RR 0.99 [0.89-1.10]; p=0.84). For the incidence (hospitalisation or death) rates of specific diseases, RRs were as follows: pulmonary embolus 1.87 (95% CI 1.13−3.07, $p=0.01$ [including 0.2% mortality in both treatment groups]), stroke 1.06 (0.83−1.36), ischaemic heart disease 0.76 (0.60-0.95, $p=0.02$), and endometrial cancer 1.74 (1.30-2.34, $p=0.0002$). The cumulative risk of endometrial cancer during years 5−14 was 3.1% (mortality 0.4%) for women allocated to continue versus 1.6% (mortality 0.2%) for controls (absolute mortality increase 0.2%).

Interpretation.—For women with ER-positive disease, continuing tamoxifen to 10 years rather than stopping at 5 years produces a further reduction in recurrence and mortality, particularly after year 10. These results, taken together with results from previous trials of 5 years of tamoxifen treatment versus none, suggest that 10 years of tamoxifen treatment can approximately halve breast cancer mortality during the second decade after diagnosis.

▶ More than 15 years ago, the National Surgical Adjuvant Breast and Bowel Project completed a trial of 5 vs 10 years of tamoxifen as adjuvant therapy in breast cancer patients who were estrogen receptor positive and had negative lymph nodes.[1] This study randomly assigned 1153 patients, who had no evidence of recurrence after 5 years of tamoxifen, to either observation or 5 additional years of tamoxifen. The trial showed through 4 years of the additional therapy that there was a disease-free and distant disease-free survival advantage for those who discontinued tamoxifen after 5 years. Overall survival was not significantly different. Those continuing tamoxifen experienced more thromboembolic events and endometrial cancers. The conclusion was reached that 10 years of tamoxifen therapy actually offered no advantage and some potential disadvantages. The Adjuvant Tamoxifen: Longer Against Shorter study sought to confirm or refute these observations in a much larger patient population. The study involved 12 894 women, in particular, 6846 women with estrogen receptor—positive disease. Women assigned to the additional 5 years of tamoxifen showed a reduced risk of breast cancer recurrence, a reduced breast cancer mortality, and a reduced overall mortality at the expense of more pulmonary emboli, more endometrial cancer, and less ischemic heart disease. Much of the advantage for the additional 5 years appears in the second decade after initiation of the 10 years of tamoxifen; hence, longer-term follow-up is needed to appreciate the full effects. Based on these data from a much larger trial with longer follow-up, 10 years of tamoxifen appears to be the new standard.

J. T. Thigpen, MD

Reference

1. Fisher B, Dignam J, Bryant J, et al. Five versus more than five years of tamoxifen therapy for breast cancer patients with negative lymph nodes and estrogen receptor-positive tumors. *J Natl Cancer Inst.* 1996;88:1529-1542.

Diagnostic Imaging

Evaluation of breast amorphous calcifications by a computer-aided detection system in full-field digital mammography

Scaranelo AM, Eiada R, Bukhanov K, et al (Univ of Toronto, Ontario, Canada)
Br J Radiol 85:517-522, 2012

Objectives.—The purpose of this study was to evaluate the performance of a direct computer-aided detection (d-CAD) system integrated with full-field digital mammography (FFDM) in assessment of amorphous calcifications.

Methods.—From 1438 consecutive stereotactic-guided biopsies, FFDM images with amorphous calcifications were selected for retrospective evaluation by d-CAD in 122 females (mean age, 56 years; range, 35—84 years). The sensitivity, specificity, accuracy and false-positive rate of the d-CAD system were calculated in the total group of 124 lesions and in the subgroups based on breast density, mammographic lesion distribution and extension. Logistic regression analysis was used to stratify the risk of malignancy by patient risk factors and age.

Results.—The d-CAD marked all (36/36) breast cancers, 85% (11/13) of the high-risk lesions and 80% (60/75) of benign amorphous calcifications ($p < 0.01$) correctly. The sensitivity, specificity and diagnostic accuracy for the combined malignant and "high-risk" lesions was 96, 80 and 86%, respectively. The likelihood of malignancy was 29%. There was no significant difference between the marking of fatty or dense breasts ($p > 0.05$); however, d-CAD marks showed differences for small (< 7 mm) lesions ($p = 0.02$) and clustered calcifications ($p = 0.03$). The false-positive rate of d-CAD was 1.76 marks per full examination.

Conclusion.—The d-CAD system correctly marked all biopsy-proven breast cancers and a large number of biopsy-proven high-risk lesions that presented as amorphous calcifications. Given our 29% likelihood of malignancy, imaging-guided biopsy appears to be a reasonable recommendation in cases of amorphous calcifications marked by d-CAD.

▶ This interesting study by Scaranelo and colleagues describes the effectiveness of d-CAD in identifying amorphous calcifications with FFDM. This is important because amorphous calcifications can be among the more challenging lesions to identify on mammography, yet they are associated with a substantial risk of malignancy. What this study demonstrates is that like indirect CAD, that is, film screen mammography (FSM) images that are digitized and then analyzed with CAD, d-CAD can be used to detect amorphous calcifications with high sensitivity. In fact, the sensitivity for the detection of amorphous calcifications with d-CAD seems to be higher than that with indirect CAD. Perhaps more importantly, the consistency of d-CAD as compared with that of CAD from FSM images not only allows for more accurate detection but also potentially allows for improved differentiation between benign and malignant amorphous calcifications. This could alter the use of CAD from detecting the presence of a lesion to determining the likelihood of malignancy. Certainly, adding determination of the likelihood of malignancy will be a significant step forward in improving mammographic specificity. A lesion with a 3% likelihood of malignancy will be approached differently than one with a 93% likelihood of malignancy. In this study, 100% of malignant amorphous calcifications, 85% of high-risk lesions, and 80% of benign amorphous calcifications were detected. The detection rate difference is based on objective morphologic differences, the basis for ultimately determining the likelihood of malignancy.

There are other advantages to the implementation of d-CAD. The number of "distracting" marks on the images is lower than that reported for indirect CAD. With the increasing interest in breast density and the need to detect cancer in this intermediate-risk population of women, the finding that there was no statistically significant difference in the detection of amorphous calcifications in women with dense versus fatty breasts is important as well. The ability to detect cancer in this mammographically challenging population is yet another advantage of CAD.

Several points in this study are noteworthy. The positive predictive value (PPV) of biopsy of amorphous calcifications in this study was 29%, higher than that previously reported.[1] This further emphasizes the need to optimize the detection of amorphous calcifications to detect the earliest of breast cancers. However, the majority of cancers detected in this study were found to be ductal carcinoma in situ (DCIS), albeit high-grade DCIS. The importance of detecting DCIS remains controversial. However, until we have biological markers to distinguish DCIS that is clinically significant from DCIS that is not, we must identify and treat DCIS to ensure that the progression to invasive cancer is stopped. Finally, it is important to note that although the number of such cancers was limited, no cancers presenting as amorphous calcifications were missed with d-CAD in this study.

In summary, this is an interesting study that contributes to the literature by demonstrating that d-CAD has very high sensitivity for the detection of amorphous calcifications, that the PPV of amorphous calcifications detected with d-CAD is higher than that reported for indirect CAD, that the rate of distracting "false-positive" marks per image is lower with d-CAD, and that the rate of cancers manifesting as amorphous calcifications is not statistically different in women with dense or fatty breasts. Excitingly, the differential detection rates of malignant, high-risk, and benign amorphous calcifications may bode well for the implementation of d-CAD that not only detects lesions but also determines the likelihood of malignancy based on objective morphologic assessment of the lesion characteristics. It seems that the future may be here after all.

R. F. Brem, MD

J. A. Rapelyea, MD

J. Torrente, MD

Reference

1. Soo MS, Rosen EL, Xia JQ, Ghate S, Baker JA. Computer-aided detection of amorphous calcifications. *AJR Am J Roentgenol.* 2005;184:887-892.

Locally Advanced Breast Cancer: MR Imaging for Prediction of Response to Neoadjuvant Chemotherapy—Results from ACRIN 6657/I-SPY TRIAL

Hylton NM, For the ACRIN 6657 Trial Team and I-SPY 1 TRIAL Investigators (Univ of California, San Francisco; et al)

Radiology 263:663-672, 2012

Purpose.—To compare magnetic resonance (MR) imaging findings and clinical assessment for prediction of pathologic response to neoadjuvant chemotherapy (NACT) in patients with stage II or III breast cancer.

Materials and Methods.—The HIPAA-compliant protocol and the informed consent process were approved by the American College of Radiology Institutional Review Board and local-site institutional review boards.

Women with invasive breast cancer of 3 cm or greater undergoing NACT with an anthracycline-based regimen, with or without a taxane, were enrolled between May 2002 and March 2006. MR imaging was performed before NACT (first examination), after one cycle of anthracyline-based treatment (second examination), between the anthracycline-based regimen and taxane (third examination), and after all chemotherapy and prior to surgery (fourth examination). MR imaging assessment included measurements of tumor longest diameter and volume and peak signal enhancement ratio. Clinical size was also recorded at each time point. Change in clinical and MR imaging predictor variables were compared for the ability to predict pathologic complete response (pCR) and residual cancer burden (RCB). Univariate and multivariate random-effects logistic regression models were used to characterize the ability of tumor response measurements to predict pathologic outcome, with area under the receiver operating characteristic curve (AUC) used as a summary statistic.

Results.—Data in 216 women (age range, 26—68 years) with two or more imaging time points were analyzed. For prediction of both pCR and RCB, MR imaging size measurements were superior to clinical examination at all time points, with tumor volume change showing the greatest relative benefit at the second MR imaging examination. AUC differences between MR imaging volume and clinical size predictors at the early, mid-, and posttreatment time points, respectively, were 0.14, 0.09, and 0.02 for prediction of pCR and 0.09, 0.07, and 0.05 for prediction of RCB. In multivariate analysis, the AUC for predicting pCR at the second imaging examination increased from 0.70 for volume alone to 0.73 when all four predictor variables were used. Additional predictive value was gained with adjustments for age and race.

Conclusion.—MR imaging findings are a stronger predictor of pathologic response to NACT than clinical assessment, with the greatest advantage observed with the use of volumetric measurement of tumor response early in treatment.

▶ This prospective study by Hylton and colleagues of 216 patients was a companion imaging study to the Cancer and Leukemia Group B 150007 trial and compared magnetic resonance imaging (MRI) findings and clinical assessment for the prediction of pathologic response to NACT in patients with stage II or III breast cancer. The American College of Radiology Imaging Network 6657 study showed that MRI findings are a stronger predictor of pathologic response to NACT than is clinical assessment at all time points, and the advantage was greatest when MRI was used to measure tumor volume at the early treatment time point. The strengths of the study include the prospective design, patient sample size, standardization of time points for assessing tumor response by MRI, and impressive compliance rate of enrolled patients who returned for repeat imaging.

In the setting of locally advanced breast cancer, NACT is introduced with the aim of reducing the size of the primary tumor and achieving breast conservation at surgery. In addition to reducing the overall tumor burden, NACT allows for the direct and early observation of the response to treatment, thereby allowing for treatment plan modifications early in the course of the disease, which leads to better clinical outcomes. After treatment, the primary tumor bed is surgically excised to verify tumor response and to obtain negative margins prior to the initiation of radiation therapy.

The literature supports MRI as the most specific, yet relatively less sensitive, modality for predicting pCR when compared with mammography, sonography, and clinical examination.[1] Moreover, a prospective study by Yeh and colleagues showed that although MRI demonstrated the best pathologic correlation, residual disease was either overestimated or underestimated in 26% of patients[2]; these findings were corroborated in a companion study by Shin and colleagues in 2011.[3]

In the present study by Hylton and colleagues, contrast-enhanced images at all imaging time points were analyzed using the single-enhancement ratio technique, with voxel-based comparison of both early and late contrast enhancement, a technique that is considered somewhat outdated and has recently been supplanted by dynamic contrast-enhanced high-temporal-resolution imaging that allows for the exploitation of pharmacokinetic modeling.[4] Moreover, the criteria used for estimating the greatest extent of disease accounted for intervening areas of nonenhancing tissue on baseline MRI, an approach that may overestimate the overall tumor size.

From a technological standpoint, it should be acknowledged that this study formally began nearly 10 years ago, using the nascent technology provided by vendors of breast MRI systems. Since that time, there have been substantial technological advancements in MRI systems that specifically affect breast MRI protocols. Improvements in static magnetic field homogeneity, radiofrequency amplifiers, and encoding gradients over the large, off-isocenter fields of view needed for breast MRI, as well as in the number of channels and the design of breast MRI—specific phased-array coils, have helped to improve image quality substantially. Additionally, 3-tesla systems have shown promise for breast MRI compared with the 1.5-tesla systems used in this study. An array of more advanced acquisition and image reconstruction techniques, such as parallel imaging for increased temporal resolution and Dixon techniques for more uniform fat suppression across large fields of view, may also increase breast MRI quality in modern systems. Additionally, postprocessing algorithms seek to reduce the impact of motion on subtracted images. Such techniques could affect the measurements reported in this study using both T2-weighted and 3-dimensional T1-weighted images, particularly those describing lesion size and enhancement kinetics. These comments do not detract from the current study but rather bolster the authors' conclusions. The results reported here using nascent breast MRI technology support further investigation of the effect of modern MRI approaches on the assessment of response to NACT.

Although MRI is quickly emerging as a powerful tool for monitoring disease response to NACT, it has several limitations. While MRI has been shown to be a stronger predictor of pathologic response to NACT when compared with clinical assessment at all time points, a multivariate analysis including histologic subtype and receptor status was not performed in this study, and these are emerging variables that should be considered when assessing tumor response. Loo and colleagues recently reported statistically significant differences in the presence of residual tumor on pathologic analysis when tumors were categorized by histologic subtype.[5] Residual tumor was most often documented at surgical excision following NACT in patients with estrogen receptor (ER)-positive/human epidermal growth factor receptor 2 (HER2)-negative subtypes. Furthermore, imaging findings closely correlated with pathologic outcome in triple-negative and HER2-positive tumors and less predictively in ER-positive/HER2-negative tumors.[6,7]

The results reported in the present study by Hylton and colleagues substantiate the body of literature supporting MRI as the most specific and sensitive modality for image-based prediction of response to NACT. The study underscores the importance of continued investigation into how various histologic subtypes of breast carcinoma respond both histologically and radiographically to NACT and may help identify a subset of patients who would benefit most from MRI monitoring of chemotherapy response.

M. Kalambo, MD
J. Stafford, PhD
W. T. Yang, MD

References

1. Yuan Y, Chen XS, Liu SY, Shen KW. Accuracy of MRI in prediction of pathologic complete remission in breast cancer after preoperative therapy: a meta-analysis. *AJR Am J Roentgenol.* 2010;195:260-268.
2. Yeh E, Slanetz P, Kopans DB, et al. Prospective comparison of mammography, sonography, and MRI in patients undergoing neoadjuvant chemotherapy for palpable breast cancer. *AJR Am J Roentgenol.* 2005;184:868-877.
3. Shin HJ, Kim HH, Ahn JH, et al. Comparison of mammography, sonography, MRI and clinical examination in patients with locally advanced or inflammatory breast cancer who underwent neoadjuvant chemotherapy. *Br J Radiol.* 2011;84: 612-620.
4. Hylton NM. Vascularity assessment of breast lesions with gadolinium-enhanced MR imaging. *Magn Reson Imaging Clin N Am.* 1999;7:411-420.
5. Loo CE, Straver ME, Rodenhuis S, et al. Magnetic resonance imaging response monitoring of breast cancer during neoadjuvant chemotherapy: relevance of breast cancer subtype. *J Clin Oncol.* 2011;29:660-666.
6. Lips EH, Mukhtar RA, Yau C, et al; I-SPY TRIAL Investigators. Lobular histology and response to neoadjuvant chemotherapy in invasive breast cancer. *Breast Cancer Res Treat.* 2012;136:35-43.
7. Esserman LJ, Berry DA, DeMichele A, et al. Pathologic complete response predicts recurrence-free survival more effectively by cancer subset: results from the I-SPY 1 TRIAL—CALGB 150007/150012, ACRIN 6657. *J Clin Oncol.* 2012;30:3242-3249.

Preoperative Breast MRI Can Reduce the Rate of Tumor-Positive Resection Margins and Reoperations in Patients Undergoing Breast-Conserving Surgery

Obdeijn I-M, Tilanus Linthorst MMA, Spronk S, et al (Erasmus MC Rotterdam, The Netherlands)
AJR Am J Roentgenol 200:304-310, 2013

Objective.—In breast cancer patients eligible for breast-conserving surgery, we evaluated whether the information provided by preoperative MRI of the breast would result in fewer tumor-positive resection margins and fewer reoperations.

Subjects and Methods.—The study group consisted of 123 consecutive patients diagnosed with either breast cancer or ductal carcinoma in situ eligible for breast-conserving surgery between April 2007 and July 2010. For these patients, a first plan for breast-conserving surgery was made on the basis of clinical examination and conventional imaging. The final surgical plan was made with knowledge of the preoperative breast MRI. The rates of tumor-positive resection margins and reoperations were compared with those of a historical control group consisting of 119 patients who underwent 123 breast-conserving procedures between January 2005 and December 2006. The percentage of change in the surgical plan was recorded.

Results.—Preoperative breast MRI changed the surgical plan to more extensive surgery in 42 patients (34.1%), mainly to mastectomy (29 patients, 23.6%). Ninety-four patients underwent 95 breast-conserving procedures. Significantly fewer patients had tumor-positive resection margins than in the control group (15.8%, 15/95 versus 29.3%, 36/123; $p < 0.01$). Patients in the study group underwent significantly fewer reoperations compared with the historical control group (18.9%, 18/95 vs 37.4%, 46/123; $p < 0.01$).

Conclusion.—Preoperative breast MRI can substantially decrease the rate of tumor-positive resection margins and reoperations in breast cancer patients eligible for breast-conserving surgery.

▶ Published outcomes with preoperative breast MRI have been highly variable, perhaps too variable to establish guidelines based on high-quality evidence as of yet. In fact, there has been such a wide array of methodology, technology, and expertise (or lack thereof) that it may be more appropriate to reserve the use of preoperative MRI for those institutions that can demonstrate improvement in outcomes, rather than deal with the multifactorial issues that hamper strict guidelines. Such a broad range in outcomes is not a unique problem for breast surgeons trying to establish quality measures. Consider the proposal that multifactorial issues likely preclude the use of reoperation rates as a measure of quality in breast cancer surgery.[1]

While the words "prospective" and "randomized" lull some observers into believing high-quality evidence against using MRI already exists, we hold an opposing view: Multiple possible endpoints remain untested, and the 2 randomized trials[2,3] were composed of highly selected cohorts, not the general breast cancer population. High-quality evidence in its purest form, using principles borrowed from pharmaceutical trials, also includes "placebo-controlled" and "blinded," critical features to harness bias that cannot be used in the study of preoperative MRI, in which the approach depends on the radiologist's eyes transmitting information to the surgeon's fingertips, all while depending on large variations in the technology used. Prospective, randomized trials for preoperative MRI, both past and future, are inevitably vulnerable to unblinded bias or confounding variables. Trying to overcome this challenge using meta-analyses that include nonrandomized trials only churns the weak with the strong, dragging centers of excellence into a lowest common denominator while using the semantically more acceptable term of "generalizability."

Although well-defined guidelines for MRI seem desirable owing to the high cost of this preoperative assessment, high reoperation rates are even more costly than MRI on a per-patient basis, and if the reoperation rate is high enough in a cohort, it will exceed the cost of preoperative MRI. The challenge has been demonstrating that preoperative MRI can lower reoperation rates to a degree that translates to an overall cost savings. Moreover, for some, the more pressing question is whether preoperative MRI results in a decrease in reoperation rates at all. If reoperation rates are taken to be the only endpoint, then many seem satisfied with the "no benefit" or "adverse" outcome seen in the COMICE[2] and MONET[3] trials, respectively.

That being said, individual institutions have described significant reductions in reoperation rates. In this article from the Netherlands by Obdeijn and colleagues, a statistically significant reoperation rate reduction from 37.4% to 18.9% invites an immediate appraisal of cost-effectiveness. Given 100 patients newly diagnosed with breast cancer, what would be the actual cost (as opposed to charges) of 100 MRIs, including resultant biopsies, and what would be the savings from performing 19 fewer reoperations? No matter what numbers are used, the differential is not as great as one's bias might dictate.

An acknowledgment is due to the Netherlands for that country's role in contributing to the breast MRI literature. One of the 6 high-risk MRI screening trials upon which the American Cancer Society based its 2007 guidelines was the Magnetic Resonance Imaging Screening Study Group (MRISC) trial from the Netherlands, which revealed that MRI identified more than twice the number of cancers revealed by mammography, where sensitivity was only 33%.[4] From participating researchers in this multi-institutional cooperative group, with investigators working subsequently from their respective institutions, this article by Obdeijn and colleagues (predominantly from the Erasmus Medical Center in Rotterdam) represents the third Dutch study of preoperative MRI in which a benefit has been claimed. In contrast, the MONET trial,[3] in which reoperation outcomes trended worse after MRI, was based in Utrecht and Dordrecht and did not include investigators who participated in the MRISC trial.

The first article on preoperative MRI from the Netherlands came from the Netherlands Cancer Institute in Amsterdam. In that study, the overall successful primary excision rate trended toward benefit ($P = .17$) with MRI, whereas patients with the most common tumor type—invasive ductal carcinoma—experienced a statistically significant improvement in complete excision rate

($P = .02$) with the remarkably low probability of positive margins being 1.6%.[5] In order to form a larger cohort and draw conclusions about invasive lobular carcinoma as well, some of these investigators in Amsterdam joined with others in Nijmegen and Maastricht who had participated in the MRISC trial, ultimately finding that patients with invasive lobular carcinoma who underwent preoperative MRI showed a statistically significant lowering of reoperation rates from 27% to 9% ($P = .01$) as well as a trend toward *fewer* mastectomies.[6]

The response by critics of preoperative MRI in the United States (prior to the MONET trial) was a pervasive "no benefit" from studies in the Netherlands. This interpretation was so distanced from the apparent reality that we wrote Gilhuijs, senior author of the first publication and a participant in the second study as well, to ask if he understood how these studies were being depicted in the United States. In a personal communication (November 10, 2010, email from Kenneth G.A. Gilhuijs, PhD, to Alan B. Hollingsworth, MD), Dr Gilhuijs expressed awareness of the "no benefit" depiction, stating that he was "puzzled." He went on to state, "We have therefore now demonstrated (level 2) significance on surgical impact in both IDC [invasive ductal carcinoma] and ILC sub-groups."

Now, in this third article that shows a lower reoperation rate and includes some of the MRISC investigators, what are the strengths and weaknesses? The fact that this is not a prospective, randomized trial will, for some, exclude the study from any consideration. Instead, the MONET trial[3] is held out as high-quality evidence because of those key words, "prospective, randomized," that obscure the underlying reality. The MONET was a trial of screen-detected mammographic cancers and is thus heavily skewed with DCIS (50%), the only histology for which nearly all investigators are in agreement that MRI is of questionable benefit for the index lesion (Note: We have demonstrated that preoperative MRI in patients with DCIS may not be justified through the index lesion but through findings of invasion at other sites that exceed the yields from the high-risk screening trials.[7]). Furthermore, even after significant problems with their 3 T approach had been resolved, there was still a remarkably high false-negative rate with MRI in patients with DCIS (50%), translating to half the volume excised by surgeons when the MRI was falsely negative, all in such a small population of patients ($n = 74$ with cancer + MRI) that the overall "harm" caused by MRI did not reach statistical significance. This is not, in our opinion, high-quality evidence.

In general, written guidelines for preoperative MRI focus on women with dense mammograms and lobular histology; however, the MONET trial (and for that matter, the COMICE trial, in which 70% of conservation-bound candidates were excluded or refused participation) addressed a different population. Thus, we are currently operating under the inexplicable situation in which no prospective, randomized trials have addressed the patient population that MRI is said to benefit per current guidelines, while condemning preoperative MRI based on 2 prospective trials that accrued patients who do not fit the guidelines.

In the present article, Obdeijn and colleagues have the advantage of a consecutive series of patients, thus avoiding the selection bias that is so prevalent in many nonrandomized studies in which the MRI group is composed of patients who are younger, with dense mammograms, lobular histology, and positive margins after surgical biopsy, and are then compared to women with none of these features. When "no difference" is the conclusion, in spite of remarkable differences in the 2 groups (with group differences often confirmed by *P* values), a possible benefit to breast MRI is obscured. The unanswered question from such studies is: What would have been the reoperation rate in the MRI group had the MRI not been performed?

Although studies using historical controls are often dismissed without thought, consider how, in the assessment of preoperative breast MRI, these studies are likely to offer more reliable information than those with built-in selection bias, as long as there has been no change in surgical personnel or other variables. In this article by Obdeijn and colleagues, the control group was drawn from the 2 years immediately prior to starting the consecutive MRIs. The authors noted no major changes in physician personnel or policy.

We would argue that this retrospective study design is far preferable to the retrospective approaches that create 2 sharply unequal groups in the name of "concurrency." Whenever concurrency requires specific patient/tumor characteristics in a retrospective study, there is going to be selection bias. It will be more reliable to use consecutive series of patients, as long as there have been no other known changes, as was done in this article under review. Prospective randomization of *all* newly diagnosed breast cancer patients would be preferable, of course, and would capture the "mastectomy-to-conservation" patients. So far, this global approach has eluded investigators who seem intent on defining conservation-bound patients prior to accrual, allowing only 1 of 2 vectors to be quantified (ie, conservation-to-mastectomy).

Other strengths to this study include a thoughtful attempt to define clear margins, appreciating the difference between focal positivity (which, according to Dutch guidelines, is not an indication for reexcision) and gross positivity. Another strength is the fact that the authors appreciated that one of the chief problems in translating MRI results to surgical outcomes is the difference in patient positioning—prone in the MRI suite, supine in surgery. Close consultation between radiologist and surgeon was described in detail—a far greater focus than was placed in the prospective randomized COMICE trial of generalizability.[2] In the Obdeijn and colleagues study, the magnetic resonance images were reviewed in the operating room during the procedure.

The authors identified the primary weakness of this particular study in the fact that 7.3% underwent a "medically unnecessary" mastectomy. There is a relationship between reoperation rates and mastectomy rates. Taken to its extreme, if one performs mastectomy on all, there will be no reoperations. Thus, reoperation rates do not exist independently of all other issues. The authors concluded that histologic verification of the "presumed more-extended malignancy is mandatory before converting from conservation to mastectomy."

As an initial ground rule in our program, before seeing our first patient for preoperative MRI over 10 years ago, we established the need for biopsy confirmation before surgical action was taken on additional areas of enhancement on MRI. We subsequently altered our protocol to even more aggressive use of preoperative biopsy to include patients who have an "extension" or a large area of non-mass enhancement surrounding the index lesion. As a result of this policy together with our routine performance of preoperative MRI immediately following diagnosis and prior to the first visit with the surgeon,[8] we have achieved the unique combination of fewer reoperations coupled with fewer mastectomies. This unique combination of outcomes is further supported by the counterintuitive outcome of an even higher rate of breast conservation (70%) after false-positive MRI.[9]

With regard to that issue of reoperation rates being related to conservation rates, the weakness of this study was the overall conversion rate of 23.6% to mastectomy, a number inflated by a lack of histologic confirmation of additional sites of malignancy. Even if biopsies had been performed and if the reported "unnecessary" 7.3% had instead undergone conservation, however, the conversion rate to mastectomy still exceeds local recurrence rates, and this is the primary reason for the extended controversy about preoperative MRI. Here, we would be on the side of the critics who note the disparity between "conversion-to-mastectomy" rates and modern recurrence rates.

So again, as we have outlined in detail with regard to "pivotal" and "non-pivotal" MRI,[8] if MRI is performed up front and all false-positive issues are settled before pretreatment conference and before meeting with the surgeon, the power of false positives is lost and the true-positive benefits of MRI are allowed to emerge. Furthermore, and of critical importance in our view, the patient who has previously convinced herself to undergo mastectomy can be converted to conservation when she sees the well-defined tumor extent on MRI, a phenomenon we believe has occurred in our cohort, which includes a larger number than the MRI conversions to mastectomy. We again draw attention to this phenomenon, as it is a scenario that is *impossible to measure* when prospective, randomized trials begin by accruing patients who are already chosen and cleared for conservation through conventional measures.

We do not believe that preoperative MRI should be the standard at all facilities. The studies with neutral or adverse outcomes have demonstrated that preoperative MRI is a delicate tool that must be used with great care or not at all. On the other hand, we do not believe that results from poorly designed or poorly executed studies, or meta-analyses of the same, should be used to prompt global condemnation of preoperative MRI when some sites are consistently demonstrating improved outcomes. If "evidence-based medicine" is groomed only for "generalizability," it will squelch aspirations of excellence.

A. B. Hollingsworth, MD

R. G. Stough, MD

References

1. Morrow M, Katz SJ. The challenge of developing quality measures for breast cancer surgery. *JAMA.* 2012;307:509-510.
2. Turnbull L, Brown S, Harvey I, et al. Comparative effectiveness of MRI in breast cancer (COMICE) trial: a randomized controlled trial. *Lancet.* 2010;375:563-571.
3. Peters NH, van Esser S, van den Bosch MA, et al. Preoperative MRI and surgical management in patients with nonpalpable breast cancer: the MONET - randomized controlled trial. *Eur J Cancer.* 2011;47:879-886.
4. Kriege M, Brekelmans CTM, Boetes C, et al; Magnetic Resonance Imaging Screening Study Group. Efficacy of MRI and mammography for breast-cancer screening in women with a familial or genetic predisposition. *N Engl J Med.* 2004;351:427-437.

5. Pengel KE, Loo CE, Teertstra HJ, et al. The impact of preoperative MRI on breast-conserving surgery of invasive cancer: a comparative cohort study. *Breast Cancer Res Treat.* 2009;116:161-169.
6. Mann RM, Loo CE, Wobbes T, et al. The impact of preoperative breast MRI on the re-excision rate in invasive lobular carcinoma of the breast. *Breast Cancer Res Treat.* 2010;119:415-422.
7. Hollingsworth AB, Stough RG. Multicentric and contralateral invasive tumors identified with preoperative MRI in patients newly diagnosed with ductal carcinoma in situ of the breast. *Breast J.* 2012;18:420-427.
8. Hollingsworth AB, Stough RG. Conflicting outcomes with preoperative breast MRI: differences in technology or methodology? *Breast Dis Year Bk Q.* 2010; 21:109-112.
9. Hollingsworth AB, Stough RG, O'Dell CA, Brekke CE. Breast magnetic resonance imaging for preoperative locoregional staging. *Am J Surg.* 2008;196:389-397.

Computer-aided Detection of Masses at Mammography: Interactive Decision Support Versus Prompts

Hupse R, Samulski M, Lobbes MB, et al (Radboud Univ Nijmegen Med Centre, the Netherlands; Maastricht Univ Med Ctr, the Netherlands; et al)
Radiology 266:123-129, 2013

Purpose.—To compare effectiveness of an interactive computer-aided detection (CAD) system, in which CAD marks and their associated suspiciousness scores remain hidden unless their location is queried by the reader, with the effect of traditional CAD prompts used in current clinical practice for the detection of malignant masses on full-field digital mammograms.

Materials and Methods.—The requirement for institutional review board approval was waived for this retrospective observer study. Nine certified screening radiologists and three residents who were trained in breast imaging read 200 studies (63 studies containing at least one screen-detected mass, 17 false-negative studies, 20 false-positive studies, and 100 normal studies) twice, once with CAD prompts and once with interactive CAD. Localized findings were reported and scored by the readers. In the prompted mode, findings were recorded before and after activation of CAD. The partial area under the location receiver operating characteristic (ROC) curve for an interval of low false-positive fractions typical for screening, from 0 to 0.2, was computed for each reader and each mode. Differences in reader performance were analyzed by using software.

Results.—The average partial area under the location ROC curve with unaided reading was 0.57, and it increased to 0.62 with interactive CAD, while it remained unaffected by prompts. The difference in reader performance for unaided reading versus interactive CAD was statistically significant ($P = .009$).

Conclusion.—When used as decision support, interactive use of CAD for malignant masses on mammograms may be more effective than the current use of CAD, which is aimed at the prevention of perceptual oversights.

▶ This article by Hupse and colleagues may be the most significant article published on computer-aided diagnosis since the seminal article by Chan and colleagues in 1990.[1] The study by Chan and colleagues showed for the first time that an automated computer detection scheme could improve radiologists' ability to detect clustered microcalcifications on mammograms. Since that article, very few studies in mammography have replicated that result. Furthermore, when implemented clinically, CAD systems have been only mildly successful.[2]

The premise when CAD was developed was that if a radiologist overlooked a cancer on a mammogram, the program's placement of a marker on the image would prompt the radiologist to recognize the cancer and recall the patient for a diagnostic workup. This is the second-reader paradigm. The systems were touted as a sort of "spellchecker"—the radiologist would see prompts at all locations at which the computer found a suspicious lesion. It has been noted somewhat anecdotally that, clinically, radiologists would not always recognize a correct CAD prompt. Nishikawa and colleagues showed that radiologists ignore 70% of correct CAD prompts.[3] The reason for the error is not known.

In this article, Hupse and colleagues report on an observer study that compared CAD used as a second reader and CAD used in an interactive mode. They showed no significant improvement in radiologists' ability to detect breast cancer on mammograms when CAD was used as a second reader, but they did show a significant improvement when interactive CAD was used. For interactive CAD, radiologists are only shown CAD output when they query a specific location in the mammogram. If the location being queried has a CAD detection, a marker is shown and the likelihood that the lesion is malignant is displayed numerically and with a color contour around the lesion. This study shows that the second-reader paradigm is not as effective as the interactive paradigm; in fact, it indicates that the second-reader paradigm is not very helpful to radiologists.

Why might this be the case? Wolfe and colleagues[4] have shown that at a very low prevalence, such as in screening mammography, humans tend to have lower sensitivity. That is, a radiologist would be more likely to overlook a cancer when reading at low prevalence than at high prevalence. The false-detection rate with CAD is approximately 2 per case (0.5 per image). In a typical screening population, where the cancer prevalence is approximately 4 per 1000, there would be 2000 false detections with 7 true detections (assuming a CAD sensitivity of 90%). Thus, the prevalence of true CAD detection is low: 286 false marks for every true mark. Extrapolating Wolfe and colleagues' result, then, it seems that radiologists ignore true computer prompts because the chance that a CAD prompt is marking a cancer is very low. Another way of looking at it is that there are too many false CAD detections. With the current iteration of CAD—the second-reader paradigm—radiologists are shown all CAD detections. In the interactive mode, radiologists do not see any CAD detections unless they query an area that has a CAD detection. This explains why second-reader CAD is suboptimal.

Another possible explanation is that cancers that are clinically missed by radiologists are not overlooked but are visualized and considered to be benign—an interpretation error, not a search or perception error. If this were true, radiologists would not necessarily benefit from seeing the location of lesions that the computer believes may be a cancer, since it is likely that the radiologist has already examined these lesions. Instead, information about the likelihood that the lesion is malignant may be more beneficial, and this is the information that the radiologist can view, if he or she so desires. Radiologists are likely to query only lesions that are of uncertain pathology. Because the sensitivity of CAD is high (90%), the negative predictive value of CAD is also high. That is, if a radiologist queries a lesion and there is no CAD detection, it is highly probable that the lesion is not a cancer. This suggests that interactive CAD is superior to second-reader CAD.

One major limitation of the study by Hupse and colleagues was that it was conducted in the Netherlands with Dutch screening radiologists reading screening mammograms from Dutch women. The Dutch program has a very low recall rate relative to other screening programs worldwide—less than 2%, compared with 5% in Sweden and the United Kingdom and 8% or higher in the United States.[5] It is unlikely that Dutch radiologists are overlooking suspicious lesions more than are US radiologists (which might have explained the difference in recall rates). It must be that Dutch radiologists have a higher threshold for recalling women than do U.S. radiologists. Thus, interpretation errors would be the major cause of screening error in the Netherlands. Operating at a higher threshold for recall would lower the number of interpretation errors by the U.S. radiologists, leading to a higher percentage of missed cancer being a result of an incomplete search (i.e., overlooking a cancer). If this were true, U.S. radiologists may receive less benefit than do Dutch radiologists when using interactive CAD.

The results of Hupse and colleagues' study challenge the CAD-as-a-second-reader paradigm. If their results hold true clinically, changing CAD to be used interactively could lead to significant improvements in cancer detection in screening. More research is needed to understand the differences between second-reader CAD and interactive CAD. Ultimately, it is important for others to evaluate interactive CAD, particularly in the United States, and to perform clinical trials using interactive CAD.

R. M. Nishikawa, PhD

References

1. Chan HP, Doi K, Vyborny CJ, et al. Improvement in radiologists' detection of clustered microcalcifications on mammograms: the potential of computer-aided diagnosis. *Invest Radiol.* 1990;25:1102-1110.
2. Taylor P, Potts HW. Computer aids and human second reading as interventions in screening mammography: two systematic reviews to compare effects on cancer detection and recall rate. *Eur J Cancer.* 2008;44:798-807.
3. Nishikawa RM, Schmidt RA, Linver MN, Edwards AV, Papaioannou J, Stull MA. Clinically missed cancer: how effectively can radiologists use computer-aided detection? *AJR Am J Roentgenol.* 2012;198:708-716.
4. Wolfe JM, Horowitz TS, Kenner NM. Cognitive psychology: rare items often missed in visual searches. *Nature.* 2005;435:439-440.

5. Elmore JG, Nakano CY, Koepsell TD, Desnick LM, D'Orsi CJ, Ransohoff DF. International variation in screening mammography interpretations in community-based programs. *J Natl Cancer Inst.* 2003;95:1384-1393.

Breast Cancer: Assessing Response to Neoadjuvant Chemotherapy by Using US-guided Near-Infrared Tomography

Zhu Q, DeFusco PA, Ricci A Jr, et al (Univ of Connecticut, Storrs; Hartford Hosp, CT; et al)
Radiology 266:433-442, 2013

Purpose.—To assess initial breast tumor hemoglobin (Hb) content before the initiation of neoadjuvant chemotherapy, monitor the Hb changes at the end of each treatment cycle, and correlate these fndings with tumor pathologic response.

Materials and Methods.—The HIPAA-compliant study protocol was approved by the institutional review boards of both institutions. Written informed consent was obtained from all patients. Patients who were eligible for neoadjuvant chemotherapy were recruited between December 2007 and May 2011, and their tumor Hb content was assessed by using a near-infrared imager coupled with an ultrasonography (US) system. Thirty-two women (mean age, 48 years; range, 32–82 years) were imaged before treatment, at the end of every treatment cycle, and before definitive surgery. The patients were graded in terms of their final pathologic response on the basis of the Miller-Payne system as nonresponders and partial responders (grades 1–3) and near-complete and complete responders (grades 4 and 5). Tumor vascularity was assessed from total Hb (tHb), oxygenated Hb (oxyHb), and deoxygenated Hb (deoxyHb) concentrations. Tumor vascularity changes during treatment were assessed from percentage tHb normalized to the pretreatment level. A two-sample two-sided t test was used to calculate the P value and to evaluate statistical significance between groups. Bonferroni-Holm correction was applied to obtain the corrected P value for multiple comparisons.

Results.—There were 20 Miller-Payne grade 1–3 tumors and 14 grade 4 or 5 tumors. Mean maximum pretreatment tHb, oxyHb, and deoxyHb levels were significantly higher in grade 4 and 5 tumors than in grade 1–3 tumors ($P=.005$, $P=.008$, and $P=.017$, respectively). The mean percentage tHb changes were significantly higher in grade 4 or 5 tumors than in grade 1–3 tumors at the end of treatment cycles 1–3 ($P=.009$ and corrected $P=.009$, $P=.002$ and corrected $P=.004$, and $P<.001$ and corrected $P<.001$, respectively).

Discussion.—These findings indicate that initial tumor Hb content is a strong predictor of final pathologic response. Additionally, the tHb changes during early treatment cycles can further predict final pathologic response.

▶ In patients with breast cancer more advanced than stage II who need chemotherapy in the course of treatment, the benefit of receiving neoadjuvant chemotherapy (NAC) before surgery is well established. The goal of NAC is to achieve pathologic complete response (pCR), which is proven to be associated with favorable prognosis. Many cytotoxic chemotherapeutic agents and targeted agents can be used to treat breast cancer, and with the promising research in this field, more agents may gradually become available. One great advantage of NAC is that it allows in vivo assessment of tumor response for timely adjustment of regimens, thereby not only avoiding unnecessary toxicity, but also allowing the effective regimen to work more quickly. Therefore, it would be very helpful to find a reliable early response indicator that can guide the change of regimens. The clinical examination and standard clinical breast imaging modalities—mammography, US, and magnetic resonance imaging (MRI)—rely on a change in tumor size, and they cannot provide a reliable, early response indicator before tumor shrinkage occurs. Many MRI-based studies have tried to investigate whether other parameters (eg, vascular parameters measured by dynamic contrast-enhanced MRI, proliferation markers measured by magnetic resonance spectroscopy, cellular density markers measured by diffusion-weighted imaging) can be used as early markers for predicting final response; however, these studies have produced inconclusive findings.

Over the past 2 decades, a substantial research effort has been devoted to developing optical imaging technology for the breast so as to provide an alternative or complementary imaging modality. This imaging technology's advantages over existing modalities include its lack of radiation, the fact that it is not limited by breast density, its relatively low cost, and its portability as a bedside device that can be used to image the patient frequently. Among all optical imaging systems, US-guided diffuse optical tomography developed by Zhu and colleagues is a unique system that can provide anatomic information as well as tomographic optical images without being limited by the depth of the lesion. The system has been successfully applied in a large clinical study to test its diagnostic performance in differentiating between malignant lesions (early Tis-T1 stage and more advanced T2-T4 stage) and benign lesions (proliferating and non-proliferating) and has yielded very interesting results. The maximum tHb within the lesion was measured. It was found that when a tHb cutoff value of 82 µmol/L was chosen, sensitivity and specificity were 92% and 93%, respectively, for Tis-T1 tumors, and 75% and 93%, respectively, for T2-T4 tumors. For more advanced tumors, although the sensitivity is not high, when complementary optical imaging is used to rule out possible malignancy, a high specificity that can aid in avoiding unnecessary biopsy is most important.

In the present article, Zhu and colleagues used a refined system with 4 wavelengths (740, 780, 808, and 830 nm) to measure oxyHb, deoxyHb, and tHb in tumors undergoing NAC at different times before and after 1, 2, and 3 cycles of treatment. Several studies published earlier[1-6] have demonstrated the potential role of optical imaging in distinguishing good from poor responders, but all were pilot studies that analyzed only a very small number of subjects. The present study enrolled a total of 35 patients, with 32 complete data sets available for analysis. Only Hb parameters (including tHb, oxyHb, and deoxyHb) were considered. The maximum value within the tumor was measured, and the averaged value from volumetric zone exceeding 50% of the maximum value was calculated. The baseline values and the percent changes at different cycles during the treatment were used to differentiate tumors showing a good response from those showing a poor response. With the improved NAC regimens, most tumors will respond to some extent, and the traditional way of separating them into responders and non-responders may not be applicable anymore. Although pCR is known to be associated with favorable prognosis, tumors that show a very close to complete response are also known to have a good prognosis, and in this study they are combined as a good response group. The authors used the MP grade system based on the cellularity of the residual disease to separate tumors into 2 response groups: MP1-3 (less than 90% change in cellularity) and MP4-5 (less than 90% change in cellularity and pCR). The results showed a significantly higher tHb in the MP4-5 group than in the MP1-3 group, suggesting that tumors with higher vascularity (more Hb) have a better response, presumably through better delivery of therapeutic agents into the tumors. The percentage changes from the baseline value in tHb after 1 cycle, 2 cycles, and 3 cycles were all greater in the MP4-5 group than in the MP1-3 group. Since the system has an integrated US, the tumor size measured by US was also used to differentiate between the 2 response groups. The US tumor size could only be measured in 21 of the 32 patients. The size difference between these 2 groups was not significant after 1 or 2 cycles, but it became significant after 3 cycles. These results suggest that US may not be applied to evaluate tumor sizes in some cases and that early size change cannot be used to predict final treatment outcome. The best imaging modality for evaluating the extent of residual disease is MRI, but given that most patients had only 1 MRI done after completing NAC, it is not possible to compare the predictive value of MRI size with other parameters measured by the US-diffuse optical tomography system.

Although Zhu and colleagues present very encouraging results, processing optical imaging data to generate tHb maps requires sophisticated experience and is thus operator-dependent. The ROI used in the reconstruction was based on the segmentation of the lesion seen on the pretreatment US examination, and the same ROI was used for processing all data sets obtained at different treatment cycles while the tumor was shrinking. The reason for using the same ROI throughout the treatment period was not explained. A possible reason was that it would minimize variation resulting from the use of different ROIs; however, it is necessary to evaluate the extent to which the reconstructed parameter is dependent on the choice of ROI, particularly when the tumor is shrinking substantially. For those patients whose tumor size cannot be measured on US, tumor size determined on MRI was used in the reconstruction. In general, it will be interesting for authors to investigate how the obtained results are dependent on the data-processing methods, as Jiang and colleagues have done,[4] as well as the dependence on the operators who perform the optical imaging acquisition and data analysis. For this imaging system to become clinically feasible, a more automated procedure that minimizes operator variations needs to be developed. In a recently optical imaging study, Ueda and colleagues[7] analyzed 41 patients receiving NAC and reported that none of the Hb parameters (tHb, oxyHb, and deoxyHb) measured at baseline before treatment showed a significant difference between the pCR and non-pCR groups. Moreover, only oxygen saturation showed a significant difference (higher in pCR than in non-pCR, also explained by delivery of therapeutic agents, less in hypoxic tumors). Many reasons may account for different findings that were reported in different studies, but overall, the variation of optical imaging parameters measured by different imaging systems using different data analysis procedures may be the main reason. This needs to be investigated further.

One great advantage of optical imaging in NAC management is the technology's capacity for frequent measurements, even within hours or days after administration of agents to assess flare response. In a recent study published by Roblyer and colleagues,[6] the authors reported a statistically significant increase (a flare) of oxyHb measured on day 1 after the first infusion in partial responders (n = 11) and patients who had shown pCR (n = 8), whereas non-responders (n = 5) showed no flare and a subsequent decrease in oxyHb on day 1. Whether the initial flare on day 1 can serve as a reliable indicator of response, at least for partial response, needs to be further evaluated. If it is proven true, optical imaging can provide unique information that cannot be measured by any other breast imaging modality. Moreover, this will have a great impact on improving the management of patients undergoing NAC, with the ultimate goal of reaching pCR with the lowest level of toxicity.

M.-Y. L. Su, PhD

References

1. Zhou C, Choe R, Shah N, et al. Diffuse optical monitoring of blood flow and oxygenation in human breast cancer during early stages of neoadjuvant chemotherapy. *J Biomed Opt.* 2007;12:051903.
2. Cerussi A, Hsiang D, Shah N, et al. Predicting response to breast cancer neoadjuvant chemotherapy using diffuse optical spectroscopy. *Proc Natl Acad Sci U S A.* 2007;104:4014-4019.
3. Zhu Q, Tannenbaum S, Hegde P, Kane M, Xu C, Zurtzman SH. Noninvasive monitoring of breast cancer during neoadjuvant chemotherapy using optical tomography with ultrasound localization. *Neoplasia.* 2008;10:1028-1040.
4. Jiang S, Pogue BW, Carpenter CM, et al. Evaluation of breast tumor response to neoadjuvant chemotherapy with tomographic diffuse optical spectroscopy: case studies of tumor region-of-interest changes. *Radiology.* 2009;252:551-560.
5. Soliman H, Gunasekara A, Rycroft M, et al. Functional imaging using diffuse optical spectroscopy of neoadjuvant chemotherapy response in women with locally advanced breast cancer. *Clin Cancer Res.* 2010;16:2605-2614.
6. Roblyer D, Ueda S, Cerussi A, et al. Optical imaging of breast cancer oxyhemoglobin flare correlates with neoadjuvant chemotherapy response one day after starting treatment. *Proc Natl Acad Sci U S A.* 2011;108:14626-14631.
7. Ueda S, Roblyer D, Cerussi A, et al. Baseline tumor oxygen saturation correlates with a pathologic complete response in breast cancer patients undergoing neoadjuvant chemotherapy. *Cancer Res.* 2012;72:4318-4328.

Sentinel Node Biopsy

High risk of non-sentinel node metastases in a group of breast cancer patients with micrometastases in the sentinel node

Tvedskov TF, Jensen M-B, Lisse IM, et al (Copenhagen Univ Hosp, Denmark; Danish Breast Cancer Cooperative Group, Copenhagen, Denmark; Herlev Hosp, Copenhagen, Denmark)
Int J Cancer 131:2367-2375, 2012

Axillary lymph node dissection (ALND) in breast cancer patients with positive sentinel nodes is under debate. We aimed to establish two models to predict non-sentinel node (NSN) metastases in patients with micrometastases or isolated tumor cells (ITC) in sentinel nodes, to guide the decision for ALND. A total of 1,577 breast cancer patients with micrometastases and 304 with ITC in sentinel nodes, treated by sentinel lymph node dissection and ALND in 2002–2008 were identified in the Danish Breast Cancer Cooperative Group database. Risk of NSN metastases was calculated according to clinicopathological variables in a logistic regression analysis. We identified tumor size, proportion of positive sentinel nodes, lymphovascular invasion, hormone receptor status and location of tumor in upper lateral quadrant of the breast as risk factors for NSN metastases in patients with micrometastases. A model based on these risk factors identified 5% of patients with a risk of NSN metastases on nearly 40%. The model was however unable to identify a subgroup of patients with a very low risk of NSN metastases. Among patients with ITC, we identified tumor size, age and proportion of positive sentinel nodes as risk factors. A model based on these risk factors identified 32% of patients with risk of NSN metastases on only 2%. Omission of ALND would be acceptable in this group of patients. In contrast, ALND may still be beneficial in the subgroup of patients with micrometastases and a high risk of NSN metastases.

▶ Micrometastases have been perceived in various ways since their introduction into breast cancer staging by Huvos et al,[1] and changes in perception reflect a pendulum effect. At the beginning, they were considered prognostically insignificant and negligible; later, they were reported to represent a minor prognostic disadvantage.[2] And currently, several guidelines suggest ignoring them or approaching them as node-negative cases in terms of both staging (ie, stage IB rather than stage II disease with the tumor not larger than 2 cm, according to the latest edition of the TNM staging system[3]) and locoregional and systemic treatment.[4,5] A generalization without consideration of other clinical and pathologic parameters may be wrong.

A number of multivariable predictive models have been built to identify the subset of patients with low risk of NSN metastasis to follow on the idea that ALND can be omitted not only in patients with a negative sentinel node (SN) but also in a subset of patients with a positive SN, and SN metastasis size is one of the factors that are often found to influence the risk of NSN involvement.[6,7] The logic behind creating these models and predictive tools was the finding that most patients with a positive SN had no further lymph node involvement identified after ALND; therefore, ALND had only potential morbidity but no benefit for them. Importantly, these multivariable models demonstrate that having one factor that diminishes the risk of NSN involvement may be compensated or even overrun by other factors increasing this risk.

The results of the American College of Surgeons Oncology Group trial Z0011 have gone further by suggesting that many patients with metastatic SNs need no further axillary surgery,[8] and the surgical approach to patients meeting the entry criteria of the Z0011 trial has substantially changed: intraoperative assessment is less frequent, fewer patients are undergoing ALND despite their positive SN(s), and immunohistochemical analysis allowing for a higher detection rate of low-volume metastases has been abandoned.[9] On the basis of the ALND arm of the Z0011 trial, 27% of all patients and 10% of the 137 patients with SN micrometastases had NSN involvement, and this rate of NSN metastasis translated into only a 1% regional recurrence rate in the SN biopsy-only arm after 6.3 years of median follow-up.[8] Alternately worded, it seems that residual axillary disease after surgery did not translate into disease recurrence or adverse outcome in most patients enrolled.

In a recent Spanish trial in which patients with SN micrometastases were randomized to ALND or observation, 13% of the patients in the ALND arm had NSN involvement, but only 2.5% of the patients in the SN biopsy-only arm experienced a recurrence after a median follow-up of 62 months, which is very much in keeping with the results of the Z0011 trial.[10] It is clear that the numbers in the trial are relatively low to allow specific subgroup analyses. Although the conclusions may be true in general, limited SN and NSN involvement left behind after surgery (but subjected to non-targeted axillary effects of whole-breast irradiation and systemic therapy) does not influence disease-free survival in the short term. However, there might be subsets of patients with a high risk of NSN metastasis or more massive NSN involvement in whom ALND could be beneficial.

The existing predictive models can also be used to identify patients with a high risk of NSN metastasis but seem to perform less reliably than when used to identify low-risk patients.[11] Therefore, new models have been generated to delineate this group of patients.[12] Several NSN status predictive models devised for patients with SN micrometastases have shown that the worst combination of factors included in them may lead to considerable risks of NSN involvement. The highest predictable risk on the basis of the original 4-variable-based French micrometastasis nomogram is 51%, although 0/2 (95% confidence interval [CI]: 0% to 84%) such patients had NSN involvement in the relevant report.[13] The highest predicted risk in the Helsinki nomogram is 32.5% (with a theoretical multifocal tumor of 6 cm),[14] and this value is above 50% in the revised, 5-variable-based French micrometastasis nomogram.[15] Finally, 40% (23/57; 95% CI: 29% to 53%) of the patients with SN micrometastases also had NSN involvement when at least 4 of 5 predictive factors in the model described by Tvedskov and colleagues were present. These predictive tools perform differently at different institutions, which is not surprising owing to the differences in the proportions of patients having one or the other feature included in the models.[11,16] In our hands, the 4-variable-based French micrometastasis nomogram was one of the best performing models in tumors measuring up to 15 mm in the greatest dimension[13]; 66% of the patients were predicted to have less than 10% NSN involvement, and only 2/36 (5%; 95% CI: 2% to 18%) in this group had real involvement of NSNs, whereas 6/20 (30%; 95% CI: 15% to 52%) of those predicted to have more than 10% involvement had NSN metastasis.[17] After this validation, we introduced the model to predict the risk of NSN metastasis and also communicated the results to the patients while advising them on treatment possibilities. Although the number of patients was very small in this prospective series, several patients were afraid of having additional positive nodes that were left in situ and therefore chose to undergo ALND even when their risk was perceived low by doctors.[18] Patient information should probably forgo these risk estimates as much as possible and concentrate more on real outcome data available from the relevant studies[8,10] to avoid overtreatment.

Tvedskov and colleagues found no subgroup with sufficiently low risk of NSN involvement in the largest population-based series of breast cancer patients with SN micrometastases analyzed to date. This does not seem to matter in the setting of the Z0011 and the Spanish trials.[8,10] On the other hand, they identified a small subgroup of patients with sufficiently high (40%) risk of further lymph node involvement in a group of patients generally perceived as "node negative" according to current conceptions. Of course, the prediction is not perfect, as with other similar models, but the relatively rare unfavorable combination of factors influencing the risk of NSN metastasis, or a higher risk of more massive axillary involvement, could still be taken into account when deciding about further treatment of the axilla. This is why predictive models may still be of value, even in the micrometastatic setting.

G. Cserni, MD, PhD, DSc

References

1. Huvos AG, Hutter RV, Berg JW. Significance of axillary macrometastases and micrometastases in mammary cancer. *Ann Surg.* 1971;173:44-46.
2. Dowlatshahi K, Fan M, Snider HC, Habib FA. Lymph node micrometastases from breast carcinoma: reviewing the dilemma. *Cancer.* 1997;80:1188-1197.
3. Edge SB, Byrd DR, Compton CC, et al, eds. *AJCC Cancer Staging Handbook: From the AJCC Cancer Staging Manual.* 7th edition. New York: Springer; 2009.
4. Goldhirsch A, Wood WC, Coates AS, et al. Strategies for subtypes—dealing with the diversity of breast cancer: highlights of the St. Gallen International Expert Consensus on the Primary Therapy of Early Breast Cancer 2011. *Ann Oncol.* 2011;22:1736-1747.
5. National Comprehensive Cancer Network. NCCN Clinical Practice Guidelines in Oncology. Breast Cancer. Version 1. 2013. http://www.nccn.org/professionals/physician_gls/pdf/breast.pdf. Accessed March 5, 2013.
6. Cserni G. Sentinel node biopsy and nodal staging. In: Kahán Z, Tot T, eds. *Breast Cancer, a Heterogeneous Disease Entity. The Very Early Stages.* New York: Springer; 2011:149-184.
7. van la Parra RF, Peer PG, Ernst MF, Bosscha K. Meta-analysis of predictive factors for non-sentinel lymph node metastases in breast cancer patients with a positive SLN. *Eur J Surg Oncol.* 2011;37:290-299.
8. Giuliano AE, McCall L, Beitsch P, et al. Locoregional recurrence after sentinel lymph node dissection with or without axillary dissection in patients with sentinel lymph node metastases: the American College of Surgeons Oncology Group Z0011 randomized trial. *Ann Surg.* 2010;252:426-432 [discussion: 432-433].

9. Cody HS III, Houssami N. Axillary management in breast cancer: what's new for 2012? *Breast.* 2012;21:411-415.

10. Solá M, Alberro JA, Fraile M, et al. Complete axillary lymph node dissection versus clinical follow-up in breast cancer patients with sentinel node micrometastasis: final results from the multicenter clinical trial AATRM 048/13/2000. *Ann Surg Oncol.* 2013;20:120-127.

11. Cserni G, Bori R, Maráz R, et al. Multi-institutional comparison of non-sentinel lymph node predictive tools in breast cancer patients with high predicted risk of further axillary metastasis. *Pathol Oncol Res.* 2013;19:95-101.

12. Meretoja TJ, Audisio RAA, Heikkilä P, et al. International multicenter tool to predict the risk of four or more tumor-positive axillary lymph nodes in breast cancer patients with sentinel node macrometastases. *Breast Cancer Res Treat.* 2013;138:817–827.

13. Houvenaeghel G, Nos C, Giard S, et al. A nomogram predictive of non-sentinel lymph node involvement in breast cancer patients with a sentinel lymph node micrometastasis. *Eur J Surg Oncol.* 2009;35:690-695.

14. Meretoja TJ, Strien L, Heikkilä PS, Leidenius MH. A simple nomogram to evaluate the risk of nonsentinel node metastases in breast cancer patients with minimal sentinel node involvement. *Ann Surg Oncol.* 2012;19:567-576.

15. Houvenaeghel G, Bannier M, Nos C, et al. Non sentinel node involvement prediction for sentinel node micrometastases in breast cancer: nomogram validation and comparison with other models. *Breast.* 2012;21:204-209.

16. Cserni G, Boross G, Maráz R, et al. Multicentre validation of different predictive tools of non-sentinel lymph node involvement in breast cancer. *Surg Oncol.* 2012; 21:59-65.

17. Cserni G, Bori R, Sejben I, et al. Analysis of predictive tools for further axillary involvement in patients with sentinel-lymph-node-positive, small (< or =15 mm) invasive breast cancer. *Orv Hetil.* 2009;150:2182-2188 [in Hungarian].

18. Cserni G, Bezsenyi I, Markó L. Patients' choice on axillary lymph node dissection following sentinel lymph node micrometastasis - first report on prospective use of a nomogram in very low risk patients. *Pathol Oncol Res.* 2013;19:211-216.

Surgical Treatment

An Updated Meta-Analysis on the Effectiveness of Preoperative Prophylactic Antibiotics in Patients Undergoing Breast Surgical Procedures

Sajid MS, Hutson K, Akhter N, et al (Worthing Hosp, West Sussex, UK)
Breast J 18:312-317, 2012

To systematically analyze published randomized trials on the effectiveness of preoperative prophylactic antibiotics in patients undergoing breast surgical procedures. Trials on the effectiveness of preoperative prophylactic antibiotics in patients undergoing breast surgery were selected and analyzed to generate summated data (expressed as risk ratio [RR]) by using RevMan 5.0. Nine randomized controlled trials encompassing 3720 patients undergoing breast surgery were retrieved from the electronic databases. The antibiotics group comprised a total of 1857 patients and non-antibiotics group, 1863 patients. There was no heterogeneity [$\chi^2 = 7.61$, d.f. = 7, $p < 0.37$; $I^2 = 8\%$] amongst trials. Therefore, in the fixed-effects model (RR, 0.64; 95% CI, 0.50–0.83; z = 3.48; $p < 0.0005$), the use of preoperative prophylactic antibiotics in patients undergoing breast surgical procedures was statistically significant in reducing the incidence of surgical site infection (SSI). Furthermore, in the fixed-effects model (RR, 1.30; 95%

CI, $0.89-1.90$; $z = 1.37$; $p < 0.17$), adverse reactions secondary to the use of prophylactic antibiotics was not statistically significant between the two groups. Preoperative prophylactic antibiotics significantly reduce the risk of SSI after breast surgical procedures. The risk of adverse reactions from prophylactic antibiotic administration is not significant in these patients. Therefore, preoperative prophylactic antibiotics in breast surgery patients may be routinely administered. Further research is required, however, on risk stratification for SSI, timing and duration of prophylaxis, and the need for prophylaxis in patients undergoing breast reconstruction versus no reconstruction.

▶ "Clean procedures" do not generally warrant presurgical antibiotic prophylaxis, as the risk of SSI is low, but there are compelling reasons to consider its use in patients undergoing surgery for breast cancer. For one, SSI rates (3% to 15%) are higher in this patient group than the 3.4% SSI rate reported for other clean procedures.[1] In addition, the morbidity, increased healthcare costs, and potential delay in adjuvant chemotherapy and/or breast reconstruction associated with incurring an infection are not inconsequential. However, results from individual studies investigating the utility and safety of preoperative prophylaxis in this patient population have been inconclusive until now.

This well-done meta-analysis by Sajid et al incorporated 9 randomized controlled trials that included 3720 patients undergoing breast cancer surgery in Australia, Finland, Hong Kong, Italy, Norway, the United Kingdom, and the United States. Procedures ranged from excisional biopsy to axillary lymph node dissection to mastectomy. Prophylactic details were unavailable for one study and pre- and postoperative prophylaxis were used in 2 studies, but the majority employed a single preoperative dose of a beta-lactam ($n = 5$) or macrolide ($n = 1$) that would cover skin flora. The use of antimicrobial prophylaxis statistically reduced the incidence of SSI when compared with placebo or no treatment. Interestingly, an updated 2012 Cochrane review[2] examined the same question, using 8 of the 9 studies identified by Sajid and colleagues, and reached the same conclusion — preoperative prophylaxis reduces the risk of SSI in patients undergoing surgery for breast cancer. Sajid and colleagues also addressed whether there was a downside to prophylaxis, but they did not find one.

These 2 systematic reviews provide convincing evidence of the value of surgical prophylaxis, but the results are limited to non-reconstructive breast cancer surgery only. Insertion of a breast implant or tissue expander is a well-known risk factor for SSI, and clinical studies are needed to address whether prophylaxis would be beneficial for this particular subgroup. Another area of uncertainty is the optimal duration of prophylaxis. National guidelines[3] favor no more than 24 hours, but a common practice is to prescribe postoperative antibiotics for patients going home with a new prosthesis or drains. Because of the potential for adverse effects associated with antibiotic use, further evaluation is necessary. Finally, there is a growing understanding of other risk factors for SSI (eg, prior chest irradiation, active smoking, and suboptimal dosing in obese patients),[4] some of which are potentially modifiable. The possibility of developing a risk-stratification tool to predict SSI risk and/or strategies to prevent infection in patients undergoing surgery for breast cancer poses an additional area for research.

S. K. Seo, MD

References

1. Vazquez-Aragon P, Lizan-Garcia M, Cascales-Sanchez P, Villar-Canovas MT, Garcia-Olmo D. Nosocomial infection and related risk factors in a general surgery service: a prospective study. *J Infect.* 2003;46:17-22.
2. Bunn F, Jones DJ, Bell-Syer S. Prophylactic antibiotics to prevent surgical site infection after breast cancer surgery. *Cochrane Database Syst Rev.* 2012;(1):CD005360.
3. Antimicrobial prophylaxis in surgery. *Treat Guidel Med Lett.* 2012;10:73-78.
4. Olsen MA, Lefta M, Dietz JR, et al. Risk factors for surgical site infection after major breast operation. *J Am Coll Surg.* 2008;207:326-335.

Axillary Dissection Versus No Axillary Dissection in Older Patients With T1N0 Breast Cancer: 15-Year Results of a Randomized Controlled Trial
Martelli G, Boracchi P, Ardoino I, et al (Fondazione IRCCS Istituto Nazionale dei Tumori, Milan, Italy; Univ of Milan, Italy; et al)
Ann Surg 256:920-924, 2012

Objective.—To assess the role of axillary dissection in older breast cancer patients with a clinically clear axilla.

Background.—Axillary dissection, once standard treatment for breast cancer, is associated with considerable morbidity. It has been substituted by sentinel node biopsy with dissection only if the sentinel node is positive. We aimed to determine whether axillary surgery can be omitted in older women, thereby sparing them morbidity, without compromising long-term disease control.

Methods.—We carried out a randomized clinical trial on 238 older (65–80 years) breast cancer patients, with clinically N0 disease of radiographic diameter 2 cm or less. Patients were randomized to quadrantectomy with or without axillary dissection. All received radiotherapy to the residual breast but not the axilla; all were prescribed tamoxifen for 5 years. Main outcome measures were overall survival and breast cancer mortality. We also assessed overt axillary disease in those who did not receive axillary dissection.

Results.—After 15 years of follow-up, distant metastasis rate, overall survival, and breast cancer mortality in the axillary dissection and no axillary dissection arms were indistinguishable. The 15-year cumulative incidence of overt axillary disease in the no axillary dissection arm was only 6%.

Conclusions.—Older patients with early breast cancer and a clinically clear axilla treated by conservative surgery, postoperative radiotherapy,

TABLE 1.—Randomized Controlled Trials Avoiding Axillary Lymph Node Dissection in Patients With Metastatic Axillary Lymph Nodes

Trial	No-ALND Group (cN0)	Further LN Met ALND Group (%)	Follow-up	Axillary Disease (% Overall)	Axillary Disease (% With LN Met)
Martelli[7]	Age >65 yrs: BCS + WBRT + Tam (n = 110)	23%	5 yrs / 12.5 yrs	1.8% / 3.6%	7.9% / 16%
NSABP B-04[4,8]	Total mast: No RT, no Sys Rx (n = 365)	40%	3 yrs / 25 yrs	14% / 19%	36% / 47%
IBCSG 10-93[3]	Age >60 yrs: Surg ± RT + Tam (n = 239)	27%	6.6 yrs	2.5%	9.2%
ACOSOG Z0011[5]	SLN met: BCS + WBRT + Sys Rx (n = 446)	27%	6.3 yrs	0.9%	3.3%
IBCSG 23-01[1]	SLN micromet: BCS + RT + Sys Rx (n = 469)	13%	5 yrs	1.9%	13%

ALND, axillary lymph node dissection; cN0, clinically node negative; met, metastasis; yrs, years; LN, lymph node; SLN, sentinel lymph node; RT, radiation therapy; BCS, breast-conserving surgery; WBRT, whole-breast radiotherapy; Tam, tamoxifen; NSABP, National Surgical Adjuvant Breast and Bowel Project; mast, mastectomy; sys Rx, systemic therapy; IBCSG, International Breast Cancer Study Group; ACOSOG, American College of Surgeons Oncology Group; micromet, micrometastasis.

Editor's Note: Please refer to original journal article for full references.

and adjuvant tamoxifen do not benefit from axillary dissection. This study was registered at clinicaltrials.gov (ID NCT00002720) (Table 1).

▶ Martelli et al recently published their 15-year follow-up of a study in which women between 65 and 80 years old with clinically lymph node-negative breast cancers less than 2 cm on mammography who underwent breast-conserving surgery (BCS) were randomized to undergo axillary lymph node dissection (ALND) or no axillary surgery. In this study, from 1996 to 2000, before the widespread use of sentinel lymph node biopsy (SLNB), all patients received adjuvant whole-breast radiation therapy (WBRT) and tamoxifen for 5 years. The authors acknowledge that accrual was slow, and only 238 of the targeted 642 patients were recruited. Nonetheless, after a median follow-up of 150 months, there were no differences in overall survival or disease-specific survival between patients who had undergone ALND and those who had not. Only 4 patients (3.6%) who had not undergone axillary surgery developed overt axillary metastatic disease.

Previously, ALND was the standard of care for all patients with breast cancer. Following the introduction of SLNB, it became the standard treatment for those with sentinel lymph node (SLN) metastases. This important study is part of the growing evidence that not all patients with axillary lymph node metastasis are required to undergo ALND with its associated morbidity (Table 1). In 4 other randomized controlled trials,[1-4] the avoidance of ALND in patients who were clinically node negative (with limited SLN metastasis in 2 of these studies)[1,2] did not compromise overall survival or disease-specific survival.

Surgeons have also performed ALND in patients with known lymph node metastases to avoid the morbidity of uncontrolled axillary disease. In the National

Surgical Adjuvant Breast and Bowel Project B-04 study, after 25 years of follow-up, fewer than half of the 40% of patients with axillary lymph node metastasis treated without ALND, radiation therapy (RT), or systemic treatment developed obvious axillary disease.[4] In more recent studies, with the use of adjuvant systemic treatment and RT, after 5 years of follow-up, axillary disease was reported in only 3.3% to 13% of the 13% to 27% of patients who had axillary lymph node metastasis treated without ALND.[1,3,5] Clinically evident axillary disease developed in only 0.9% to 2.5% of all patients who avoided ALND. One criticism in particular, levied against the American College of Surgeons Oncology Group Z0011 trial, is that the 6.3 years of follow-up is too short to detect differences in survival or locoregional recurrence between groups with mainly estrogen receptor-positive breast cancer. Martelli and colleagues have rebutted this argument: after 150 months of follow-up without ALND, only 16% of the patients with axillary lymph node metastasis (3.6% of all patients) developed overt axillary disease.

Because of these trials, we can now omit ALND in patients with early-stage breast cancer and clinically negative axillary lymph nodes (including those with limited SLN metastasis) who are undergoing BCS, RT, and systemic treatment. With the advent of genomic analysis, axillary staging in early breast cancer has become less important in deciding which adjuvant systemic therapies should be used. The necessity of even performing SLNB in patients with early-stage breast cancer and negative axillary lymph nodes by clinical examination and ultrasonography who are undergoing BCS and RT is now being investigated.[6-8] Overall, 1560 patients who meet the eligibility criteria for this trial will be randomized to SLNB (with ALND for macrometastasis) or no axillary staging surgery. The accrual and results of this trial will be watched with great anticipation.

J. O. Murphy, MD

V. S. Sacchini, MD

References

1. Galimberti V, Cole BF, Zurrida S, et al; International Breast Cancer Study Group Trial 23-01 investigators. Axillary dissection versus no axillary dissection in patients with sentinel-node micrometastases (IBCSG 23-01): a phase 3 randomised controlled trial. *Lancet Oncol.* 2013;14:297-305.
2. Giuliano AE, Hunt KK, Ballman KV, et al. Axillary dissection vs no axillary dissection in women with invasive breast cancer and sentinel node metastasis: a randomized clinical trial. *JAMA.* 2011;305:569-575.
3. International Breast Cancer Study Group, Rudenstam CM, Zahrieh D, Forbes JF, et al. Randomized trial comparing axillary clearance versus no axillary clearance in older patients with breast cancer: first results of International Breast Cancer Study Group Trial 10-93. *J Clin Oncol.* 2006;24:337-344.
4. Fisher B, Jeong JH, Anderson S, Bryant J, Fisher ER, Wolmark N. Twenty-five-year follow-up of a randomized trial comparing radical mastectomy, total mastectomy, and total mastectomy followed by irradiation. *N Engl J Med.* 2002;347:567-575.
5. Giuliano AE, McCall L, Beitsch P, et al. Locoregional recurrence after sentinel lymph node dissection with or without axillary dissection in patients with sentinel lymph node metastases: the American College of Surgeons Oncology Group Z0011 randomized trial. *Ann Surg.* 2010;252:426-432. discussion, 432-433.

6. Gentilini O, Veronesi U. Abandoning sentinel lymph node biopsy in early breast cancer? A new trial in progress at the European Institute of Oncology of Milan (SOUND: sentinel node vs Observation after axillary UltraSouND). *Breast.* 2012;21:678-681.
7. Martelli G, Boracchi P, De Palo M, et al. A randomized trial comparing axillary dissection to no axillary dissection in older patients with T1N0 breast cancer: results after 5 years of follow-up. *Ann Surg.* 2005;242:1-6. discussion, 7-9.
8. Fisher B, Montague E, Redmond C, et al. Comparison of radical mastectomy with alternative treatments for primary breast cancer. A first report of results from a prospective randomized clinical trial. *Cancer.* 1977;39:2827-2839.

Reduced Incidence of Breast Cancer–Related Lymphedema following Mastectomy and Breast Reconstruction versus Mastectomy Alone

Card A, Crosby MA, Liu J, et al (Univ of Texas MD Anderson Cancer Ctr, Houston)
Plast Reconstr Surg 130:1169-1178, 2012

Background.—As breast cancer survivorship has increased, so has an awareness of the morbidities associated with its treatment. The incidence of breast cancer–related lymphedema has been reported to be 8 to 30 percent in all breast cancer survivors. To determine whether breast cancer reconstruction has an impact on the incidence of breast cancer–related lymphedema, the authors compared its incidence in patients who underwent mastectomy with reconstruction versus mastectomy alone.

Methods.—All patients who underwent mastectomy, with or without immediate breast reconstruction, between 2001 and 2006, were identified through a search of prospective institutional databases. To reduce variation caused by known predictive factors, the individuals were cross-matched for age, axillary intervention, and postoperative axillary irradiation. The incidence of lymphedema was based on the presence of arm edema that lasted more than 6 months and was documented clinically.

Results.—Of the 574 cross-matched patients included in the study, 78 (6.8 percent) developed lymphedema (21 with reconstructed breasts and 57 with unreconstructed breasts). Patients who did not undergo reconstruction were significantly more likely to develop breast cancer–related lymphedema (9.9 percent versus 3.7 percent; $p < 0.001$). Postoperative axillary radiation therapy ($p < 0.001$), one or more positive lymph nodes ($p = 0.010$), and body mass index of 25 or greater ($p = 0.021$) were also associated with an increased incidence of lymphedema. Reconstruction patients developed lymphedema significantly later than nonreconstruction patients ($p < 0.001$).

Conclusion.—Patients who undergo breast reconstruction have a lower incidence and a delay in onset of breast cancer–related lymphedema compared with patients who undergo mastectomy alone.

Clinical Question/Level of Evidence.—Therapeutic, III.

▶ In this article, the authors from The University of Texas MD Anderson Cancer Center retrospectively reviewed the incidence of lymphedema in women with breast cancer who underwent mastectomy and reconstruction or mastectomy alone. They included patients treated between 2001 and 2006 to have sufficient follow-up available for lymphedema development. Patients were cross-matched between groups for age, axillary intervention, and postoperative axillary radiation therapy. The incidence of breast cancer-related lymphedema was reported for each group based on "subjective data" documented in the prospectively maintained institutional database and on arm circumference measurements. Patients who had had preoperative radiation therapy or for whom measurements were not available were excluded. In the final analysis, 574 patient pairs (1148 breasts) were analyzed with an average follow-up of 59 ± 26.9 months.

Overall, 6.8% of all patients in the study developed lymphedema (78 patients, 21 of whom had reconstruction and 57 of whom did not). Patients who did not undergo reconstruction had a higher incidence of lymphedema (9.9%) than did those who underwent reconstruction (3.7%). This difference in the rate of lymphedema persisted even when the authors performed multivariate logistic regression analysis controlling for body mass index, lymph node dissection, and radiation therapy. In addition, using a univariate Cox proportional hazards regression analysis, the authors found that the development of lymphedema in women who underwent reconstruction was significantly slower than in women who did not have reconstruction.

The results reported in this article are interesting; when taken at face value, they suggest that reconstruction after mastectomy may have a protective effect vis-a-vis the development of lymphedema. However, this conclusion should be tempered until prospective data are available. The most significant weakness of this article is the fact that even though the groups were cross-matched for a few variables, they were significantly different in a number of important ways. For example, the non-reconstructed group was significantly older, significantly heavier (body mass index 28.6 vs 25.7), and had significantly more lymph nodes removed than did the group that underwent mastectomy and reconstruction. These factors are all known risk variables for developing lymphedema; therefore, the finding that women who did not have reconstruction were more likely to develop lymphedema may simply reflect the fact that this group was also older, sicker, and heavier than was the reconstructed group. This explanation is further supported by the finding that patients in the non-reconstructed group also had a higher incidence of diabetes and hypertension and were more likely to smoke. The multivariate logistic regression analysis in this study did help to control for some of these factors; however, it is difficult to control for multiple comorbid conditions when the index number of outcomes is relatively low (ie, 78 patients overall who developed lymphedema). In addition, it is impossible to control for all these outcomes using this analysis.

Another issue is the diagnosis of lymphedema in this study. Although the authors stated that this was based on subjective measures (undefined) and circumference measurements, it is unclear what criteria were used to define lymphedema (eg, differences in affected and unaffected arms, preoperative vs postoperative measurements). In addition, the use of circumference measurements is somewhat problematic owing to inter- and intra-user variability.

Overall, this is an interesting article and a step forward in the lymphedema literature. Additional prospective studies are needed, however, to test the hypothesis that reconstruction after mastectomy has a protective effect in terms of postmastectomy lymphedema.

B. Mehrara, MD, PhD

Tumor Biology

Clinically Used Breast Cancer Markers Such As Estrogen Receptor, Progesterone Receptor, and Human Epidermal Growth Factor Receptor 2 Are Unstable Throughout Tumor Progression
Lindström LS, Karlsson E, Wilking UM, et al (Karolinska Institutet and Karolinska University Hospital, Solna, Sweden; et al)
J Clin Oncol 30:2601-2608, 2012

Purpose.—To investigate whether hormonal receptors and human epidermal growth factor receptor 2 (HER2) change throughout tumor progression, because this may alter patient management.

Patients and Methods.—The study cohort included female patients with breast cancer in the Stockholm health care region who relapsed from January 1, 1997, to December 31, 2007. Either biochemical or immunohistochemical (IHC)/immunocytochemical (ICC) methods were used to determine estrogen receptor (ER), progesterone receptor (PR), and HER2 status, which was then confirmed by fluorescent in situ hybridization for IHC/ICC 2+ and 3+ status.

Results.—ER (459 patients), PR (430 patients), and HER2 (104 patients) from both primary tumor and relapse were assessed, revealing a change in 32.4% (McNemar's test $P < .001$), 40.7% ($P < .001$), and 14.5% ($P = .44$) of patients, respectively. Assessment of ER (119 patients), PR (116 patients), and HER2 (32 patients) with multiple (from two to six) consecutive relapses showed an alteration in 33.6%, 32.0%, and 15.7% of patients, respectively. A statistically significant differential overall survival related to intraindividual ER and PR status in primary tumor and relapse (log-rank $P < .001$) was noted. In addition, women with ER-positive primary tumors that changed to ER-negative tumors had a significant 48% increased risk of death (hazard ratio, 1.48; 95% CI, 1.08 to 2.05) compared with women with stable ER-positive tumors.

Conclusion.—Patients with breast cancer experience altered hormone receptor and HER2 status throughout tumor progression, possibly influenced by adjuvant therapies, which significantly influences survival.

Hence, marker investigations at relapse may potentially improve patient management and survival.

▶ Breast cancer treatment is determined by the tumor subtype; knowledge of the ER, PR, and HER2 status is fundamental for treatment selection among not only patients with early-stage breast cancer but also for those with metastatic disease.[1] The lack of stability in the expression of the hormone receptors and HER2 has been described by several groups,[2-6] but the frequency of discordance, its relationship to changes in treatment, its prognostic implications, and whether this change is influenced by adjuvant therapies remain areas of great interest.

In this study, Lindström et al assessed intraindividual ER, PR, and HER2 status in a large cohort of breast cancer patients by contrasting primary tumor and relapse marker status and by comparing intra-individual marker status in consecutive relapses. The authors identified a total of 459, 430, and 104 patients with paired determination of ER, PR, and HER2, respectively. A very high frequency of discordance was observed. Among patients with positive ER, PR, and HER2 status in the primary tumor, a change to negative status was observed in 24.6%, 33.0%, and 8.7% of relapses, respectively. Of less magnitude but similar interest, the ER, PR, and HER2 status changed from negative in the primary tumor to positive in the relapse in 7.8%, 7.7%, and 5.8% of patients, respectively. The absolute discordance rate was 32.4%, 40.7%, and 14.5% for ER, PR, and HER2, respectively. Among the patients with multiple relapses, the authors evaluated the discrepancy among relapses and found that the discrepancy rate was 33.6%, 32.0%, and 15.7% for ER, PR, and HER2, respectively. Furthermore, the proportion of patients who lost ER positivity was highest in the group who underwent endocrine therapy compared with those who underwent chemotherapy alone or received no treatment. In addition, the risk of death was higher in patients whose ER status changed from positive to negative than in patients whose positive ER status was stable.

Despite its retrospective nature, this study was strengthened by the inclusion of a large cohort of prospectively identified patients at an institution where performing biopsies at the time of relapse is considered standard practice. The frequent change in the biomarkers observed between primary tumors and relapses highlights the fact that tumor progression is a dynamic process and that intratumor heterogeneity can be affected by treatment, resulting in clonal selection. Considering how important the previously discussed biomarkers are in treatment selection, the data presented by Lindström and colleagues should strongly influence our practice. Biopsies at the time of relapse should become part of the standard of care. Information on biomarkers at the time of relapse will help us expand our understanding of the biology of disease progression and metastasis and, most importantly, will help us to better tailor and personalize our treatment decisions.

M. Chavez-MacGregor, MD, MSc
V. Valero, MD

References

1. NCCN Clinical Practice Guidelines in Oncology. Breast Cancer. Version 1. 2013. http://www.nccn.org/professionals/physician_gls/pdf/breast.pdf. Accessed February 21, 2013.
2. Amir E, Ooi WS, Simmons C, et al. Discordance between receptor status in primary and metastatic breast cancer: an exploratory study of bone and bone marrow biopsies. *Clin Oncol (R Coll Radiol)*. 2008;20:763-768.
3. Guarneri V, Giovannelli S, Ficarra G, et al. Comparison of HER-2 and hormone receptor expression in primary breast cancers and asynchronous paired metastases: impact on patient management. *Oncologist*. 2008;13:838-844.
4. Idirisinghe PK, Thike AA, Cheok PY, et al. Hormone receptor and c-ERBB2 status in distant metastatic and locally recurrent breast cancer. Pathologic correlations and clinical significance. *Am J Clin Pathol*. 2010;133:416-429.
5. Simmons C, Miller N, Geddie W, et al. Does confirmatory tumor biopsy alter the management of breast cancer patients with distant metastases? *Ann Oncol*. 2009; 20:1499-1504.
6. Wilking U, Karlsson E, Skoog L, et al. HER2 status in a population-derived breast cancer cohort: discordances during tumor progression. *Breast Cancer Res Treat*. 2011;125:553-561.

CHEK2*1100delC Heterozygosity in Women With Breast Cancer Associated With Early Death, Breast Cancer–Specific Death, and Increased Risk of a Second Breast Cancer

Weischer M, Nordestgaard BG, Pharoah P, et al (Univ of Copenhagen, Denmark; Univ of Cambridge, UK; et al)
J Clin Oncol 30:4308-4316, 2012

Purpose.—We tested the hypotheses that *CHEK2*1100delC heterozygosity is associated with increased risk of early death, breast cancer–specific death, and risk of a second breast cancer in women with a first breast cancer.

Patients and Methods.—From 22 studies participating in the Breast Cancer Association Consortium, 25,571 white women with invasive breast cancer were genotyped for *CHEK2*1100delC and observed for up to 20 years (median, 6.6 years). We examined risk of early death and breast cancer-specific death by estrogen receptor status and risk of a second breast cancer after a first breast cancer in prospective studies.

Results.—*CHEK2*1100delC heterozygosity was found in 459 patients (1.8%). In women with estrogen receptor–positive breast cancer, multifactorially adjusted hazard ratios for heterozygotes versus noncarriers were 1.43 (95% CI, 1.12 to 1.82; log-rank $P = .004$) for early death and 1.63 (95% CI, 1.24 to 2.15; log-rank $P < .001$) for breast cancer–specific death. In all women, hazard ratio for a second breast cancer was 2.77 (95% CI, 2.00 to 3.83; log-rank $P < .001$) increasing to 3.52 (95% CI, 2.35 to 5.27; log-rank $P < .001$) in women with estrogen receptor–positive first breast cancer only.

Conclusion.—Among women with estrogen receptor-positive breast cancer, *CHEK2*1100delC heterozygosity was associated with a 1.4-fold risk of early death, a 1.6-fold risk of breast cancer-specific death, and a 3.5-fold risk of a second breast cancer. This is one of the few examples of a genetic factor that influences long-term prognosis being documented in an extensive series of women with breast cancer.

▶ In contrast to the high risk associated with highly penetrant mutations in the tumor suppressors *BRCA1* and *BRCA2*, individuals heterozygous for the *CHEK2*1100delC* variant in the *CHEK2* cell cycle checkpoint gene have a modestly increased risk of breast cancer.[1-3] *CHEK2*1100delC* is a rare dysfunctional variant primarily carried by individuals of Northern and Eastern European descent. Previously, it was reported that *CHEK2*1100delC* heterozygotes with breast cancer had a 2-fold increased risk of developing secondary breast cancer and a lower recurrence-free survival rate.[4] However, the retrospective nature of this cohort study and the relatively small number of carriers call for more precise estimates.

In this article, Weischer and colleagues analyzed 22 studies from 12 countries participating in the Breast Cancer Association Consortium (BCAC), a large collection of studies with prospective design that included 25 571 women with early mortality information, including 459 *CHEK2*1100delC* heterozygotes. The authors found that *CHEK2*1100delC* carriers were more likely to have estrogen receptor (ER)—positive breast cancer compared to noncarriers and that among ER-positive patients, *CHEK2*1100delC* heterozygotes had a 1.4-fold higher risk of early death, a 1.6-fold higher risk of breast cancer—specific death, and a 3.5-fold higher risk of a second breast cancer.

The 2- to 4-fold increase in the risk of a second breast cancer reported in these 2 studies is similar to the increased risk of primary cancer associated with *CHEK2*1100delC*, suggesting that inherited susceptibility likely persists due to haploinsufficiency of the *CHEK2* gene. It is interesting that, unlike the effect of the variant on breast cancer risk, the association between *CHEK2*1100delC* and early and breast cancer—specific deaths is found only in ER-positive patients; however, the underlying biological mechanism of this association is unclear and additional confirmation in independent studies may be necessary.

Using the same study population from the BCAC, Fasching and colleagues[5] recently examined the prognostic relevance of 11 common single-nucleotide polymorphisms identified from genome-wide association studies of risk. The authors found that only one variant of the *TOX3* gene was moderately associated with breast cancer survival, suggesting that survival may be influenced by a distinct set of genetic variants. *CHEK2* belongs to a class of medium- to high-risk breast cancer genes whose rare variants (minor allele frequency = 0.1% to 0.5%) contribute to a 3- to 5-fold increased risk of breast cancer. The same gene class also includes *p53*, *PTEN*, *ATM*, *NBS1*, *RAD50*, *BRIP1*, and *PALB2*. Rare variants in these genes have been linked to breast cancer prognosis (eg, survival, recurrence, and second cancers) in a variety of studies, although none of them, except *CHEK2*1100delC*, has been tested in large studies such as the BCAC study. It is possible that rare variants of this gene class contribute to the heritability of breast cancer survival and/or second cancers; some of these variants are awaiting future discovery by further fine mapping and targeted deep sequencing.

As mentioned by the authors, there are several limitations to this study. Most of them are directly related to missing key clinical data. For example, 25% to 30% of the study subjects did not have ER status information, and 40% to 45% were missing lymph node status. In addition, the treatment information was completely absent. Although there was no direct evidence to suggest that the missing clinical data would alter the overall conclusions, it is possible that they might change the interpretation of specific results. For example, if treatment information were available, one might investigate whether radiation-based adjuvant therapy could affect the association between *CHEK2**1100delC and survival and second cancer occurrence. Since *CHEK2* is activated by double-strand DNA breaks and is involved in cell cycle control, DNA repair, and apoptosis, it is plausible that this rare genetic variant could function as a predictive factor for treatment outcome. Missing clinical information is not an infrequent occurrence in consortium-based epidemiologic studies because of the logistic difficulty of collecting comprehensive clinical data from various study sites that are often in different countries. Besides geographic and administrative barriers, the clinical data from disparate sites may be difficult to merge due to differences in recording systems for clinical variables. Moreover, there may be variations in treatment options and treatment quality that could confound the clinical outcomes. Thus, despite concerted efforts to minimize missing data, the collection and management of clinical information still pose a significant challenge in the consortium-based approach to studying cancer outcomes. Nevertheless, the large sample size of this study and the lengthy duration of prospective follow-up provide confidence that the dysfunctional *CHEK2* variant in women with breast cancer plays a prognostic role.

X. Wu, MD, PhD

H. Zhao, PhD

References

1. Meijers-Heijboer H, van den Ouweland A, Klijn J, et al; CHEK2-Breast Cancer Consortium. Low-penetrance susceptibility to breast cancer due to CHEK2(*) 1100delC in noncarriers of BRCA1 or BRCA2 mutations. *Nat Genet.* 2002;31: 55-59.
2. CHEK2 Breast Cancer Case-Control Consortium. CHEK2*1100delC and susceptibility to breast cancer: a collaborative analysis involving 10,860 breast cancer cases and 9,065 controls from 10 studies. *Am J Hum Genet.* 2004;74:1175-1182.
3. Weischer M, Bojesen SE, Ellervik C, Tybjaerg-Hansen A, Nordestgaard BG. CHEK*1100delC genotyping for clinical assessment of breast cancer risk: meta-analyses of 26,000 patient cases and 27,000 controls. *J Clin Oncol.* 2008;26: 542-548.
4. Schmidt MK, Tollenaar RA, de Kemp SR, et al. Breast cancer survival and tumor characteristics in premenopausal women carrying the CHEK2*1100delC germline mutation. *J Clin Oncol.* 2007;25:64-69.
5. Fasching PA, Pharoah PD, Cox A, et al. The role of genetic breast cancer susceptibility variants as prognostic factors. *Hum Mol Genet.* 2012;21:3926-3929.

Breast Conserving Therapy

Variability in Reexcision Following Breast Conservation Surgery

McCahill LE, Single RM, Aiello Bowles EJ, et al (Michigan State Univ, Grand Rapids; Univ of Vermont, Burlington; Group Health Res Inst, Seattle, WA; et al)
JAMA 307:467-475, 2012

Context.—Health care reform calls for increasing physician accountability and transparency of outcomes. Partial mastectomy is the most commonly performed procedure for invasive breast cancer and often requires reexcision. Variability in reexcision might be reflective of the quality of care.

Objective.—To assess hospital and surgeon-specific variation in reexcision rates following partial mastectomy.

Design, Setting, and Patients.—An observational study of breast surgery performed between 2003 and 2008 intended to evaluate variability in breast cancer surgical care outcomes and evaluate potential quality measures of breast cancer surgery. Women with invasive breast cancer undergoing partial mastectomy from 4 institutions were studied (1 university hospital [University of Vermont] and 3 large health plans [Kaiser Permanente Colorado, Group Health, and Marshfield Clinic]). Data were obtained from electronic medical records and chart abstraction of surgical, pathology, radiology, and outpatient records, including detailed surgical margin status. Logistic regression including surgeon-level random effects was used to identify predictors of reexcision.

Main Outcome Measure.—Incidence of reexcision.

Results.—A total of 2206 women with 2220 invasive breast cancers underwent partial mastectomy and 509 patients (22.9%; 95% CI, 21.2%-24.7%) underwent reexcision (454 patients [89.2%; 95% CI, 86.5%-91.9%] had 1 reexcision, 48 [9.4%; 95% CI, 6.9%-12.0%] had 2 reexcisions, and 7 [1.4%; 95% CI, 0.4%-2.4%] had 3 reexcisions). Among all patients undergoing initial partial mastectomy, total mastectomy was performed in 190 patients (8.5%; 95% CI, 7.2%-9.5%). Reexcision rates for margin status following initial surgery were 85.9% (95% CI, 82.0%-89.8%) for initial positive margins, 47.9% (95% CI, 42.0%-53.9%) for less than 1.0 mm margins, 20.2% (95% CI, 15.3%-25.0%) for 1.0 to 1.9 mm margins, and 6.3% (95% CI, 3.2%-9.3%) for 2.0 to 2.9 mm margins. For patients with negative margins, reexcision rates varied widely among surgeons (range, 0%-70%; $P = .003$) and institutions (range, 1.7%-20.9%; $P < .001$). Reexcision rates were not associated with surgeon procedure volume after adjusting for case mix ($P = .92$).

Conclusion.—Substantial surgeon and institutional variation were observed in reexcision following partial mastectomy in women with invasive breast cancer.

▶ The goals of breast-conserving therapy (defined as lumpectomy and postoperative radiation therapy) in the management of invasive breast cancer are 2-fold:

First and foremost is the need to eradicate the disease so as to maintain maximal quantity of life. Given that this technique has been tested in multiple prospective, randomized, phase III trials against mastectomy, we know that this technique does preserve quantity of life. The second role, and truly a vital role of this therapy, is maintenance of quality of life (ie, preserving the breast as close to the original as possible).

Pivotal to the second role is the amount of surgery done. Lumpectomy followed by one or more re-excisions can definitely decrease the quality of the second goal, not to mention issues of increased cost. These data looking at the variability of re-excision following breast conservation surgery reveal a wide array of practices regarding re-excision that are not all related to patient or cancer factors. These data beg for some standardization. This standardization could be done via coordination between breast surgeons and breast radiation oncologists to develop some consensus guidelines to enhance the quality of care for these patients.

C. Lawton, MD

Hormonal Therapy

Everolimus in Postmenopausal Hormone-Receptor–Positive Advanced Breast Cancer

Baselga J, Campone M, Piccart M, et al (Massachusetts General Hosp Cancer Ctr, Boston, MA; Institut de Cancérologie de l'Ouest/René Gauducheau, Nantes Saint Herblain, France; Inst Jules Bordet, Brussels; et al)
N Engl J Med 366:520-529, 2012

Background.—Resistance to endocrine therapy in breast cancer is associated with activation of the mammalian target of rapamycin (mTOR) intracellular signaling pathway. In early studies, the mTOR inhibitor everolimus added to endocrine therapy showed antitumor activity.

Methods.—In this phase 3, randomized trial, we compared everolimus and exemestane versus exemestane and placebo (randomly assigned in a 2:1 ratio) in 724 patients with hormone-receptor-positive advanced breast cancer who had recurrence or progression while receiving previous therapy with a nonsteroidal aromatase inhibitor in the adjuvant setting or to treat advanced disease (or both). The primary end point was progression-free survival. Secondary end points included survival, response rate, and safety. A preplanned interim analysis was performed by an independent data and safety monitoring committee after 359 progression-free survival events were observed.

Results.—Baseline characteristics were well balanced between the two study groups. The median age was 62 years, 56% had visceral involvement, and 84% had hormone-sensitive disease. Previous therapy included letrozole or anastrozole (100%), tamoxifen (48%), fulvestrant (16%), and chemotherapy (68%). The most common grade 3 or 4 adverse events were stomatitis (8% in the everolimus-plus-exemestane group vs. 1% in the placebo-plus-exemestane group), anemia (6% vs. <1%), dyspnea

(4% vs. 1%), hyperglycemia (4% vs. <1%), fatigue (4% vs. 1%), and pneumonitis (3% vs. 0%). At the interim analysis, median progression-free survival was 6.9 months with everolimus plus exemestane and 2.8 months with placebo plus exemestane, according to assessments by local investigators (hazard ratio for progression or death, 0.43; 95% confidence interval [CI], 0.35 to 0.54; $P < 0.001$). Median progression-free survival was 10.6 months and 4.1 months, respectively, according to central assessment (hazard ratio, 0.36; 95% CI, 0.27 to 0.47; $P < 0.001$).

Conclusions.—Everolimus combined with an aromatase inhibitor improved progression-free survival in patients with hormone-receptor-positive advanced breast cancer previously treated with nonsteroidal aromatase inhibitors. (Funded by Novartis; BOLERO-2 ClinicalTrials.gov number, NCT00863655.)

▶ The birth of targeted therapy for breast cancer was arguably in 1896, when Beatson described the successful treatment of advanced breast cancer with oophorectomy.[1] This discovery ultimately led to the recognition that the majority of breast cancers are hormonally driven and may be effectively managed with directed therapies, including selective estrogen receptor modulators, and, more recently, aromatase inhibitors (AIs). Although these drugs significantly improve clinical outcomes for patients with hormone receptor (HR)-positive cancer, the vast majority of patients with metastatic disease demonstrate either de novo or acquired resistance to these therapies.[2] Thus, although effective treatments exist for HR-positive disease, understanding the mechanisms of tumor resistance to hormonally directed therapies may facilitate the development of a new generation of medications to circumvent resistance and improve patient outcomes.

One proposed mechanism of endocrine resistance supported by preclinical work is the activation of alternative pathways, such as the PI3K/AKT/mTOR pathway.[3,4] In preclinical models, inhibition of the PI3K pathway reversed anti-estrogen resistance.[5] Clinically, phase I[6-8] and phase II[9] studies in the neoadjuvant[10] and metastatic settings have shown the activity of everolimus, an oral mTOR inhibitor, as a single agent or in combination with tamoxifen or an AI. Based on these promising preclinical and early clinical results, the Breast Cancer Trials of Oral Everolimus-2 (BOLERO-2) trial was undertaken. In this randomized phase III study, 724 postmenopausal women with metastatic HR-positive, human epidermal growth factor receptor 2-negative breast cancer who had refractory or progressive disease after or while receiving a nonsteroidal aromatase inhibitor (NSAI) were randomly assigned to exemestane with everolimus or exemestane with placebo. Patients in the everolimus arm had a significantly longer progression-free survival (PFS) duration than did those in the control arm. Exploratory subgroup analysis by factors such as age, performance status, geographic region, previous hormonal therapy or chemotherapy, and number of prior therapies showed similar benefits in all subgroups.

The impressive improvement in PFS associated with everolimus came at the cost of an increase in adverse events. In the combination arm, 23% of patients experienced serious adverse events, compared with 12% in the control arm. Moreover, more patients in the everolimus arm than in the control group discontinued therapy because of adverse events (19% vs 4%, respectively). Interestingly, although the incidence of adverse effects was higher in the everolimus arm, the authors reported no difference in quality of life between the 2 arms (data not shown). It should be noted, however, that within the context of a clinical trial, study participants tend to be monitored more closely for adverse events and receive protocol-mandated dose reductions or supportive measures as appropriate. As clinicians begin to widely adopt the use of everolimus as the standard of care outside the clinical trial setting, they must recognize the more common and more serious adverse events and, in turn, have the resources and training to provide the proper management. The more notable side effects of everolimus include stomatitis, anemia, hyperglycemia, fatigue, and pneumonitis. Although most of these events are reversible via dose adjustments and appropriate supportive care, a course of steroids may be necessary in patients with grade 3 or higher pneumonitis.

Several questions remain regarding the addition of everolimus to endocrine therapy. One question is the optimal timing for the initiation of everolimus plus exemestane. Based on these phase III data, everolimus should be used in the setting of resistance to an NSAI. An appropriate standard treatment in this setting is fulvestrant. Although low-dose (250 mg monthly) fulvestrant has been found to have equivalent efficacy when compared with exemestane,[11] the more efficacious high-dose[12] (500 mg) fulvestrant has not been compared directly with exemestane. Interestingly, 17% of patients in the BOLERO-2 study had previously received fulvestrant. Therefore, it appears that exemestane plus everolimus can be used after fulvestrant, although the benefit of the reverse order is not known at this time. Another question relates to whether everolimus should be used in combination with other hormonally directed therapies. Although phase II data support the use of everolimus in combination with tamoxifen,[9] the relative benefit of adding everolimus to other endocrine agents, including fulvestrant and NSAIs, is not yet known. Other questions relating to its relative benefits compared with chemotherapy and its use in premenopausal patients and in the less treatment-resistant settings (ie, the adjuvant setting and the AI-naive metastatic setting) remain but will likely be addressed in future studies.

Since the results of the BOLERO-2 study were published, we have used everolimus in combination with exemestane for suitable patients whose disease has demonstrated resistance to an NSAI. When prescribing everolimus, however, we educate patients regarding the possible side effects and provide recommendations for good oral care and guidelines for reporting new dyspnea, cough, fever, rash, or mouth sores. As an alternative, it is also reasonable in our opinion to try high-dose, single-agent fulvestrant before switching to everolimus and exemestane.

Over a century after Beatson's discovery, and more than 30 years since tamoxifen began to be used to treat advanced breast cancer, we are now seeing the birth of new classes of medications that promise to dramatically improve upon the successes of hormonally targeted agents. Although the toxicity of everolimus must not be ignored, and many questions regarding its use naturally remain, the data presented in this article represent an important milestone, as they provide evidence that targeting the mTOR pathway is a viable option for reversing or at least slowing the natural course of endocrine-resistant breast cancer.

S. A. Hurvitz, MD

P. F. Peddi, MD

References

1. Beatson GT. On the treatment of inoperable cases of carcinoma of the mamma: suggestions for a new method of treatment, with illustrative cases. *Lancet.* 1896; 148:162-165.
2. Hurvitz SA, Pietras RJ. Rational management of endocrine resistance in breast cancer: a comprehensive review of estrogen receptor biology, treatment options, and future directions. *Cancer.* 2008;113:2385-2397.
3. Sun M, Paciga JE, Feldman RI, et al. Phosphatidylinositol-3-OH kinase (PI3K)/AKT2, activated in breast cancer, regulates and is induced by estrogen receptor alpha (ERalpha) via interaction between ERalpha and PI3K. *Cancer Res.* 2001;61:5985-5991.
4. Schiff R, Massarweh SA, Shou J, Bharwani L, Mohsin SK, Osborne CK. Cross-talk between estrogen receptor and growth factor pathways as a molecular target for overcoming endocrine resistance. *Clin Cancer Res.* 2004;10:331S-336S.
5. Boulay A, Rudloff J, Ye J, et al. Dual inhibition of mTOR and estrogen receptor signaling in vitro induces cell death in models of breast cancer. *Clin Cancer Res.* 2005;11:5319-5328.
6. O'Donnell A, Faivre S, Burris HA 3rd, et al. Phase I pharmacokinetic and pharmacodynamic study of the oral mammalian target of rapamycin inhibitor everolimus in patients with advanced solid tumors. *J Clin Oncol.* 2008;26:1588-1595.
7. Awada A, Cardoso F, Fontaine C, et al. The oral mTOR inhibitor RAD001 (everolimus) in combination with letrozole in patients with advanced breast cancer: results of a phase I study with pharmacokinetics. *Eur J Cancer.* 2008;44:84-91.
8. Tabernero J, Rojo F, Calvo E, et al. Dose- and schedule-dependent inhibition of the mammalian target of rapamycin pathway with everolimus: a phase I tumor pharmacodynamic study in patients with advanced solid tumors. *J Clin Oncol.* 2008;26:1603-1610.
9. Bachelot T, Bourgier C, Cropet C, et al. Randomized phase II trial of everolimus in combination with tamoxifen in patients with hormone receptor-positive, human epidermal growth factor receptor 2-negative metastatic breast cancer with prior exposure to aromatase inhibitors: a GINECO study. *J Clin Oncol.* 2012;30:2718-2724.
10. Baselga J, Semiglazov V, van Dam P, et al. Phase II randomized study of neoadjuvant everolimus plus letrozole compared with placebo plus letrozole in patients with estrogen receptor-positive breast cancer. *J Clin Oncol.* 2009;27:2630-2637.
11. Chia S, Gradishar W, Mauriac L, et al. Double-blind, randomized placebo controlled trial of fulvestrant compared with exemestane after prior nonsteroidal aromatase inhibitor therapy in postmenopausal women with hormone receptor-positive, advanced breast cancer: results from EFECT. *J Clin Oncol.* 2008;26: 1664-1670.
12. Di Leo A, Jerusalem G, Petruzelka L, et al. Results of the CONFIRM phase III trial comparing fulvestrant 250 mg with fulvestrant 500 mg in postmenopausal women with estrogen receptor-positive advanced breast cancer. *J Clin Oncol.* 2010;28:4594-4600.

Follow-up Care

A Prospective Surveillance Model for Physical Rehabilitation of Women With Breast Cancer: Chemotherapy-Induced Peripheral Neuropathy

Stubblefield MD, McNeely ML, Alfano CM, et al (Memorial Sloan-Kettering Cancer Ctr, NY; Univ of Alberta and Cross Cancer Inst, Edmonton, Canada; Natl Cancer Inst/Natl Insts of Health, Bethesda, MD; et al)
Cancer 118:2250-2260, 2012

Chemotherapy-induced peripheral neuropathy (CIPN) results from damage to or dysfunction of the peripheral nerves. The development of CIPN is anticipated for the majority of breast cancer patients who receive neurotoxic chemotherapy, depending on the agent used, dose, and schedule. Sensory symptoms often predominate and include numbness, tingling, and distal extremity pain. Weakness, gait impairment, loss of functional abilities, and other deficits may develop with more severe CIPN. This article outlines a prospective surveillance model for physical rehabilitation of women with breast cancer who develop CIPN. Rehabilitative efforts for CIPN start at the time of breast cancer diagnosis and treatment planning. The prechemotherapy evaluation identifies patients with preexisting peripheral nervous system disorders that may place them at higher risk for the development of CIPN. This clinical evaluation should include a history focusing on symptoms and functional activities as well as a physical examination that objectively assesses the patient's strength, sensation, reflexes, and gait. Ongoing surveillance following the initiation of a neurotoxic agent is important to monitor for the development and progression of symptoms associated with CIPN, and to ensure its resolution over the long term. CIPN is managed best by a multidisciplinary team approach. Early identification of symptoms will ensure appropriate referral and timely symptom management. The prospective surveillance model promotes a patient-centered approach to care, from pretreatment through survivorship and palliative care. In this way, the model offers promise in addressing and minimizing both the acute and long-term morbidity associated with CIPN.

▶ Chemotherapy-induced peripheral neuropathy (CIPN) is a debilitating complication for tens of thousands of women and men across the world who are survivors of cancer. In breast cancer alone, CIPN occurs in more than half of the patients treated, as the drugs of choice today almost always include neurotoxic agents such as the taxanes.

The neuropathy symptoms can be permanent and include numbness, tingling, pain, cold sensitivity, and more. Unfortunately, there are no current medications available to prevent or reverse the neuropathy. But many patients will have spontaneous resolution or mitigation of the symptoms over time.

Given the magnitude of this problem, assessing the risk for CIPN as outlined in this rehabilitation model is essential. It will help to understand the risk of

CIPN development and allow patients and their physicians to be proactive in trying to mitigate CIPN effects on the quality of life of these cancer patients.

C. Lawton, MD

Efficacy of Cognitive Behavioral Therapy and Physical Exercise in Alleviating Treatment-Induced Menopausal Symptoms in Patients With Breast Cancer: Results of a Randomized, Controlled, Multicenter Trial
Duijts SFA, van Beurden M, Oldenburg HSA, et al (Netherlands Cancer Inst, Amsterdam; Antoni van Leeuwenhoek Hosp, Amsterdam, The Netherlands; et al)
J Clin Oncol 30:4124-4133, 2012

Purpose.—The purpose of our study was to evaluate the effect of cognitive behavioral therapy (CBT), physical exercise (PE), and of these two interventions combined (CBT/PE) on menopausal symptoms (primary outcome), body image, sexual functioning, psychological well-being, and health-related quality of life (secondary outcomes) in patients with breast cancer experiencing treatment-induced menopause.

Patients and Methods.—Patients with breast cancer reporting treatment-induced menopausal symptoms (N = 422) were randomly assigned to CBT (n = 109), PE (n = 104), CBT/PE (n = 106), or to a waiting list control group (n = 103). Self-report questionnaires were completed at baseline, 12 weeks, and 6 months. Multilevel procedures were used to compare the intervention groups with the control group over time.

Results.—Compared with the control group, the intervention groups had a significant decrease in levels of endocrine symptoms (Functional Assessment of Cancer Therapy—Endocrine Symptoms; $P < .001$; effect size, 0.31-0.52) and urinary symptoms (Bristol Female Lower Urinary Tract Symptoms Questionnaire; $P = .002$; effect size, 0.29-0.33), and they showed an improvement in physical functioning (36-Item Short Form Health Survey physical functioning subscale; $P = .002$; effect size, 0.37-0.46). The groups that included CBT also showed a significant decrease in the perceived burden of hot flashes and night sweats (problem rating scale of the Hot Flush Rating Scale; $P < .001$; effect size, 0.39-0.56) and an increase in sexual activity (Sexual Activity Questionnaire habit subscale; $P = .027$; effect size, 0.65). Most of these effects were observed at both the 12-week and 6-month follow-ups.

Conclusion.—CBT and PE can have salutary effects on endocrine symptoms and, to a lesser degree, on sexuality and physical functioning of patients with breast cancer experiencing treatment-induced menopause. Future work is needed to improve the design and the planning of these interventions to improve program adherence.

▶ There has been much interest in using a technique designed to improve cognitive function (cognitive behavioral therapy) together with physical exercise in the treatment of patients with cancer. This particular study examines various combinations of cognitive behavioral therapy and physical exercise to alleviate treatment-induced menopausal symptoms in 422 patients. The cognitive behavioral therapy intervention consisted of 6 weekly group sessions of 90 minutes each and one follow-up booster session 6 weeks after the program was completed and included relaxation exercises. Symptoms focused on in these sessions were primarily hot flashes and night sweats. The physical exercise program was a 12-week, individually tailored, home-based, self-directed exercise program of 2.5 to 3 hours per week, including exercises such as swimming, running, and cycling, and it asked that the individual achieve a targeted heart rate during the sessions. Women were randomly assigned to none, one, or both of these approaches. The intervention groups showed a statistically significant decrease in levels of endocrine symptoms and urinary symptoms and showed an improvement in physical functioning, including sexual activity. The biggest problem was ensuring compliance with the intervention programs. Similar programs are being looked at in ovarian cancer patients as well. The exact role of such programs for the management of patients with breast cancer is as yet undetermined.

J. T. Thigpen, MD

Prognostic Factors

Prognostic Impact of Pregnancy After Breast Cancer According to Estrogen Receptor Status: A Multicenter Retrospective Study
Azim HA Jr, Kroman N, Paesmans M, et al (Université Libre de Bruxelles, Brussels, Belgium; Rigshospitalet, Copenhagen, Denmark; et al)
J Clin Oncol 31:73-79, 2013

Purpose.—We questioned the impact of pregnancy on disease-free survival (DFS) in women with history of breast cancer (BC) according to estrogen receptor (ER) status.

Patients and Methods.—A multicenter, retrospective cohort study in which patients who became pregnant any time after BC were matched (1:3) to patients with BC with similar ER, nodal status, adjuvant therapy, age, and year of diagnosis. To adjust for guaranteed time bias, each nonpregnant patient had to have a disease-free interval at least equal to the time elapsing between BC diagnosis and date of conception of the matched pregnant one. The primary objective was DFS in patients with ER-positive BC. DFS in the ER-negative cohort, whole population, and overall survival (OS) were secondary objectives. Subgroup analyses included DFS according to pregnancy outcome and BC–pregnancy interval. With a two-sided $\alpha = 5\%$ and $\beta = 20\%$, 645 ER-positive patients were required to detect a hazard ratio (HR) = 0.65.

Results.—A total of 333 pregnant patients and 874 matched nonpregnant patients were analyzed, of whom 686 patients had an ER-positive disease. No difference in DFS was observed between pregnant and nonpregnant patients in the ER-positive (HR = 0.91; 95% CI, 0.67 to 1.24, $P = .55$) or the ER-negative (HR = 0.75; 95% CI, 0.51 to 1.08, $P = .12$) cohorts. However, the pregnant group had better OS (HR = 0.72; 95% CI, 0.54 to 0.97, $P = .03$), with no interaction according to ER status ($P = .11$).

Pregnancy outcome and BC—pregnancy interval did not seem to impact the risk of relapse.

Conclusion.—Pregnancy after ER-positive BC does not seem to reduce the risk of BC recurrence.

▶ There will never be a randomized controlled trial or meta-analysis with level-1 evidence to demonstrate the impact of pregnancy on BC recurrence risk and mortality in patients treated successfully for primary BC. Nevertheless, patients who have been successfully treated for primary BC may remain interested in maintaining fertility and having a subsequent pregnancy. The American Society of Clinical Oncology recognized this issue and sponsored a clinical practice guideline to address patient and physician concerns.[1] A number of studies of varied design, including registry studies, clinical trials, and population-based studies,[2-5] have assessed pregnancy impact on BC recurrence risk and patient survival. These studies have not demonstrated an increase in BC recurrence or mortality for women who have had a pregnancy after BC diagnosis. However, none of the studies adequately addressed the potential impact of pregnancy on BC recurrence in women with hormone receptor—positive primary BCs. Anecdotal evidence suggests that patients and physicians remain skeptical about the desirability and safety of becoming pregnant in the context of a prior BC, especially one that is hormone receptor positive.

Azim and colleagues, the authors of this article, are to be commended for developing their retrospective case-control study of pregnancy subsequent to a diagnosis of BC. Their processes for matching pregnant with nonpregnant BC survivors not only accounted for the usual clinical and tumor variables of concern but also provided details of hormone receptor status and could be adjusted for time from diagnosis and time to pregnancy to attempt to control selection biases. Their use of multicenter databases makes their findings broadly generalizable to populations of women with BC. This study examined DFS in patients with ER-positive BC as a primary objective. Secondary objectives included DFS in the ER-negative group and OS in the 2 cohorts. The results are encouraging for patients, and the clinicians who care for them, as they face the decision of whether to have a child.

Azim and colleagues' detailed analyses showed no difference in DFS between pregnant and nonpregnant BC survivors with respect to ER-positive or ER-negative tumors. OS in the pregnant group was better (HR = 0.72; 95% confidence interval, 0.54-0.97) and had no interaction with ER values. The authors concluded that "pregnancy after ER-positive BC does not seem to reduce the risk of BC recurrence." An alternative interpretation might be that pregnancy has no influence on BC recurrence, whether the primary tumor was ER positive or ER negative, and that patients who experienced a pregnancy after BC treatment had better survival than those who did not. Although there has been concern about the potential of the charged hormonal environment of pregnancy accelerating BC recurrence and death from BC, this study adds to those previously published that have reached the conclusion that this concern is not warranted.

How physicians and patients will use these data is yet to be seen; however, the strong proscription against pregnancy for BC survivors does not seem tenable.

R. L. Theriault, DO, MBA, FACP

References

1. Lee SJ, Schover LR, Partridge AH, et al; American Society of Clinical Oncology. American Society of Clinical Oncology recommendations on fertility preservation in cancer patients. *J Clin Oncol.* 2006;24:2917-2931.
2. Ives A, Saunders C, Bulsara M, Semmens J. Pregnancy after breast cancer: population based study. *BMJ.* 2007;334:194.
3. Mueller BA, Simon MS, Deapen D, Kamineni A, Malone KE, Daling JR. Childbearing and survival after breast carcinoma in young women. *Cancer.* 2003;98:1131-1140.
4. Velentgas P, Daling JR, Malone KE, et al. Pregnancy after breast carcinoma: outcomes and influence on mortality. *Cancer.* 1999;85:2424-2432.
5. von Schoultz E, Johansson H, Wilking N, Rutqvist LE. Influence of prior and subsequent pregnancy on breast cancer prognosis. *J Clin Oncol.* 1995;13:430-434.

Economic, Legal, and Social Issues

Cost Effectiveness of Fracture Prevention in Postmenopausal Women Who Receive Aromatase Inhibitors for Early Breast Cancer

Ito K, Blinder VS, Elkin EB (Brigham and Women's Hosp, Boston, MA; Memorial Sloan-Kettering Cancer Ctr, NY)

J Clin Oncol 30:1468-1475, 2012

Purpose.—Aromatase inhibitors (AIs) increase the risk of osteoporosis and related fractures in postmenopausal women who receive adjuvant AIs for hormone receptor (HR) —positive early breast cancer (EBC). We compared the cost effectiveness of alternative screening and treatment strategies for fracture prevention.

Methods.—We developed a Markov state transition model to simulate clinical practice and outcomes in a hypothetical cohort of women age 60 years with HR-positive EBC starting a 5-year course of AI therapy after primary surgery for breast cancer. Outcomes were quality-adjusted life-years (QALYs), lifetime cost, and incremental cost-effectiveness ratio (ICER). We compared the following strategies: no intervention; one-time bone mineral density (BMD) screening and selective bisphosphonate therapy in women with osteoporosis or osteopenia; annual BMD screening and selective bisphosphonate therapy in women with osteoporosis or osteopenia; and universal bisphosphonate therapy.

Results.—ICERs for annual BMD screening followed by oral bisphosphonates for those with osteoporosis, annual BMD screening followed by oral bisphosphonates for those with osteopenia, and universal treatment with oral bisphosphonates were $87,300, $129,300, and $283,600 per QALY gained, respectively. One-time BMD screening followed by oral bisphosphonates for those with osteoporosis or osteopenia was dominated. Our results were sensitive to age at the initiation of AI therapy, type of bisphosphonates, post-treatment residual effect of bisphosphonates, and a potential adjuvant benefit of intravenous bisphosphonates.

Conclusion.—In postmenopausal women receiving adjuvant AIs for HR-positive EBC, a policy of baseline and annual BMD screening followed by selective treatment with oral bisphosphonates for those diagnosed with osteoporosis is a cost-effective use of societal resources.

▶ In this study, Ito et al estimated the cost-effectiveness of several commonly used fracture prevention strategies among postmenopausal women who received AIs as adjuvant therapy for HR-positive EBC. Adjuvant therapy with AIs, unless otherwise contraindicated, is considered the standard of care for these patients.[1,2] However, AIs are associated with greater loss of BMD and fractures[2]; therefore, baseline assessment (including BMD studies) and, possibly, subsequent pharmacologic interventions have been recommended for AI users.[3] Clinical management in this setting is complex, as clinicians must consider the combination of a history of breast cancer and the possibility of disease progression, the underlying condition of osteoporosis, and an elevated risk of osteoporosis from the use of AIs and its associated risk of fractures. The clinical contribution of this study was highlighted in the accompanying editorial in the *Journal of Clinical Oncology*,[4] which applauded the authors' effort to apply an analytical framework to complex clinical scenarios in the evaluation of the cost-effectiveness of fracture prevention strategies.

The analytical framework employed in the study by Ito and colleagues is known as the Markov state transition model,[5] which allowed the authors to model the progression of breast cancer while taking into account changes in BMD over time due to AI or aging and the associated risk of fractures. The structure of this decision model is clever and captures key events with nontrivial clinical or economic implications. The authors further established the credibility of the model by presenting the findings of model validations, which are rarely found in published cost-effectiveness analyses. For modeling parameters with a wide range of uncertainties, the authors erred on the conservative side to avoid biasing in favor of any particular fracture prevention strategy. In addition, 1-way sensitivity analyses were performed for an array of key modeling parameters to inform readers of the effect of each parameter. The authors concluded that the most cost-effective fracture prevention strategy for postmenopausal women with HR-positive EBC was BMD screening at baseline and annually for the duration of adjuvant AI therapy, followed by oral bisphosphonates for those with osteoporosis.

Can this cost-effectiveness analysis be further improved to provide more information to decision makers? Yes: our review of this study suggested that 2 major modifications are worth considering. First, expand the model from a deterministic to a probabilistic cost-effectiveness analysis. Presenting the findings of a cost-effectiveness analysis as a point estimate of ICER ignores the precision of the estimated ratio, whereas 1-way sensitivity analyses, by isolating 1 parameter at a time and keeping all remaining parameters at their baseline values, tend to underestimate uncertainties.[6] Thus, probabilistic analysis has become the recommended approach to addressing parameter uncertainties in recent textbooks and good practice guidelines for decision modeling.[7,8] Given the multitude of uncertainties around several clinical parameters in this study, it is highly possible that the estimated ICER would be of poor precision (ie, it would have a wide confidence interval). Under this circumstance, information such as which prevention strategy has the highest probability of cost-effectiveness at a predetermined threshold value (eg, $100 000 per QALY) will likely be more useful to decision makers.

Second, the strategy of "universal bisphosphonates" should consider the possibility of a substantial reduction in drug cost when generic formulations become available in the United States market. All 3 agents considered in the model (risedronate, ibandronate, and zoledronic acid) have reached or are approaching patent expiration.[9] Reductions in the costs of bisphosphonates as a result of the availability of generic formulations will lower the costs, and thus the ICER, of the universal bisphosphonates prevention strategy and possibly change the cost-effectiveness of this strategy. Unfortunately, this potentially influential modeling parameter was overlooked in the 1-way sensitivity analysis.

Other modifications to consider include replacing the Sweden-based health utility values of fractures with those from a systematic review published more recently[10] and expanding the comparators to other emerging pharmaceutical agents, such as denosumab,[11] which has demonstrated efficacy in protecting against AI-induced bone loss. The modification to include better-quality health utility data for various types of fractures is unlikely to change the main conclusion of this study because 1-way sensitivity analysis showed that the findings from this study remained robust within a wide range of changes (ie, ±50%) in the disutility of fractures. It is difficult to project whether expanding the fracture prevention strategy to include denosumab, a monoclonal antibody, would change the relative cost-effectiveness of strategies examined in this study because of the mixed findings in published cost-effectiveness analyses comparing denosumab and bisphosphonates.[12,13]

In summary, this study by Ito and colleagues is a well-conducted and clearly presented cost-effectiveness analysis, and the authors paid attention to many important details. Based on the evidence presented in this study, it is reasonable to conclude that annual BMD screening and selective use of oral bisphosphonates for osteoporosis is the most cost-effective fracture prevention strategy, although the universal bisphosphonates strategy could become cost-effective owing to generic drug use and synergistic interactions with cytotoxic drugs, which may lead to a reduction in cancer recurrence, especially bone metastasis, among postmenopausal women.[14]

Y. C. T. Shih, PhD

C. R. Chien, MD, PhD

Y. Shen, PhD

References

1. National Comprehensive Cancer Network. NCCN clinical practice guidelines in oncology. Breast cancer. Version 3.2012. http://www.nccn.org/professionals/physician_gls/pdf/breast.pdf. Accessed December 11, 2012.

2. Burstein HJ, Prestrud AA, Seidenfeld J, et al; American Society of Clinical Oncology. American Society of Clinical Oncology clinical practice guideline: update on adjuvant endocrine therapy for women with hormone receptor-positive breast cancer. *J Clin Oncol.* 2010;28:3784-3796.

3. Hadji P, Aapro MS, Body JJ, et al. Management of aromatase inhibitor-associated bone loss in postmenopausal women with breast cancer: practical guidance for prevention and treatment. *Ann Oncol.* 2011;22:2546-2555.

4. Dhesy-Thind SK. Screening for osteoporosis in postmenopausal women with breast cancer receiving aromatase inhibitors: less is more? *J Clin Oncol.* 2012; 30:1408-1410.

5. Grusenmeyer PA, Wong YN. Interpreting the economic literature in oncology. *J Clin Oncol.* 2007;25:196-202.

6. Briggs AH, Goeree R, Blackhouse G, O'Brien BJ. Probabilistic analysis of cost-effectiveness models: choosing between treatment strategies for gastroesophageal reflux disease. *Med Decis Making.* 2002;22:290-308.

7. Weinstein MC, O'Brien B, Hornberger J, et al; ISPOR Task Force on Good Research Practices—Modeling Studies. Principles of good practice for decision analytic modeling in health-care evaluation: report of the ISPOR Task Force on Good Research Practices—Modeling Studies. *Value Health.* 2003;6:9-17.

8. Briggs A, Claxton K, Sculpher M. *Decision Modelling for Health Economic Evaluation.* New York, NY: Oxford University Press; 2006.

9. U.S. Food and Drug Administration. Orange Book: Approved Drug Products with Therapeutic Equivalence Evaluations. http://www.accessdata.fda.gov/scripts/cder/ob/default.cfm. Accessed December 10, 2012.

10. Peasgood T, Herrmann K, Kanis JA, Brazier JE. An updated systematic review of Health State Utility Values for osteoporosis related conditions. *Osteoporos Int.* 2009;20:853-868.

11. Ellis GK, Bone HG, Chlebowski R, et al. Randomized trial of denosumab in patients receiving adjuvant aromatase inhibitors for nonmetastatic breast cancer. *J Clin Oncol.* 2008;26:4875-4882.

12. Jönsson B, Ström O, Eisman JA, et al. Cost-effectiveness of denosumab for the treatment of postmenopausal osteoporosis. *Osteoporos Int.* 2011;22:967-982.

13. Snedecor SJ, Carter JA, Kaura S, Botteman MF. Cost-effectiveness of denosumab versus zoledronic acid in the management of skeletal metastases secondary to breast cancer. *Clin Ther.* 2012;34:1334-1349.

14. Coleman RE, Marshall H, Cameron D; AZURE Investigators. Breast-cancer adjuvant therapy with zoledronic acid. *N Engl J Med.* 2011;365:1396-1405.

6 Genitourinary

Bladder

Radiotherapy with or without Chemotherapy in Muscle-Invasive Bladder Cancer

James ND, for the BC2001 Investigators (Univ of Birmingham, UK; et al)
N Engl J Med 366:1477-1488, 2012

Background.—Radiotherapy is an alternative to cystectomy in patients with muscle-invasive bladder cancer. In other disease sites, synchronous chemoradiotherapy has been associated with increased local control and improved survival, as compared with radiotherapy alone.

Methods.—In this multicenter, phase 3 trial, we randomly assigned 360 patients with muscle-invasive bladder cancer to undergo radiotherapy with or without synchronous chemotherapy. The regimen consisted of fluorouracil (500 mg per square meter of body-surface area per day) during fractions 1 to 5 and 16 to 20 of radiotherapy and mitomycin C (12 mg per square meter) on day 1. Patients were also randomly assigned to undergo either whole-bladder radiotherapy or modified-volume radiotherapy (in which the volume of bladder receiving full-dose radiotherapy was reduced) in a partial 2-by-2 factorial design (results not reported here). The primary end point was survival free of locoregional disease. Secondary end points included overall survival and toxic effects.

Results.—At 2 years, rates of locoregional disease–free survival were 67% (95% confidence interval [CI], 59 to 74) in the chemoradiotherapy group and 54% (95% CI, 46 to 62) in the radiotherapy group. With a median follow-up of 69.9 months, the hazard ratio in the chemoradiotherapy group was 0.68 (95% CI, 0.48 to 0.96; $P = 0.03$). Five-year rates of overall survival were 48% (95% CI, 40 to 55) in the chemoradiotherapy group and 35% (95% CI, 28 to 43) in the radiotherapy group (hazard ratio, 0.82; 95% CI, 0.63 to 1.09; $P = 0.16$). Grade 3 or 4 adverse events were slightly more common in the chemoradiotherapy group than in the radiotherapy group during treatment (36.0% vs. 27.5%, $P = 0.07$) but not during follow-up (8.3% vs. 15.7%, $P = 0.07$).

Conclusions.—Synchronous chemotherapy with fluorouracil and mitomycin C combined with radiotherapy significantly improved locoregional control of bladder cancer, as compared with radiotherapy alone, with no significant increase in adverse events. (Funded by Cancer Research U.K.; BC2001 Current Controlled Trials number, ISRCTN68324339.)

▶ Organ preservation with quality organ function should be a goal for all cancer patients. Often this requires scientific study of the surgical options vs the radiation plus or minus chemotherapy options, as has been successfully documented in breast and many other cancers. Interestingly, bladder cancer, whose mainstay of treatment in the United States is surgical, is treated differently in Western Europe. Organ preservation with radiation is the primary form of treatment for invasive bladder cancer and has been successfully performed in Europe for decades. The underpinning of these different treatment approaches can be debated, but radiation therapy can result in the cure of bladder cancer with good organ function and has been proven both in the US and in Europe.

The question of the role of adding chemotherapy to radiation has been addressed from a retrospective perspective, suggesting a benefit to radiation and chemotherapy over radiation alone. This prospective, randomized trial examined this question and gives us new insights into the benefits of adding fluorouracil and mitomycin-C to radiation therapy for bladder cancer patients. The results show a clear benefit to the addition of chemotherapy in terms of local regional control with some increased acute toxicity, but no increase in late toxicity. Overall survival was not statistically improved, yet there was an absolute difference of 13% (48% vs 35%) in 5-year survival rates. These data add significantly to the available science in treating bladder cancer patients with an organ preservation approach.

C. Lawton, MD

Prostate

Diagnostic Performance of PCA3 to Detect Prostate Cancer in Men with Increased Prostate Specific Antigen: A Prospective Study of 1,962 Cases
Crawford ED, Rove KO, Trabulsi EJ, et al (Univ of Colorado, Aurora; Thomas Jefferson Univ, Philadelphia, PA; et al)
J Urol 188:1726-1731, 2012

Purpose.—The detection of prostate cancer relies primarily on abnormal digital rectal examination or increased serum prostate specific antigen concentration. However, low positive predictive values result in many men with increased prostate specific antigen and/or suspicious digital rectal examination having a negative biopsy. We investigated the value of the PCA3 (prostate cancer gene 3) urine test in predicting the likelihood of diagnosis of cancer before biopsy.

Materials and Methods.—We performed a prospective, community based clinical trial to evaluate PCA3 score before any biopsy. This trial was conducted at 50 urology practices in the United States. Samples were obtained from 1,962 men with increased serum prostate specific antigen (greater than 2.5 ng/ml) and/or abnormal digital rectal examination before transrectal prostate needle biopsy. Study samples (urinary PCA3 and biopsies) were processed and analyzed by a central laboratory. Sensitivity-specificity analyses were conducted.

Results.—A total of 1,913 urine samples (97.5%) were adequate for PCA3 testing. Of 802 cases diagnosed with prostate cancer 222 had high grade prostatic intraepithelial neoplasia or atypical small acinar proliferation and were suspicious for cancer, whereas 889 cases were benign. The traditional PCA3 cutoff of 35 reduced the number of false-positives from 1,089 to 249, a 77.1% reduction. However, false-negatives (missed cancers) increased significantly from 17 to 413, an increase of more than 2,300%. Lowering the PCA3 cutoff to 10 reduced the number of false-positives 35.4% and false-negatives only increased 5.6%.

Conclusions.—Urinary PCA3 testing in conjunction with prostate specific antigen has the potential to significantly decrease the number of unnecessary prostate biopsies.

▶ Despite the fact that approximately 28 000 men in the United States die of prostate cancer each year, the current recommendation from the US Preventive Services Task Force is against routine prostate-specific antigen (PSA) screening. This would never be tolerated in the breast cancer community, but sadly it is being tolerated in the prostate cancer world. The argument against PSA screening is that it costs too much in terms of overdiagnosis in the elderly and overtreatment for patients who could simply be monitored.

Given that PSA screening is not recommended routinely now and, therefore, not paid for, we as physicians must develop better tests to identify patients with significant prostate cancer to avoid overbiopsying. And we have to develop better ways to ensure that overtreatment is not done for patients with the disease who are best served with active surveillance.

These data attempt to help further select patients with elevated PSA levels or abnormal digital rectal examination results. The urine PCA3 test is not perfect, either. It did, however, help better identify patients with prostate cancer and represents the kind of work that we need to do to help better screen patients for this important disease.

C. Lawton, MD

Cost-effectiveness analysis of SBRT versus IMRT: an emerging initial radiation treatment option for organ-confined prostate cancer
Hodges JC, Lotan Y, Boike TP, et al (Univ of Texas Southwestern, Dallas)
Am J Manag Care 18:e186-e193, 2012

Objectives.—The purpose of this study is to compare the cost-effectiveness of 2 external beam radiation therapy techniques for treatment of low to intermediate-risk prostate cancer: stereotactic body radiation therapy (SBRT) and intensity modulated radiation therapy (IMRT).

Materials and Methods.—A Markov decision analysis model with probabilistic sensitivity analysis was designed with the various disease states of a 70-year-old patient with organ-confined prostate cancer to evaluate the cost-effectiveness of 2 external beam radiation treatment options.

Results.—The Monte Carlo simulation revealed that the mean cost and quality-adjusted life-years (QALYs) for SBRT and IMRT were $22,152 and 7.9 years and $35,431 and 7.9 years, respectively. The sensitivity analysis revealed that if the SBRT cohort experienced a decrease in quality of life of 4% or a decrease in efficacy of 6%, then SBRT would no longer dominate IMRT in cost-effectiveness. In fact, with these relaxed assumptions for SBRT, the incremental cost-effectiveness ratio of IMRT met the societal willingness to pay threshold of $50,000 per QALY.

Conclusions.—Compared with IMRT, SBRT for low-to intermediate-risk prostate cancer has great potential cost savings for our healthcare system payers and may improve access to radiation, increase patient convenience, and boost quality of life for patients. Our model suggests that the incremental cost-effectiveness ratio of IMRT compared with SBRT is highly sensitive to quality-of-life outcomes, which should be adequately and comparably measured in current and future prostate SBRT studies.

▶ In the era of trying to attain medical cost containment, methods to decrease the cost of treating common cancers, such as prostate and breast cancer, are at the forefront of consideration. In both diseases, radiation therapy plays a curative/noninvasive role and, therefore, is often the option of choice for the patient. Yet, coming for treatment for 8 weeks or more, which has been the standard for prostate cancer patients for decades, is inconvenient and costly for the patient.

Since the understanding of the probable lower α/β ratio for prostate cancer (likely in the range of 1.5 to 3.0), the role of hypofractionation has come to the fore as a potentially better (more effective) way of radiation therapy delivery. Of course, any time that hypofractionation is considered, the question of toxicity is immediately raised. Given the very close proximity of the rectum and bladder, all radiation oncologists should pause as they consider doses of more than 7 Gy per fraction. Yet with the excellent image-guided radiation therapy available as well as intrafractionation monitoring, it may be possible to deliver such large doses safely.

These authors have analyzed the cost of stereotactic body radiation therapy (SBRT), which is extreme hypofractionation, vs standard intensity-modulated radiation therapy, and a large benefit can be found assuming that the toxicity for SBRT is not large. The clear message within this analysis is that we need good data with significant follow-up to ensure that SBRT is, in fact, safe so that the potential cost savings can be realized.

C. Lawton, MD

Radical Prostatectomy in Austria From 1992 to 2009: An Updated Nationwide Analysis of 33,580 Cases

Wehrberger C, Berger I, Willinger M, et al (Donauspital and Austrian Health Inst (MW), Vienna, Austria)
J Urol 187:1626-1631, 2012

Purpose.—We analyzed the demographics and outcome of radical prostatectomy in Austria in a nationwide series.

Materials and Methods.—We analyzed the records of all 33,580 patients who underwent radical prostatectomy at a public hospital, including 95% of all surgical procedures, in Austria between 1992 and 2009. Patient demographics, perioperative mortality, interventions for anastomotic strictures and urinary incontinence, and overall survival were determined. Data were provided by the Austrian Health Institute.

Results.—The annual number of radical prostatectomies increased 688% from 396 in 1992 to 3,123 in 2007 and gradually decreased to 2,612 in 2009. Mean ± SD patient age at surgery decreased slightly from 64.4 ± 6.3 years in 1992 to 62.0 ± 6.7 years in 2003. Age has remained at that level since then. Endourological intervention for anastomotic stricture and urinary incontinence was done in 7.5% and 2.8% of cases, respectively. The risk of each intervention increased with patient age and decreased in patients treated within the last 10 years compared to those treated before 2000. The 30-day mortality rate was 0.1%, which increased threefold from the youngest to the oldest age group. Ten-year overall survival decreased from 93% in patients 45 to 49 years old to 63% in those 70 years old or older at surgery.

Conclusions.—This nationwide analysis of a country that has had a public, equal access health care system for decades describes some current radical prostatectomy trends. Since 2007, the absolute number of radical prostatectomies has decreased. Data on morbidity, perioperative mortality and overall survival raise caution about performing radical prostatectomy in elderly men, eg those 70 years old or older.

▶ The role of surgery for prostatic adenocarcinoma is well established. All other treatments, such as external-beam radiation therapy, current low-dose rate (LDR) and high-dose rate brachytherapy, cryotherapy, and so forth, are compared with radical prostatectomy to establish their role in this disease. In doing these comparisons, it has been well established that for patients with localized prostate cancer, surgery, external-beam radiation therapy, and LDR brachytherapy result in equivalent outcomes.

But there is often a question in the minds of both surgical oncologists and radiation oncologists as to which procedures might be best suited for which subset of prostate cancer patients. This concern has resulted in the recommendation for surgery for younger patients and radiation therapy of either form for older patients. However, large-quality data for these recommendations have been sparse.

The data from the Austria Health Institute dataset have added significantly to this discussion. Their data, from over 33 000 men treated with surgery for prostate cancer, would suggest caution when using a surgical approach in patients over 70 years of age. Morbidity rates and perioperative mortality appear to be higher in these older patients, who could just as effectively have been treated with a radiation approach.

C. Lawton, MD

Interval to Biochemical Failure as a Biomarker for Cause-Specific and Overall Survival After Dose-Escalated External Beam Radiation Therapy for Prostate Cancer

Kapadia NS, Olson K, Sandler HM, et al (Univ of Michigan Med Ctr, Ann Arbor; Cedars Sinai Med System, Los Angeles, CA)
Cancer 118:2059-2068, 2012

Background.—After external beam radiation therapy (EBRT) for prostate cancer, a short interval to biochemical failure of <18 months has been proposed as a surrogate for cause-specific survival. Because EBRT dose influences biochemical failure, the authors investigated the interval to biochemical failure in a cohort of patients treated with dose-escalated EBRT.

Methods.—From 1998 to 2008, 710 patients were treated with EBRT (≥75 grays) ± androgen deprivation therapy (ADT) at the University of Michigan. Biochemical failure was defined using the Phoenix consensus definition (nadir + 2 ng/mL). A short interval to biochemical failure was defined as <18 months after completing radiotherapy and/or ADT. The associations between biochemical failure, the interval to biochemical failure, and clinical factors with cause-specific survival (CSS) and overall survival (OS) were evaluated.

Results.—There were 149 biochemical failures (21%), and short interval to biochemical failure accounted for 14% and 40% of biochemical failures in those with intermediate-risk or high-risk disease, respectively. Biochemical failure impacted CSS ($P < .0001$) but not OS ($P = .36$). However, a short interval to biochemical failure predicted decreased CSS ($P < .0001$; hazard ratio [HR], 5.6; 95% confidence interval [CI], 2.4-13.0) and OS ($P < .0001$; HR, 4.8; 95% CI, 2.3-10.3) when compared with a long interval to biochemical failure. The 8-year OS was 78% without biochemical failure, compared with 87% with a long interval to biochemical failure ($P = .1$; HR, 0.7; 95% CI, 0.4-1.1) and 38% with a short interval to biochemical failure ($P < .0001$; HR, 3.7; 95% CI, 2.3-5.9). On multivariate analysis, a short interval to biochemical failure increased the risk of prostate cancer death ($P < .0001$; HR, 18.1; 95% CI, 8.4-39) and all cause mortality ($P = .0027$; HR, 1.5; 95% CI, 1.2-2.1), whereas a long interval to biochemical failure did not.

Conclusions.—The relation between the interval to biochemical failure, CSS, and OS was independently validated in patients treated with dose-escalated EBRT. Further evaluation of the interval to biochemical failure as a surrogate endpoint is warranted.

▶ Given the relatively long duration of the natural history of prostate cancer and the age of the patients who receive this diagnosis, it is imperative that we try to find surrogates to overall survival and cause-specific survival. Both patients and their treating physicians need answers to treatment questions as soon as they are available. So looking to endpoints such as time to prostate-specific antigen failure, as seen in this analysis, is potentially important information.

Clearly, these data are representative of only one institution and are a retro-spective review. But given the lack of large registries, these are exactly the type of data that we need to utilize to find the surrogate endpoints. The findings here of a short interval to biochemical failure (ie, < 18 months) being associated with both cause-specific and overall survival make scientific sense. This endpoint needs further evaluation with multiple institutions and large patient populations. Currently, the most obvious place to find such data is within the Radiation Therapy Oncology Group. Hopefully, such an analysis is ongoing. The need for a prostate cancer registry across the United States to answer this and many other questions is obvious.

C. Lawton, MD

Conventional versus hypofractionated high-dose intensity-modulated radiotherapy for prostate cancer: preliminary safety results from the CHHiP randomised controlled trial

Dearnaley D, Syndikus I, Sumo G, et al (Royal Marsden NHS Foundation Trust, London, UK; Clatterbridge Centre for Oncology NHS Foundation Trust, Wirral, UK; The Inst of Cancer Res, London, UK; et al)
Lancet Oncol 13:43-54, 2012

Background.—Prostate cancer might have high radiation-fraction sensi-tivity, implying a therapeutic advantage of hypofractionated treatment. We present a pre-planned preliminary safety analysis of side-effects in stages 1 and 2 of a randomised trial comparing standard and hypo fractionated radiotherapy.

Methods.—We did a multicentre, randomised study and recruited men with localised prostate cancer between Oct 18, 2002, and Aug 12, 2006, at 11 UK centres. Patients were randomly assigned in a 1:1:1 ratio to receive conventional or hypofractionated high-dose intensity-modulated radio therapy, and all were given with 3—6 months of neoadjuvant androgen suppression. Computer-generated random permuted blocks were used, with risk of seminal vesicle involvement and radiotherapy-treatment centre as stratification factors. The conventional schedule was 37 fractions of 2 Gy to a total of 74 Gy. The two hypofractionated schedules involved 3 Gy treatments given in either 20 fractions to a total of 60 Gy, or 19 fractions to a total of 57 Gy. The primary endpoint was proportion of patients with grade 2 or worse toxicity at 2 years on the Radiation Therapy Oncology Group (RTOG) scale. The primary analysis included all patients who had received at least one fraction of radiotherapy and completed a 2 year assessment. Treatment allocation was not masked and clinicians were not blinded. Stage 3 of this trial completed the planned recruitment in June, 2011. This study is registered, number ISRCTN97182923.

Findings.—153 men recruited to stages 1 and 2 were randomly assigned to receive conventional treatment of 74 Gy, 153 to receive 60 Gy, and 151 to receive 57 Gy. With 50·5 months median follow-up (IQR 43·5—61·3), six (4·3%; 95% CI 1·6—9·2) of 138 men in the 74 Gy group had bowel toxicity of grade 2 or worse on the RTOG scale at 2 years, as did five (3·6%; 1·2—8·3) of 137 men in the 60 Gy group, and two (1·4%; 0·2—5·0) of 143 men in the 57 Gy group. For bladder toxicities, three (2·2%; 0·5—6·2) of 138 men, three (2·2%; 0·5—6·3) of 137, and none (0·0%; 97·5% CI 0·0—2·6) of 143 had scores of grade 2 or worse on the RTOG scale at 2 years.

Interpretation.—Hypofractionated high-dose radiotherapy seems equally well tolerated as conventionally fractionated treatment at 2 years.

▶ The use of image-guided radiotherapy (IGRT) and intensity-modulated radiation therapy (IMRT) together has allowed the radiation oncologist to deliver high doses of radiation to the prostate with relatively low toxicity profiles. In addition, the increase in dose with conventional fractionation has resulted in an increase in local control for prostate cancer patients. Yet these fractionation schemes require patients to be under treatment 5 days per week for roughly 2 months, which is a huge inconvenience, not to mention a huge cost.

The α/β data that have been developed showing a probable benefit in terms of disease control to the higher dose per fraction for prostate cancer, combined with the ability via IGRT and IMRT to safely deliver such treatments, are the basis for the hypofractionation trials that have been done, such as the data reported here. The big concern with hypofractionation is the issue of toxicity, which is the appropriate primary endpoint of this trial. These data, with a median follow-up of 50.5 months, look very promising in terms of gastrointestinal and genitourinary toxicity for these 2 hypofractionation schemes. If these favorable outcomes persist, then prostate cancer patients will be less inconvenienced when treated with external beam radiotherapy, and the cost to the patients and their insurance providers will decrease. We look forward to longer follow-up of this and other trials like it to verify these positive findings.

C. Lawton, MD

Management of Older Men With Clinically Localized Prostate Cancer: The Significance of Advanced Age and Comorbidity
Hoffman KE (The Univ of Texas MD Anderson Cancer Ctr, Houston)
Semin Radiat Oncol 22:284-294, 2012

The majority of men diagnosed with prostate cancer are diagnosed later in life. Although localized prostate cancer is often an indolent disease, older men are more frequently diagnosed with high-risk disease and are more likely to die from prostate cancer than younger men. Comorbid medical conditions are also more prevalent in the later decades of life and can impact prostate cancer treatment tolerance and the likelihood of benefiting from aggressive cancer treatment. Older men diagnosed with prostate cancer are at risk for both overtreatment of low-risk disease and undertreatment of high-risk disease. Prostate cancer management decisions for older patients should be tailored based on an individual patient's health status, coexisting medical conditions, life expectancy, and tumor characteristics.

▶ Prostate cancer is often a disease that patients die with and not of. In the older male population, however, men are more likely to have high-risk prostate cancer diagnosed. It is these higher-risk prostate cancers that are more likely to result in significant morbidity and mortality and, therefore, need to be addressed. Yet many of these older patients (ie, > 70 to 75 years of age) have other comorbidities that compete with high-risk prostate cancer with respect to morbidity and, especially, mortality.

This article is an excellent, in-depth discussion of this topic. The author presents compelling data showing insufficient treatment of older men with high-risk prostate cancer resulting in increased prostate cancer mortality and overtreatment of older men with favorable prostate cancers.

As radiation oncologists, it is imperative that we help older patients make appropriate decisions with regard to their prostate cancer diagnosis. Both undertreatment and overtreatment affect quality and quantity of life. Thus, careful evaluation of the aggressiveness of the given prostate cancer in light of existing comorbidities needs to be done to help these older men make the best decisions for their individual cases.

C. Lawton, MD

Quality-of-Life Effects of Prostate-Specific Antigen Screening
Heijnsdijk EA, Wever EM, Auvinen A, et al (Erasmus Med Ctr, Rotterdam, the Netherlands; Tampere School of Health Sciences, Finland; et al)
N Engl J Med 367:595-605, 2012

Background.—After 11 years of follow-up, the European Randomized Study of Screening for Prostate Cancer (ERSPC) reported a 29% reduction in prostate-cancer mortality among men who underwent screening for prostate-specific antigen (PSA) levels. However, the extent to which harms to quality of life resulting from overdiagnosis and treatment counter-balance this benefit is uncertain.

Methods.—On the basis of ERSPC follow-up data, we used Microsimu-lation Screening Analysis (MISCAN) to predict the number of prostate cancers, treatments, deaths, and quality-adjusted life-years (QALYs) gained after the introduction of PSA screening. Various screening strategies, effica-cies, and quality-of-life assumptions were modeled.

Results.—Per 1000 men of all ages who were followed for their entire life span, we predicted that annual screening of men between the ages of 55 and 69 years would result in nine fewer deaths from prostate cancer (28% reduction), 14 fewer men receiving palliative therapy (35% reduction), and a total of 73 life-years gained (average, 8.4 years per prostate-cancer death avoided). The number of QALYs that were gained was 56 (range, −21 to 97), a reduction of 23% from unadjusted life-years gained. To prevent one prostate-cancer death, 98 men would need to be screened and 5 cancers would need to be detected. Screening of all men between the ages of 55 and 74 would result in more life-years gained (82) but the same number of QALYs (56).

Conclusions.—The benefit of PSA screening was diminished by loss of QALYs owing to postdiagnosis long-term effects. Longer follow-up data from both the ERSPC and quality-of-life analyses are essential before universal recommendations regarding screening can be made. (Funded by the Netherlands Organization for Health Research and Development and others.)

▶ Ever since prostate-specific antigen (PSA) became a potential life-saving screening tool for prostate cancer patients, it has raised controversy. PSA screening has clearly resulted in the diagnosis of many cancers that were not likely to impact the quantity of life for certain patients. Yet there are datasets that have shown a decrease in prostate cancer mortality secondary to screening and resultant early intervention, which is the true test of any screening tool.

So the question remains, how do we best use PSA screening (if at all) for men at risk for prostate cancer? These authors looked specifically at the quality-of-life effects of PSA screening. Once diagnosed with the disease, these authors looked at both surgery and radiation therapy as potentially curative treatments, but with associated toxicities. In their analysis, these toxicities caused a decrease in quality-adjusted life-years and, thus, decreased the potential benefit of screening PSA. The good news is that rather than dumping the whole notion of PSA screening, the authors appropriately qualified their conclusions as followed:

1. We need longer follow-up regarding treatment and active surveillance and their effects on a patient's quality of life.
2. Once we have such data, then appropriate recommendations for popula-tions likely to benefit from PSA screening can be determined.

C. Lawton, MD

Intermittent Androgen Suppression for Rising PSA Level after Radiotherapy

Crook JM, O'Callaghan CJ, Duncan G, et al (British Columbia Cancer Agency, Kelowna, Canada; Queen's Univ, Kingston, Ontario, Canada; et al)
N Engl J Med 367:895-903, 2012

Background.—Intermittent androgen deprivation for prostate-specific antigen (PSA) elevation after radiotherapy may improve quality of life and delay hormone resistance. We assessed overall survival with intermittent versus continuous androgen deprivation in a noninferiority randomized trial.

Methods.—We enrolled patients with a PSA level greater than 3 ng per milliliter more than 1 year after primary or salvage radiotherapy for localized prostate cancer. Intermittent treatment was provided in 8-month cycles, with nontreatment periods determined according to the PSA level. The primary end point was overall survival. Secondary end points included quality of life, time to castration-resistant disease, and duration of nontreatment intervals.

Results.—Of 1386 enrolled patients, 690 were randomly assigned to intermittent therapy and 696 to continuous therapy. Median follow-up was 6.9 years. There were no significant between-group differences in adverse events. In the intermittent-therapy group, full testosterone recovery occurred in 35% of patients, and testosterone recovery to the trial-entry threshold occurred in 79%. Intermittent therapy provided potential benefits with respect to physical function, fatigue, urinary problems, hot flashes, libido, and erectile function. There were 268 deaths in the intermittent-therapy group and 256 in the continuous-therapy group. Median overall survival was 8.8 years in the intermittent-therapy group versus 9.1 years in the continuous-therapy group (hazard ratio for death, 1.02; 95% confidence interval, 0.86 to 1.21). The estimated 7-year cumulative rates of disease-related death were 18% and 15% in the two groups, respectively ($P = 0.24$).

Conclusions.—Intermittent androgen deprivation was noninferior to continuous therapy with respect to overall survival. Some quality-of-life factors improved with intermittent therapy. (Funded by the Canadian Cancer Society Research Institute and others; ClinicalTrials.gov number, NCT00003653.)

▶ Once a patient fails radiation for prostate cancer, whether the radiation therapy was done as the primary form of treatment or as surgical salvage, the next question is when to initiate androgen deprivation therapy (ADT). It is well understood that ADT comes with multiple side effects, from hot flashes and sexual dysfunction to weight gain and muscle mass loss. So patients naturally want to delay the onset of ADT as long as possible. In addition, once it is determined that ADT should begin, the question is raised as to the need for lifelong, continuous ADT (long considered the standard of care) vs intermittent ADT. Patients understand that with intermittent ADT there is a chance for improved quality of life because there can be testosterone recovery during the "hormone holidays."

The concern, of course, is whether intermittent ADT may not be as effective as continuous treatment in these patients and, thus, this trial is very helpful in delineating the benefits and risks of continuous vs intermittent ADT for these patients. Designed as a noninferiority, randomized trial, it is comforting to know that the intermittent ADT did not result in an increase in prostate cancer deaths in these patients. Equally comforting is the improvement in quality of life for patients who received intermittent ADT over continuous therapy. These data should solidify our practice in recommending intermittent ADT for our patients who have failed primary or salvage radiation.

C. Lawton, MD

Radical Prostatectomy versus Observation for Localized Prostate Cancer
Wilt TJ, for the Prostate Cancer Intervention versus Observation Trial (PIVOT) Study Group (Univ of Minnesota School of Medicine, Minneapolis; et al)
N Engl J Med 367:203-213, 2012

Background.—The effectiveness of surgery versus observation for men with localized prostate cancer detected by means of prostate-specific antigen (PSA) testing is not known.

Methods.—From November 1994 through January 2002, we randomly assigned 731 men with localized prostate cancer (mean age, 67 years; median PSA value, 7.8 ng per milliliter) to radical prostatectomy or observation and followed them through January 2010. The primary outcome was all-cause mortality; the secondary outcome was prostate-cancer mortality.

Results.—During the median follow-up of 10.0 years, 171 of 364 men (47.0%) assigned to radical prostatectomy died, as compared with 183 of 367 (49.9%) assigned to observation (hazard ratio, 0.88; 95% confidence interval [CI], 0.71 to 1.08; $P = 0.22$; absolute risk reduction, 2.9 percentage points). Among men assigned to radical prostatectomy, 21 (5.8%) died from prostate cancer or treatment, as compared with 31 men (8.4%) assigned to observation (hazard ratio, 0.63; 95% CI, 0.36 to 1.09; $P = 0.09$; absolute risk reduction, 2.6 percentage points). The effect of treatment on all-cause and prostate-cancer mortality did not differ according to age, race, coexisting conditions, self-reported performance status, or histologic features of the tumor. Radical prostatectomy was associated with reduced all-cause mortality among men with a PSA value greater than 10 ng per milliliter ($P = 0.04$ for interaction) and possibly among those with intermediate-risk or high-risk tumors ($P = 0.07$ for interaction). Adverse events within 30 days after surgery occurred in 21.4% of men, including one death.

Conclusions.—Among men with localized prostate cancer detected during the early era of PSA testing, radical prostatectomy did not significantly reduce all-cause or prostate-cancer mortality, as compared with observation, through at least 12 years of follow-up. Absolute differences were less than 3 percentage points. (Funded by the Department of Veterans Affairs Cooperative Studies Program and others; PIVOT ClinicalTrials. gov number, NCT00007644.)

▶ Since the era of the prostate specific antigen (PSA) test in the late 1980s and early 1990s, the question of the role of curative treatment vs active surveillance has been raised. We know that many of the prostate cancers diagnosed by PSA elevation fall into the low-risk category (PSA < 10, Gleason score < 6, clinical T2a or less disease). Many of these low-risk tumors will not benefit from curative treatment. Yet the only way to truly determine a benefit or lack thereof to definitive treatment for a PSA-detected prostate cancer is a randomized trial, such as reported in this article.

Although not confined to low-risk patients, this trial randomized localized prostate cancer patients to surgery vs observation. The conclusion of the trial with a median follow-up of 10 years is that there was no benefit to surgery in terms of all-cause or prostate cancer mortality. Yet there are important subgroups and, therefore, other messages within these data.

First, 296 of the 731 men in this trial had low-risk disease, which we know, based on current knowledge, would not likely benefit from curative intervention. If those patients were removed from the study, the findings may have been different. In addition, the incidence of bony metastasis was statistically different in the 2 groups favoring surgery. Finally, in patients with a PSA greater than 10, surgery did decrease all-cause mortality by 13.2%, which is significant. So the message here is that if we apply curative treatment to those patients who likely would benefit from it, we should be able to improve both their quantity and quality of life. The contrary is also true in that we should not apply curative treatment to patients who likely will not benefit from it so as to avoid affecting their quantity of life, but especially their quality of life.

C. Lawton, MD

Variation in Use of Androgen Suppression With External-Beam Radiotherapy for Nonmetastatic Prostate Cancer
Swisher-McClure S, Pollack CE, Christodouleas JP, et al (Univ of Pennsylvania, Philadelphia; Johns Hopkins Univ School of Medicine and the Johns Hopkins Bloomberg School of Public Health, Baltimore, MD)
Int J Radiat Oncol Biol Phys 83:8-15, 2012

Purpose.—To describe practice patterns associated with androgen suppression (AS) stratified by disease risk group in patients undergoing external-beam radiotherapy (EBRT) for localized prostate cancer.

Methods and Materials.—We identified 2,184 low-risk, 2,339 intermediate-risk, and 2,897 high-risk patients undergoing EBRT for nonmetastatic prostate cancer diagnosed between January 1, 2004, and December 31, 2005, in the linked Surveillance, Epidemiology, and End Results—Medicare database. We examined the association of patient, clinical, and demographic characteristics with AS use by multivariate logistic regression.

Results.—The proportions of patients receiving AS for low-risk, intermediate-risk, and high-risk prostate cancer were 32.2%, 56.3%, and 81.5%, respectively. AS use among men in the low-risk disease category varied widely, ranging from 13.6% in Detroit to 47.8% in Kentucky. We observed a significant decline in AS use between 2004 and 2005 within all three disease risk categories. Men aged ≥ 75 years or with elevated comorbidity levels were more likely to receive AS.

Conclusion.—Our results identified apparent overuse and underuse of AS among men within the low-risk and high-risk disease categories, respectively. These results highlight the need for clinician and patient education regarding the appropriate use of AS. Practice patterns among intermediate-risk patients reflect the clinical heterogeneity of this population and underscore the need for better evidence to guide the treatment of these patients.

▶ The role of androgen suppression (AS) with external-beam radiotherapy in nonmetastatic prostate cancer is well studied and quite clear, especially for patients with low-risk and high-risk disease. Low-risk patients do not benefit from the use of AS with external-beam radiation, and it is imperative that it is used for the best results in patients with high-risk disease.

Yet understanding if, in fact, the data have been put into practice is always a question. Given the lack of large cancer patient registries, it is difficult to assess these types of questions. In years past, the Patterns of Care and, subsequently, Quality Research in Radiation Oncology data have tried to look at these types of inquiries. With a lack funding of these important efforts, we must now rely on data such as the Surveillance, Epidemiology, and End Results—Medicare database, with all of its inherent issues, to try to assess these questions.

The data reported here show a significant use of AS in low-risk patients, and the significant lack of its use in high-risk patients is cause for concern. Clearly, education is needed to inform treating radiation oncologists and their patients on the proper and well-studied use of AS.

C. Lawton, MD

Long-Term Results of an RTOG Phase II Trial (00-19) of External-Beam Radiation Therapy Combined With Permanent Source Brachytherapy for Intermediate-Risk Clinically Localized Adenocarcinoma of the Prostate
Lawton CA, Yan Y, Lee WR, et al (Med College of Wisconsin, Milwaukee; Radiation Therapy Oncology Group Statistical Ctr, Philadelphia, PA; Duke Univ School of Medicine, Durham, NC; et al)
Int J Radiat Oncol Biol Phys 82:e795-e801, 2012

Purpose.—External-beam radiation therapy combined with low—doserate permanent brachytherapy are commonly used to treat men with localized prostate cancer. This Phase II trial was performed to document late gastrointestinal or genitourinary toxicity as well as biochemical control for this treatment in a multi-institutional cooperative group setting. This report defines the long-term results of this trial.

Methods and Materials.—All eligible patients received external-beam radiation (45 Gy in 25 fractions) followed 2—6 weeks later by a permanent iodine 125 implant of 108 Gy. Late toxicity was defined by the Radiation Therapy Oncology Group/European Organization for Research and Treatment of Cancer late radiation morbidity scoring scheme. Biochemical control was defined by the American Society for Therapeutic Radiology and Oncology (ASTRO) Consensus definition and the ASTRO Phoenix definition.

Results.—One hundred thirty-eight patients were enrolled from 20 institutions, and 131 were eligible. Median follow-up (living patients) was 8.2 years (range, 2.7—9.3 years). The 8-year estimate of late grade > 3 genitourinary and/or gastrointestinal toxicity was 15%. The most common grade > 3 toxicities were urinary frequency, dysuria, and proctitis. There were two grade 4 toxicities, both bladder necrosis, and no grade 5 toxicities. In addition, 42% of patients complained of grade 3 impotence (no erections) at 8 years. The 8-year estimate of biochemical failure was 18% and 21% by the Phoenix and ASTRO consensus definitions, respectively.

Conclusion.—Biochemical control for this treatment seems durable with 8 years of follow-up and is similar to high—dose external beam radiation alone or brachytherapy alone. Late toxicity in this multi-institutional trial is higher than reports from similar cohorts of patients treated with high—dose external-beam radiation alone or permanent low—doserate brachytherapy alone, perhaps suggesting further attention to strategies that limit doses to normal structures or to unimodal radiotherapy techniques.

▶ The role of low-dose rate (LDR) brachytherapy (prostate seed implant) in the treatment of low-risk prostate cancer (prostate specific antigen < 10, Gleason score < 6, clinical T1c-T2a disease) has become an accepted standard. It has been shown to provide excellent tumor control and a relatively favorable toxicity profile. It is also not costly relative to surgery or external-beam radiation. Expanding this treatment for intermediate-risk patients has been fraught with some concern because of the potential extension of disease beyond the gland. Thus, many radiation oncologists felt the need to combine a short course of external-beam radiation therapy with a slightly lower-dose LDR implant for the best outcomes.

In an effort to better understand the relative merit of the above approach, the Radiation Therapy Oncology Group performed its RTOG-00-19 trial, which delivered external-beam irradiation therapy and a LDR implant to patients with intermediate-risk disease. This report, with a median follow-up of 8.2 years, suggests that this approach is likely more toxic than LDR implants alone. Given that the cancer control outcomes appear no better than LDR implant as monotherapy, radiation oncologists should approach intermediate-risk patients with significant caution if they choose to treat with a combination of external-beam therapy and LDR brachytherapy boost.

C. Lawton, MD

Intensity-Modulated Radiation Therapy, Proton Therapy, or Conformal Radiation Therapy and Morbidity and Disease Control in Localized Prostate Cancer

Sheets NC, Goldin GH, Meyer AM, et al (Univ of North Carolina at Chapel Hill)
JAMA 307:1611-1620, 2012

Context.—There has been rapid adoption of newer radiation treatments such as intensity-modulated radiation therapy (IMRT) and proton therapy despite greater cost and limited demonstrated benefit compared with previous technologies.

Objective.—To determine the comparative morbidity and disease control of IMRT, proton therapy, and conformal radiation therapy for primary prostate cancer treatment.

Design, Setting, and Patients.—Population-based study using Surveillance, Epidemiology, and End Results—Medicare-linked data from 2000 through 2009 for patients with nonmetastatic prostate cancer.

Main Outcome Measures.—Rates of gastrointestinal and urinary morbidity, erectile dysfunction, hip fractures, and additional cancer therapy.

Results.—Use of IMRT vs conformal radiation therapy increased from 0.15% in 2000 to 95.9% in 2008. In propensity score—adjusted analyses (N=12 976), men who received IMRT vs conformal radiation therapy were less likely to receive a diagnosis of gastrointestinal morbidities (absolute risk, 13.4 vs 14.7 per 100 person-years; relative risk [RR], 0.91; 95% CI, 0.86-0.96) and hip fractures (absolute risk, 0.8 vs 1.0 per 100 person-years; RR, 0.78; 95% CI, 0.65-0.93) but more likely to receive a diagnosis of erectile dysfunction (absolute risk, 5.9 vs 5.3 per 100 person-years; RR, 1.12; 95% CI, 1.03-1.20). Intensity-modulated radiation therapy patients were less likely to receive additional cancer therapy (absolute risk, 2.5 vs 3.1 per 100 person-years; RR, 0.81; 95% CI, 0.73-0.89). In a propensity score—matched comparison between IMRT and proton therapy (n = 1368), IMRT patients had a lower rate of gastrointestinal morbidity (absolute risk, 12.2 vs 17.8 per 100 person-years; RR, 0.66; 95% CI, 0.55-0.79). There were no significant differences in rates of other morbidities or additional therapies between IMRT and proton therapy.

Conclusions.—Among patients with nonmetastatic prostate cancer, the use of IMRT compared with conformal radiation therapy was associated with less gastrointestinal morbidity and fewer hip fractures but more erectile dysfunction; IMRT compared with proton therapy was associated with less gastrointestinal morbidity.

▶ Given the incidence of prostate cancer in the United States and the potential revenue gained from treating it, there has been a virtual arms race in technology development. For the surgeons, it was the robot, and for radiation oncologists, it has been intensity-modulated radiation therapy (IMRT), image-guided radiation therapy, and protons.

Sadly, all of these technologies were adopted and approved by payers before there could be a clear scientific analysis of their potential benefit. Improvements in outcomes measured as increased disease control or decreased toxicity would be excellent endpoints for scientific study of any new technology. This did not happen, and now we as oncologists are trying to play catch up in defending the use of many of these costly modalities. In addition, we have become a target for the mass media, which points at our use of these expensive yet unproven technologies.

The data presented in this article attempt to correctly analyze IMRT and proton therapy vs conformal radiation therapy. The authors should be commended for this important work. The dataset used is not perfect, but it certainly should push all radiation oncologists to work toward more comparative effectiveness research so as to support or refute the adoptions of new and increasingly expensive technology.

C. Lawton, MD

Germline Mutations in *HOXB13* and Prostate-Cancer Risk

Ewing CM, Ray AM, Lange EM, et al (Johns Hopkins Univ and the James Buchanan Brady Urological Inst, Baltimore; Univ of Michigan Med School and the Univ of Michigan Comprehensive Cancer Ctr, Ann Arbor; Univ of North Carolina and the Univ of North Carolina Lineberger Comprehensive Cancer Ctr; et al)
N Engl J Med 366:141-149, 2012

Background.—Family history is a significant risk factor for prostate cancer, although the molecular basis for this association is poorly understood. Linkage studies have implicated chromosome 17q21-22 as a possible location of a prostate-cancer susceptibility gene.

Methods.—We screened more than 200 genes in the 17q21-22 region by sequencing germline DNA from 94 unrelated patients with prostate cancer from families selected for linkage to the candidate region. We tested family members, additional case subjects, and control subjects to characterize the frequency of the identified mutations.

Results.—Probands from four families were discovered to have a rare but recurrent mutation (G84E) in *HOXB13* (rs138213197), a homeobox transcription factor gene that is important in prostate development. All 18 men with prostate cancer and available DNA in these four families carried the mutation. The carrier rate of the G84E mutation was increased by a factor of approximately 20 in 5083 unrelated subjects of European descent who had prostate cancer, with the mutation found in 72 subjects (1.4%), as compared with 1 in 1401 control subjects (0.1%) ($P = 8.5 \times 10^{-7}$). The mutation was significantly more common in men with early-onset, familial prostate cancer (3.1%) than in those with late-onset, nonfamilial prostate cancer (0.6%) ($P = 2.0 \times 10^{-6}$).

Conclusions.—The novel *HOXB13* G84E variant is associated with a significantly increased risk of hereditary prostate cancer. Although the variant accounts for a small fraction of all prostate cancers, this finding has implications for prostate-cancer risk assessment and may provide new mechanistic insights into this common cancer. (Funded by the National Institutes of Health and others.)

▶ Documenting family history in patients with prostate cancer is important, and yet we know that most cases of this disease in the US male population are sporadic. But as oncologists, we all care for the occasional patient with prostate cancer whose family has a very strong history of the disease. Thus, especially for those patients and their heirs, it is important to try to elucidate the genetic basis for this.

These authors have expanded on the data already available showing a linkage between prostate cancer susceptibility and loci on chromosome 17q21-22. Their data show that a novel HOXB13-G84e variant was associated with a significant increased risk of hereditary prostate cancer.

Although admittedly this finding accounts for a small portion of all prostate cancer, it is science like this that we need to expand. These genetic abnormalities seem to be associated with disease in younger patients who are more at risk for prostate cancer mortality over their lifetime.

C. Lawton, MD

Prostate-Cancer Mortality at 11 Years of Follow-up
Schröder FH, for the ERSPC Investigators (Erasmus Univ Med Ctr, Rotterdam, the Netherlands; et al)
N Engl J Med 366:981-990, 2012

Background.—Several trials evaluating the effect of prostate-specific antigen (PSA) testing on prostate-cancer mortality have shown conflicting results. We updated prostate-cancer mortality in the European Randomized Study of Screening for Prostate Cancer with 2 additional years of follow-up.

Methods.—The study involved 182,160 men between the ages of 50 and 74 years at entry, with a predefined core age group of 162,388 men 55 to 69 years of age. The trial was conducted in eight European countries. Men who were randomly assigned to the screening group were offered PSA-based screening, whereas those in the control group were not offered such screening. The primary outcome was mortality from prostate cancer.

Results.—After a median follow-up of 11 years in the core age group, the relative reduction in the risk of death from prostate cancer in the screening group was 21% (rate ratio, 0.79; 95% confidence interval [CI], 0.68 to 0.91; $P = 0.001$), and 29% after adjustment for noncompliance. The absolute reduction in mortality in the screening group was 0.10 deaths per 1000 person-years or 1.07 deaths per 1000 men who underwent randomization. The rate ratio for death from prostate cancer during follow-up years 10 and 11 was 0.62 (95% CI, 0.45 to 0.85; $P = 0.003$). To prevent one death from prostate cancer at 11 years of follow-up, 1055 men would need to be invited for screening and 37 cancers would need to be detected. There was no significant between group difference in all-cause mortality.

Conclusions.—Analyses after 2 additional years of follow-up consolidated our previous finding that PSA-based screening significantly reduced mortality from prostate cancer but did not affect all-cause mortality. (Current Controlled Trials number, ISRCTN49127736.)

▶ Use of prostate-specific antigen (PSA) as a screening tool remains controversial. There is no question that PSA screening diagnoses prostate cancer at an earlier stage and, therefore, allows for the possibility of increased cure rates. There is also no question that almost 30 000 US men die annually of prostate cancer and that PSA screening could diagnose cancer in some of these patients earlier, potentially increasing their chances for survival. But the challenge is that PSA screening does result in the diagnosis of cancer in patients for whom prostate cancer will never be a significant problem for them in their lifetime. Many of these patients unfortunately go on to definitive treatment instead of watchful waiting/active surveillance and, thus, cost increases and quality of life decreases. Therefore, the US Preventive Services Task Force (USPSTF) recently recommended against the use of PSA for screening.

This data reinforces the fact that PSA screening does result in a statistically significant decrease in prostate cancer deaths, which actually increases over time. So, given that we cannot change the USPSTF recommendation, it is imperative that we as oncologists get the word out that PSA screening can be helpful in decreasing prostate cancer deaths. It has to be used judicially. When a diagnosis of prostate cancer is made, we must ensure that appropriate intervention or lack of intervention, such as surveillance, occurs.

C. Lawton, MD

Racial Differences in Bone Mineral Density and Fractures in Men Receiving Androgen Deprivation Therapy for Prostate Cancer

Morgans AK, Hancock ML, Barnette KG, et al (Massachusetts General Hosp Cancer Ctr, Boston; GTx Inc, Memphis, TN)
J Urol 187:889-893, 2012

Purpose.—Whether race influences bone loss and fracture risk during androgen deprivation therapy for prostate cancer is unknown. Using data from a prospective clinical trial we compared bone mineral density and fracture between African-American and Caucasian men receiving androgen deprivation therapy.

Materials and Methods.—A total of 516 subjects were in the placebo group of a 2-year randomized placebo controlled fracture prevention trial, and were African-American (68) or Caucasian (448). We compared baseline characteristics, changes in bone mineral density and rates of new fractures between races.

Results.—Compared to Caucasian men, African-American men had higher baseline hip bone mineral density (mean ± SD 0.98 ± 0.15 vs 0.91 ± 0.15 gm/m^2, $p = 0.001$) and similar spine bone mineral density

(1.09 ± 0.22 vs 1.11 ± 0.22, $p = 0.51$). There was no difference in prevalent vertebral fractures between African-American and Caucasian men (7.4% vs 15.0%, $p = 0.13$). The percentage change in hip bone mineral density at 2 years was similar between African-American and Caucasian men (mean ± SE −2.21% ± 0.59% vs −2.54% ± 0.26%, $p = 0.65$). Changes in bone mineral density of the lumbar spine were also similar between African-American and Caucasian men (−1.74% ± 0.69% vs −1.30% ± 0.33%, $p = 0.64$). No new vertebral fractures were reported in African-American men but 2 fractures were reported in Caucasian men.

Conclusions.—In a clinical trial African-American men receiving androgen deprivation therapy for prostate cancer have a greater hip bone mineral density and tended to have fewer prevalent vertebral fractures than Caucasian men. Despite a lower baseline risk of osteoporosis and fracture, African-American men experience a decrease in bone mineral density similar to that of Caucasian men.

▶ Adding hormone therapy in the form of a luteinizing hormone-releasing hormone (LHRH) agonist to definitive radiation therapy has been shown in multiple trials to be a benefit for patients with locally advanced nonmetastatic prostate cancer. This benefit is not only in terms of prostate-specific antigen and local regional control but also in terms of disease-related survival and overall survival. So its use is critical to obtaining the best results for these patients.

Yet, these medications do have associated toxicities, such as sexual dysfunction and hot flashes. For patients who need long-term hormone therapy (which is most patients with locally advanced prostate cancer) there are a number of other toxicities that need to be addressed, such as muscle mass loss and bone loss.

Assessing bone strength via a dual energy x-ray absorption scan has become a standard in evaluating the bone density of patients before, during, and after LHRH therapy. Patients with evidence of bone loss need to be evaluated for potential treatment to decrease the fracture risk. These data documenting the racial differences in that bone loss are helpful for the treating oncologist as he or she considers duration of LHRH therapy and potential interventions if bone loss occurs.

C. Lawton, MD

Long-term quality of life outcome after proton beam monotherapy for localized prostate cancer

Coen JJ, Paly JJ, Niemierko A, et al (Massachusetts General Hosp, Boston)
Int J Radiat Oncol Biol Phys 82:e201-e209, 2012

Objectives.—High-dose external radiation for localized prostate cancer results in favorable clinical outcomes and low toxicity rates. Here, we report long-term quality of life (QOL) outcome for men treated with conformal protons.

Methods.—QOL questionnaires were sent at specified intervals to 95 men who received proton radiation. Of these, 87 men reported 3- and/or 12-month outcomes, whereas 73 also reported long-term outcomes (minimum 2 years). Symptom scores were calculated at baseline, 3 months, 12 months, and long-term follow-up. Generalized estimating equation models were constructed to assess longitudinal outcomes while accounting for correlation among repeated measures in an individual patient. Men were stratified into functional groups from their baseline questionnaires (normal, intermediate, or poor function) for each symptom domain. Long-term QOL changes were assessed overall and within functional groups using the Wilcoxon signed-rank test.

Results.—Statistically significant changes in all four symptom scores were observed in the longitudinal analysis. For the 73 men reporting long-term outcomes, there were significant change scores for incontinence (ID), bowel (BD) and sexual dysfunction (SD), but not obstructive/irritative voiding dysfunction (OID). When stratified by baseline functional category, only men with normal function had increased scores for ID and BD. For SD, there were significant changes in men with both normal and intermediate function, but not poor function.

Conclusions.—Patient reported outcomes are sensitive indicators of treatment-related morbidity. These results quantitate the long-term consequences of proton monotherapy for prostate cancer. Analysis by baseline functional category provides an individualized prediction of long-term QOL scores. High dose proton radiation was associated with small increases in bowel dysfunction and incontinence, with more pronounced changes in sexual dysfunction.

▶ Successful treatment of localized prostate cancer comes in many forms. Types of surgery include either robotic or open prostatectomy, and radiation includes either external beam or brachytherapy (low-dose rate or high-dose rate). There are no convincing data that any of these options is significantly better than any other in terms of prostate cancer control. Therefore, the choices for patients need to be made based on toxicity profiles.

Within the external beam option resides standard 3-dimensional or intensity-modulated radiation therapy photon treatment and, more recently, proton therapy. The promoters of proton radiation therapy have rested their recommendation of this over photon radiation therapy in the toxicity arena. They contend that the Bragg peak is the reason that proton therapy is more precise and, therefore, less toxic. Yet data to prove this point are lacking. What is known is that proton therapy is much more expensive than photon therapy.

These authors evaluated the quality of life in approximately 80 men who received proton therapy for their localized prostate cancer. They found significant changes for incontinence and bowel and sexual dysfunction in patients with normal-functioning preproton therapy. These data are important in that they reflect patient reporting not clinician reporting and suggest that proton therapy is associated with significant changes in quality of life. More data like this are needed to determine whether the expense of protons is worth the investment in an effort to improve quality of life over photon therapy. These data suggest the opposite.

C. Lawton, MD

Long-term outcomes from a prospective trial of stereotactic body radiotherapy for low-risk prostate cancer
King CR, Brooks JD, Gill H, et al (Univ of California Los Angeles School of Medicine; Stanford Univ School of Medicine, CA)
Int J Radiat Oncol Biol Phys 82:877-882, 2012

Purpose.—Hypofractionated radiotherapy has an intrinsically different normal tissue and tumor radiobiology. The results of a prospective trial of stereotactic body radiotherapy (SBRT) for prostate cancer with long-term patient-reported toxicity and tumor control rates are presented.

Methods and Materials.—From 2003 through 2009, 67 patients with clinically localized low-risk prostate cancer were enrolled. Treatment consisted of 36.25 Gy in 5 fractions using SBRT with the CyberKnife as the delivery technology. No patient received hormone therapy. Patient self-reported bladder and rectal toxicities were graded on the Radiation Therapy Oncology Group scale (RTOG).

Results.—Median follow-up was 2.7 years. There were no grade 4 toxicities. Radiation Therapy Oncology Group Grade 3, 2, and 1 bladder toxicities were seen in 3% (2 patients), 5% (3 patients), and 23% (13 patients) respectively. Dysuria exacerbated by urologic instrumentation accounted for both patients with Grade 3 toxicity. Urinary incontinence, complete obstruction, or persistent hematuria was not observed. Rectal Grade 3, 2, and 1 toxicities were seen in 0, 2% (1 patient), and 12.5% (7 patients), respectively. Persistent rectal bleeding was not observed. Low-grade toxicities were substantially less frequent with QOD vs. QD dose regimen ($p = 0.001$ for gastrointestinal and $p = 0.007$ for genitourinary). There were two prostate-specific antigen (PSA), biopsy-proven failures with negative metastatic workup. Median PSA at follow-up was 0.5 ± 0.72 ng/mL. The 4-year Kaplan-Meier PSA relapse-free survival was 94% (95% confidence interval, 85%−102%).

Conclusion.—Significant late bladder and rectal toxicities from SBRT for prostate cancer are infrequent. PSA relapse-free survival compares favorably with other definitive treatments. The current evidence supports consideration of stereotactic body radiotherapy among the therapeutic options for localized prostate cancer.

▶ The use of hypofractionation in the treatment of localized prostate cancer is not a new concept. For decades mild hypofractionation with daily doses of approximately 2.5 Gy has been successful in the United States, Canada, and Western Europe. The Radiation Therapy Oncology Group recently completed a trial of standard fractionation of 1.8 Gy/d compared with this mild level of hypofractionation. The hypofractionation concept is based on the data suggesting a low α/β ratio for prostate cancer that has been confirmed by multiple authors and institutions.

Extreme hypofractionation for localized prostate cancer is a relatively new concept, especially for treatment within the United States. Intensity-modulated radiation therapy, image-guided radiation therapy, and the low α/β prostate models have pushed this concept to the clinic.

These authors have done an incredible job of evaluating this extreme hypofractionation called stereotactic body radiation therapy in a clinical trial. Although the follow-up is short at 2.7 years, the toxicities look promising with no grade IV and only 3 of 67 patients with grade III gastrointestinal or genitourinary toxicity. We need more data like these and longer follow-up to help understand the relative merit or lack thereof of this form of radiation for prostate cancer.

C. Lawton, MD

Adverse Effects of Robotic-Assisted Laparoscopic Versus Open Retropubic Radical Prostatectomy Among a Nationwide Random Sample of Medicare-Age Men

Barry MJ, Gallagher PM, Skinner JS, et al (Massachusetts General Hosp, Boston; Univ of Massachusetts, Boston; Dartmouth College, Hanover, NH; et al)
J Clin Oncol 30:513-518, 2012

Purpose.—Robotic-assisted laparoscopic radical prostatectomy is eclipsing open radical prostatectomy among men with clinically localized prostate cancer. The objective of this study was to compare the risks of problems with continence and sexual function following these procedures among Medicare-age men.

Patients and Methods.—A population-based random sample was drawn from the 20% Medicare claims files for August 1, 2008, through December 31, 2008. Participants had hospital and physician claims for radical prostatectomy and diagnostic codes for prostate cancer and reported undergoing either a robotic or open surgery. They received a mail survey that included self-ratings of problems with continence and sexual function a median of 14 months postoperatively.

Results.—Completed surveys were obtained from 685 (86%) of 797 eligible participants, and 406 and 220 patients reported having had robotic or open surgery, respectively. Overall, 189 (31.1%; 95% CI, 27.5% to 34.8%) of 607 men reported having a moderate or big problem with continence, and 522 (88.0%; 95% CI, 85.4% to 90.6%) of 593 men reported having a moderate or big problem with sexual function. In logistic regression models predicting the log odds of a moderate or big problem with postoperative continence and adjusting for age and educational level, robotic prostatectomy was associated with a nonsignificant trend toward greater problems with continence (odds ratio [OR] 1.41; 95% CI, 0.97 to 2.05). Robotic prostatectomy was not associated with greater problems with sexual function (OR, 0.87; 95% CI, 0.51 to 1.49).

Conclusion.—Risks of problems with continence and sexual function are high after both procedures. Medicare-age men should not expect fewer adverse effects following robotic prostatectomy.

▶ When new technology arrives in the medical market, the perception usually is that new is better. Advertising on the part of the hospitals acquiring new technology and the manufacturers that market it often push this concept despite a lack of verifying research. And as technology comes out faster than it can be scientifically vetted, it is not clear whether new is equated with better.

One example (and there are many) is the robotic-assisted laparoscopic radical prostatectomy. One cannot go to a city in the United States of any significant size without seeing billboards advertising this technology. Its adoption in the US, as seen in this article, has surpassed the traditional open prostatectomy. Yet data proving its superiority over the open radical prostatectomy are lacking. In fact, data on its use in the US actually show poorer outcomes in terms of positive margin rates.

This article looks at the issues of continence and sexual function, both touted as improved with robotic over open prostatectomy. These data show problems with both sexual functioning and continence with either open or robotic surgery based on Medicare claims.

Clearly, more data are needed to validate the continued marketing of robotic surgery as resulting in less toxicity over the traditional open procedure. Until those scientific data exist, the marketing of these nonfacts should stop.

C. Lawton, MD

Increased Survival with Enzalutamide in Prostate Cancer after Chemotherapy
Scher HI, for the AFFIRM Investigators (Memorial Sloan-Kettering Cancer Ctr, NY; et al)
N Engl J Med 367:1187-1197, 2012

Background.—Enzalutamide (formerly called MDV3100) targets multiple steps in the androgen-receptor—signaling pathway, the major driver of prostate-cancer growth. We aimed to evaluate whether enzalutamide prolongs survival in men with castration-resistant prostate cancer after chemotherapy.

Methods.—In our phase 3, double-blind, placebo-controlled trial, we stratified 1199 men with castration-resistant prostate cancer after chemotherapy according to the Eastern Cooperative Oncology Group performance-status score and pain intensity. We randomly assigned them, in a 2:1 ratio, to receive oral enzalutamide at a dose of 160 mg per day (800 patients) or placebo (399 patients). The primary end point was overall survival.

Results.—The study was stopped after a planned interim analysis at the time of 520 deaths. The median overall survival was 18.4 months (95% confidence interval [CI], 17.3 to not yet reached) in the enzalutamide group versus 13.6 months (95% CI, 11.3 to 15.8) in the placebo group (hazard ratio for death in the enzalutamide group, 0.63; 95% CI, 0.53 to 0.75; $P < 0.001$). The superiority of enzalutamide over placebo was shown with respect to all secondary end points: the proportion of patients with a reduction in the prostate-specific antigen (PSA) level by 50% or more (54% vs. 2%, $P < 0.001$), the soft-tissue response rate (29% vs. 4%, $P < 0.001$), the quality-of-life response rate (43% vs. 18%, $P < 0.001$), the time to PSA progression (8.3 vs. 3.0 months; hazard ratio, 0.25; $P < 0.001$), radiographic progression-free survival (8.3 vs. 2.9 months; hazard ratio, 0.40; $P < 0.001$), and the time to the first skeletal-related event (16.7 vs. 13.3 months; hazard ratio, 0.69; $P < 0.001$). Rates of fatigue, diarrhea, and hot flashes were higher in the enzalutamide group. Seizures were reported in five patients (0.6%) receiving enzalutamide.

Conclusions.—Enzalutamide significantly prolonged the survival of men with metastatic castrationresistant prostate cancer after chemotherapy. (Funded by Medivation and Astellas Pharma Global Development; AFFIRM ClinicalTrials.gov number, NCT00974311.)

▶ Treatment options for prostate cancer are expanding relatively rapidly. Previously, it was considered that a prostate cancer that had progressed or recurred after androgen deprivation therapy was hormone refractory. We have since learned that these cancers are often more sensitive to hormonal manipulation and that the sources of androgen in the body include not only the testes and the adrenal glands but also the prostate cancer itself. This has taught us that it is important to maintain the patient with metastatic disease at castrate levels of testosterone in the system by continued suppression of the testicular and adrenal sources. In addition, we have learned that we can further lower the testosterone level by reducing the production of testosterone from the cancer itself with the use of a blocker of the synthetic pathway for testosterone with abiraterone and achieve further response of the disease process. This article reports results in patients who have progressed after prior treatment with androgen deprivation and chemotherapy and who are treated with an inhibitor of multiple steps in the receptor-signaling pathway, enzalutamide. The trial randomly assigned patients who had received at least one prior chemotherapy to enzalutamide or placebo. As the abstract shows, this treatment resulted in a response rate of 29% in soft tissue lesions, a better than 50% reduction in the prostate-specific antigen (PSA) level, an improved quality of life, a delay in further progression of the PSA level, an improved progression-free survival, and an improved overall survival. On the basis of these data, the US Food and Drug Administration has approved enzalutamide for the treatment of metastatic prostate cancer that has not responded to one or more prior chemotherapy regimens. With the various treatment options growing by the minute (sipuleucel, abiraterone, enzalutamide, chemotherapy [multiple active agents]), we now have to ascertain the optimal way to utilize all of the options during the course of the disease.

J. T. Thigpen, MD

7 Gynecology

Cervix

ACR Appropriateness Criteria® Pretreatment Planning of Invasive Cancer of the Cervix
Siegel CL, Andreotti RF, Cardenes HR, et al (Mallinckrodt Inst of Radiology, St Louis, MO; Vanderbilt Univ Med Ctr, Nashville, TN; Indiana Univ Med Ctr, Indianapolis; et al)
J Am Coll Radiol 9:395-402, 2012

The prognosis of cervical cancer is linked to lymph node involvement, and this is predicted clinically and pathologically by the stage of the disease, as well as the volume and grade of the tumor. Staging of cervical cancer based on International Federation of Gynecology and Obstetrics (FIGO) staging uses physical examination, cystoscopy, proctoscopy, intravenous urography, and barium enema. It does not include CT or MRI. Evaluation of the parametrium is limited in FIGO staging, and lymph node metastasis, an important prognostic factor, is not included in FIGO staging. The most important role for imaging is to distinguish stages Ia, Ib, and IIa disease treated with surgery from advanced disease treated with radiation therapy with or without chemotherapy. This article reviews the current role of imaging in pretreatment planning of invasive cervical cancer.

The ACR Appropriateness Criteria® are evidence-based guidelines for specific clinical conditions that are reviewed every 2 years by a multidisciplinary expert panel. The guideline development and review include an extensive analysis of current medical literature from peer-reviewed journals and the application of a well-established consensus methodology (modified Delphi) to rate the appropriateness of imaging and treatment procedures by the panel. In those instances in which evidence is lacking or not definitive, expert opinion may be used to recommend imaging or treatment.

▶ Developing appropriateness criteria to treat myriad malignancies has been in the purview of the American College of Radiology for years. In this modified Delphi process, a panel of experts on a given topic are convened and issues related to the topic under discussion are raised. A comprehensive literature review is performed and recommendations are put forward and then voted on by the panel members to develop a consensus regarding treatments and procedures. Ratings on a scale of 1 to 9 are arrived at based on the voting, where a 1 to 3 designation is defined as usually not appropriate, a 4 to 6 rating is defined as possibly appropriate, and a 7 to 9 rating represents usually appropriate items.

This process was urgently needed in the area of cancer of the cervix, as the old Federation of Gynecology and Obstetrics (FIGO) staging system is used to classify this disease. Although this FIGO classification has been helpful in the past, it does not include important current imaging techniques, such as computed tomography and magnetic resonance imaging (MRI), to define subgroups of cervix cancer patients. These imaging techniques are routinely used in the United States and in developed worlds to help distinguish both differences in early-stage patients and locally advanced disease patients. Identifying these differences in cervix cancer patients allows them to be treated most appropriately with surgery alone, radiation alone, or some combination of chemotherapy. Congratulations should be given to this group who have recommended as appropriate the imaging of these cervix cancer patients, including MRI and positron emission tomography, so that they may receive the most appropriate therapy after better defining their disease status.

C. Lawton, MD

Incorporation of bevacizumab in the treatment of recurrent and metastatic cervical cancer: a phase III randomized trial of the Gynecologic Oncology Group
Tewari KS, Sill M, Long HJ, et al (Univ of California, Orange; Gynecologic Oncology Group Statistical and Data Ctr, Buffalo, NY; Mayo Clinic, Rochester, MN; et al)
J Clin Oncol 31, 2013

Background.—Vascular endothelial growth factor (VEGF) promotes angiogenesis, a mediator of disease progression in cervical cancer. Bevacizumab (B), a humanized anti-VEGF monoclonal antibody, has shown single-agent activity in pretreated recurrent disease. We aimed to evaluate B in chemotherapy (CTX)-naive recurrent/persistent/metastatic cervical cancer.

Methods.—Using a 2×2 factorial design, patients were randomly assigned to CTX with or without B 15 mg/kg. The CTX regimens included cisplatin 50 mg/m2 plus paclitaxel 135-175 mg/m2 and topotecan 0.75 mg/m2 d1-3 plus paclitaxel 175 mg/m2d1. Cycles were repeated every 21 days until disease progression, unacceptable toxicity, or complete response. Overall survival (OS) was the primary endpoint with a reduction in the hazard of death by 30% using anti-VEGF therapy considered important (90% power, 1-sided alpha = 2.5%). Final analysis was planned when 346 deaths were observed.

Results.—452 patients were accrued from 4/6/09 to 1/3/12. The scheduled interim analysis occurred after 174 patients had died and showed that the topotecan-paclitaxel backbone was not superior to the cisplatin-paclitaxel backbone. A second interim analysis was conducted after 271 deaths. A total of 225 patients received CTX alone and 227 patients received

CTX plus B. The randomized treatment groups were similar with regard to age, histology, performance status, previous platinum as a radiosensitizer, and recurrence, persistence, or advanced disease. The B-to-no-B hazard ratio (HR) of death was 0.71 (97.6% CI 0.54-0.95; 1-sided $p = 0.0035$). Median survival was 17 m (CTX plus B) and 13.3 m (CTX alone). The RR were 48% (CTX plus B) and 36% (CTX alone) ($p = 0.0078$). Treatment with B was associated with more grade 3-4 bleeding (5 vs 1%) thrombosis/embolism (9 vs 2%), and GI fistula (3 vs 0%).

Conclusions.—For the first time a targeted agent significantly improved OS in gynecologic cancer. The second interim analysis crossed the boundary for efficacy, warranting early release of this information. The nearly 4-month increase in median OS with the addition of B to CTX in women with recurrent cervical cancer is considered to be clinically significant. Clinical trial information: NCT00803062.

▶ The management of advanced or recurrent cervical cancer has been a major challenge because most of the patients have recurrent disease and have received prior radiation with or without cisplatin to treat their earlier-stage disease. The Gynecologic Oncology Group (GOG) has, since 1976, conducted a concerted phase II effort to identify active agents and regimens. The most active agent identified to date is cisplatin. The GOG has conducted 3 phase III trials that have shown an advantage for a doublet over single-agent cisplatin: ifosfamide/cisplatin, paclitaxel/cisplatin, and topotecan/cisplatin. A direct comparison of the latter 2 with each other and with 2 other doublets (gemcitabine/cisplatin and vinorelbine/cisplatin) showed strong trends for superior progression-free and overall survival associated with the paclitaxel/cisplatin doublet. This plenary session abstract from American Society of Clinical Oncology 2013 reports the results of the subsequent GOG trial, which sought to add bevacizumab to paclitaxel/cisplatin in advanced or recurrent disease. The data show a significant increase in response rate (48% vs 36%) and overall survival (hazard ratio = 0.71 favoring the triplet with median survivals of 17 vs 13.3 months). This establishes the triplet of paclitaxel/cisplatin plus bevacizumab followed by bevacizumab maintenance as the treatment of choice for advanced or recurrent cervical carcinoma.

J. T. Thigpen, MD

Phase II trial of nab-paclitaxel in the treatment of recurrent or persistent advanced cervix cancer: A gynecologic oncology group study
Alberts DS, Blessing JA, Landrum LM, et al (Univ of Arizona, Tucson, AZ; Roswell Park Cancer Inst, Buffalo, NY; Oklahoma Univ Health Science Ctr, Oklahoma City; et al)
Gynecol Oncol 127:451-455, 2012

Background.—Metastatic and recurrent, platinum resistant cervix cancer has an extremely poor prognosis. The Gynecologic Oncology Group has studied >20 cytotoxic drugs or drug combinations in the second-line, phase II setting of advanced, drug resistant cervix cancer.

Methods.—Nanoparticle, albumin-bound paclitaxel (nab-paclitaxel) was administered at 125 mg/m^2 IV over 30 minutes on days 1, 8 and 15 of each 28 day cycle to 37 women with metastatic or recurrent cervix cancer that had progressed or relapsed following first-line cytotoxic drug treatment. A flexible, 2-stage accrual design that allowed stopping early for lack of treatment activity was utilized. Because of slow patient accrual, the second stage was not completed.

Results.—Of 37 patients enrolled, 2 were ineligible due to no prior cytotoxic chemotherapy, which left 35 eligible patients evaluable for response and tolerability. All of the eligible patients had 1 prior chemotherapy regimen and 27 of them had prior radiation therapy with concomitant cisplatin. The median number of nab-paclitaxel cycles were 4 (range 1−15). Ten (28.6%; CI 14.6%−46.3%) of the 35 patients had a partial response and another 15 patients (42.9%) had stable disease. The median progression-free and overall survival were 5.0 and 9.4 months, respectively. The only NCI CTCAE grade 4 event was neutropenia in 2 patients (5.7%) which resolved following dose reduction. Grade 3 neurotoxicity was reported in 1 (2.9%) patient and resolved to grade 2 following dose discontinuation.

Conclusions.—Nab-paclitaxel has considerable activity and moderate toxicity in the treatment of drug resistant, metastatic and recurrent cervix cancer.

▶ The Gynecologic Oncology Group (GOG), in the last 37 years, has identified several active agents in cervical carcinoma. Those more commonly used in the treatment of the disease include the platinum compounds, in particular, cisplatin, which appears to be more active than carboplatin, paclitaxel, topotecan, and ifosfamide. A series of GOG studies led to the conclusion that the best currently available regimen is a doublet of paclitaxel plus cisplatin, and a recent report (ASCO 2013 plenary session presentation)[1] showed that the addition of bevacizumab to this doublet led to a survival advantage. Also recently, there has been interest in the newer agent nab-paclitaxel, which is a nanoparticle formulation of albumin-bound paclitaxel. This agent has some potential advantages over paclitaxel. It requires no premedication, and some have suggested that it produces less neurotoxicity. To evaluate the activity of this formulation of paclitaxel, the GOG initiated a phase II trial. The study population consisted of patients who had received one prior chemotherapy regimen not containing a taxane. Among 35 patients, 10 exhibited a partial response and another 15 exhibited stable disease with a median progression-free survival of 5.0 months and a median survival of 9.4 months. The drug was well tolerated with only one grade 3 neurotoxicity. This marks this agent active in cervical carcinoma; further trials of a randomized nature will be required to establish its place in the therapeutic armamentarium for cervical carcinoma.

J. T. Thigpen, MD

Reference

1. Tewari KS, Sill M, Long HJ, et al. Incorporation of bevacizumab in the treatment of recurrent and metastatic cervical cancer: A phase III randomized trial of the Gynecologic Oncology Group. *J Clin Oncol.* 2013; 31 no.15_suppl 3.

A systematic review of randomized trials assessing human papillomavirus testing in cervical cancer screening

Patanwala IY, Bauer HM, Miyamoto J, et al (Univ of California, San Francisco)
Am J Obstet Gynecol 208:343-353, 2013

Our objective was to assess the sensitivity and specificity of human papillomavirus (HPV) testing for cervical cancer screening in randomized trials. We conducted a systematic literature search of the following databases: MEDLINE, CINAHL, EMBASE, and Cochrane. Eligible studies were randomized trials comparing HPV-based to cytology-based screening strategies, with disease status determined by colposcopy/biopsy for participants with positive results. Disease rates (cervical intraepithelial neoplasia [CIN] 2 or greater and CIN3 or greater), sensitivity, and positive predictive value were abstracted or calculated from the articles. Six studies met inclusion criteria. Relative sensitivities for detecting CIN3 or greater of HPV testing-based strategies vs cytology ranged from 0.8 to 2.1. The main limitation of our study was that testing methodologies and screening/management protocols were highly variable across studies. Screening strategies in which a single initial HPV-positive test led to colposcopy were more sensitive than cytology but resulted in higher colposcopy rates. These results have implications for cotesting with HPV and cytology as recommended in the United States.

▶ No screening test has had more impact on mortality from disease than cervical cytology. The number of deaths in the United States has decreased from 60 000 per year in 1950 to approximately 4000 deaths per year currently as a result of the widespread use of screening cervical cytology. Because lesser changes quite often revert to normal without intervention, the real goal of screening is to detect cases that exhibit cervical intraepithelial neoplasia 3 (CIN3) or greater abnormalities. In recent years, many have suggested that adding human papillomavirus (HPV) testing to screening would improve the sensitivity of screening for CIN3. In the studies included in this review, 4 involved an active response to HPV test results, whereas 3 had a passive response if the cytology was negative. Sensitivity for CIN3 or greater was improved only if the patient was referred for colposcopy after a single positive test result. This resulted in a greater number of false-positives and a greater number of colposcopies performed per case of CIN3 or greater diagnosed. Although these observations do suggest increased sensitivity for CIN3 when HPV testing is added to screening for cervical cytology, they do not provide clear-cut guidance to add such testing because of the increased cost of multiple colposcopies and the morbidity associated with potential overtreatment. One cannot, therefore, conclude that the case for the routine addition of HPV testing has been made.

J. T. Thigpen, MD

Chemotherapy for advanced and recurrent cervical carcinoma: Results from cooperative group trials
Leath CA III, Straughn JM Jr (Univ of Alabama at Birmingham)
Gynecol Oncol 129:251-257, 2013

Objective.—To review the clinical trial experience with chemotherapy for patients with primary Stage IVB, persistent and recurrent cervical cancer.

Methods.—PubMed and cooperative group website search was performed and included clinical trials until September 2012. Emphasis was placed on the phase II and III clinical trial experience of the Gynecologic Oncology Group.

Results.—Experience and trial results with single agents and combination agents in phase II settings are reviewed. Cisplatin has been considered as the most effective agent for metastatic cervical cancer. Most patients who develop metastatic disease have received cisplatin with concurrent radiation and may no longer be sensitive to single-agent therapy. Therefore, cisplatin-based combination chemotherapy regimens have been extensively studied and eight sentinel phase III trials are discussed in this review.

Conclusion.—Based on phase III results, the combination of cisplatin and paclitaxel remains the standard of care; however, alternative combination therapies including cisplatin/topotecan and cisplatin/gemcitabine may be acceptable considerations for patients when considering potential toxicities. Further research is necessary to determine the optimal therapy for this group of patients. Final data from GOG 240 and JCOG 0505 will likely contribute to the design of future clinical trials in this disease setting.

▶ This article reviews the literature on the use of systemic therapy in advanced or recurrent cervical cancer. Much of this literature reflects the work of the Gynecologic Oncology Group (GOG) in the United States. Of particular note is a series of randomized, phase III trials of the GOC evaluating single-agent and combination chemotherapy. The most extensively tested single agent is cisplatin, which appears to be preferable to carboplatin on the basis of an enhanced response rate in GOG trials. Dose-ranging studies have found that 50 mg/m^2 every 3 weeks produces results as effective as higher doses with less toxicity. Doublets compared directly with single-agent cisplatin include ifosfamide/cisplatin, paclitaxel/cisplatin, and topotecan/cisplatin. In each instance, the doublet produced higher response rates and longer progression-free survival. Only the topotecan/cisplatin produced a superior survival in a trial in which the cisplatin arm underperformed, probably because it was the first GOG phase III trial in advanced or recurrent disease after cisplatin-based concurrent chemoradiation became the standard of care for patients with stages IB to IVA disease. Most patients on the topotecan/cisplatin trial had received prior cisplatin in an earlier disease setting. The 2 most recent GOG phase III trials in cervical cancer were GOG 204 and GOG 240. The former compared 4 cisplatin-based doublets (paclitaxel/cisplatin, topotecan/cisplatin, gemcitabine/cisplatin, and vinorelbine/cisplatin). Although there were statistically significant differences among the 4, paclitaxel/cisplatin produced substantial trends that suggested greater efficacy for this particular doublet. GOG 240 then compared paclitaxel/cisplatin with paclitaxel/cisplatin plus bevacizumab. Presented at the 2013 Association of Schools and Colleges of Optometry plenary session, this study showed both a progression-free survival and overall survival advantage for the bevacizumab arm. Currently, the evidence-based treatment of choice for advanced or recurrent cervical cancer is, therefore, paclitaxel/cisplatin plus bevacizumab.

J. T. Thigpen, MD

Endometrial

Phase II trial of combination bevacizumab and temsirolimus in the treatment of recurrent or persistent endometrial carcinoma: A Gynecologic Oncology Group study

Alvarez EA, Brady WE, Walker JL, et al (Univ of California, San Diego; Roswell Park Cancer Inst, Buffalo, NY; Univ of Oklahoma, Oklahoma City; et al)
Gynecol Oncol 129:22-27, 2013

Objective.—This two-stage phase II study was designed to assess the activity of the combination of temsirolimus and bevacizumab in patients with recurrent or persistent endometrial carcinoma (EMC).

Methods.—Eligible patients had persistent or recurrent EMC after receiving 1–2 prior cytotoxic regimens, measurable disease, and Gynecologic Oncology Group performance status ≤2. Treatment consisted of bevacizumab 10 mg/kg every other week and temsirolimus 25 mg IV weekly until disease progression or prohibitory toxicity. Primary end points were progression-free survival (PFS) at six months and overall response rate using RECIST criteria.

Results.—Fifty-three patients were enrolled. Forty-nine patients were eligible and evaluable. Median age was 63 years, and prior treatment consisted of one or two regimens in 40 (82%) and 9 (18%), respectively. Twenty (41%) received prior radiation. Adverse events were consistent with those expected with bevacizumab and temsirolimus treatment. Two gastrointestinal—vaginal fistulas, one grade 3 epistaxis, two intestinal perforations and 1 grade 4 thrombosis/embolism were seen. Three patient deaths were possibly treatment related. Twelve patients (24.5%) experienced clinical responses (one complete and 11 partial responses), and 23 patients (46.9%) survived progression free for at least six months. Median progression-free survival (PFS) and overall survival (OS) were 5.6 and 16.9 months, respectively.

Conclusion.—Combination of temsirolimus and bevacizumab is deemed active based on both objective tumor response and PFS at six months in recurrent or persistent EMC. However, this treatment regimen was associated with significant toxicity in this pretreated group. Future study will be guided by strategies to decrease toxicity and increase response rates.

▶ The Gynecologic Oncology Group (GOG) has a robust, phase II effort to identify active new agents and regimens, in particular, the major 3 gynecologic cancers: ovarian, cervical, and endometrial carcinomas. This phase II trial is the next in a logical sequence of studies that began with a phase II trial of bevacizumab. Bevacizumab exhibited a 13.5% clinical response. The 6-month progression-free rate was 40%. Both of these parameters indicated that bevacizumab had significant activity. Temsirolimus, a mammalian target of rapamycin inhibitor, was also studied by the GOG in a phase II trial. In chemo-naïve patients, temsirolimus produced a 14% response rate and a 69% 6-month progression-free rate. The next step was to combine the 2 agents in this study. The combination produced a 24.5% response rate and a 46.9% 6-month progression-free rate with median progression-free survival of 5.6 months and median overall survival of 16.9 months. These are impressive results, but the toxicity of the combination was considerable with, among the 49 patients in the analysis, 2 gastrointestinal fistulas, 1 grade 3 epistaxis, 2 intestinal perforations, and 1 grade 4 pulmonary embolism. Immediate future efforts will be aimed at ameliorating the toxicity while maintaining the activity.

J. T. Thigpen, MD

Did GOG99 and PORTEC1 change clinical practice in the United States?
Ko EM, Funk MJ, Clark LH, et al (Univ of North Carolina School of Medicine, Chapel Hill; Univ of North Carolina Gillings School of Global Public Health, Chapel Hill)
Gynecol Oncol 129:12-17, 2013

Objective.—To assess the practice of adjuvant radiation (RT) for endometrial cancer in the United States following the publication of the Post Operative Radiation Therapy in Endometrial Carcinoma (PORTEC1), and Gynecologic Oncology Group-Adjuvant Radiation for Intermediate Risk Endometrial Cancers (GOG99).

Methods.—A retrospective cohort study using the NCI SEER database compared the use of RT pre and post publication of PORTEC1 (1996—99 v 2000—03) and GOG 99 (2000—03 v 2004—07). Criteria for intermediate (IR) and high-intermediate (HIR) risk categories as defined by PORTEC1 and GOG99 were applied. Chi-squared statistics and adjusted multivariable Poisson models were used.

Results.—RT did not increase for HIR (RR 1.05, 95% CI 0.99, 1.11) or IR groups (RR 1.0, 95% CI 0.95, 1.05) following GOG99 publication, or for HIR (RR 1.01, 95% CI 0.86, 1.19) or IR groups (RR 0.88, 95% CI 0.77—1.00) following PORTEC1 publication. Radiation rates changed heterogeneously across the country without a discernible pattern of cause.

Among radiated patients, brachytherapy use increased, whereas external beam use decreased after GOG99 publication.

Conclusions.—As the debate regarding the utility of adjuvant radiation in early stage endometrial cancer continues, we found that overall, clinicians had not adopted GOG99 or PORTEC1 results into their clinical practice in the years immediately after publication. However, we did identify significant variation in practice by geographic location. Given that barely half the women deemed highest risk for recurrence received radiation, these findings illustrate that clinical practice reflects the continued controversy surrounding adjuvant radiation in the treatment of endometrial cancer.

▶ The traditional roles of radiation in the management of endometrial carcinoma have been in the postoperative adjuvant therapy setting for those thought to be at significant risk for recurrence. Pelvic or abdominopelvic radiation has been used in patients with locally advanced endometrial carcinoma stages III to IV after substantial bulk reduction or total resection of gross disease and has also been given to patients with stage I to II disease as a postoperative adjuvant for those with cervix or myometrial involvement. Brachytherapy has been used to reduce the likelihood of recurrence in the vaginal vault, particularly in those patients with cervix involvement. The plenary session presentation at American Society of Clinical Oncology 2003 of the results of the Gynecologic Oncology Group 122[1] (surgical bulk reduction followed by either abdominopelvic radiation or chemotherapy in patients with stage III—IV disease) raised significant questions about the relative roles of radiation and chemotherapy when it showed superior survival for those patients receiving chemotherapy. At the same time, the 2 studies evaluated in this article looked at the role of radiation in earlier-stage disease (essentially stage I disease with myometrial invasion or high-grade disease plus stage II patients). The bottom line for both trials was to raise questions about the role for radiation in endometrial carcinoma except for the use of brachytherapy to reduce vaginal recurrence. Although there clearly remains a controversy in the practicing community about radiation's proper role, there has been a shift in the focus of trials from examining the role of chemotherapy to examining instead whether radiation has any role to play. This shift to include chemotherapy in the management of essentially all stage III to IV cancer and to question the role of radiation in earlier-stage disease while actually evaluating chemotherapy in those settings represents a paradigm shift in our approach to endometrial carcinoma.

J. T. Thigpen, MD

Reference

1. Randall ME, Filiaci VL, Muss H, et al. Randomized phase III trial of whole-abdominal irradiation versus doxorubicin and cisplatin chemotherapy in advanced endometrial carcinoma: a Gynecologic Oncology Group study. *J Clin Oncol.* 2006;24: 36-44.

Adjuvant Radiotherapy for Stage I Endometrial Cancer: An Updated Cochrane Systematic Review and Meta-analysis

Kong A, Johnson N, Kitchener HC, et al (Univ of Oxford, UK; Royal United Hosp, Bath, UK; Univ of Manchester, UK)
J Natl Cancer Inst 104:1625-1634, 2012

Background.—The role of adjuvant radiotherapy in stage I endometrial cancer has changed in recent years. This updated Cochrane systematic review aimed to reexamine the efficacy and toxicity of adjuvant radiotherapy vs no treatment in stage I endometrial cancer.

Methods.—We searched various databases including The Cochrane Central Register of Controlled Trials (CENTRAL), MEDLINE, EMBASE, and the Specialised Register of the Cochrane Gynaecological Cancer Review Group (CGCRG) for randomized controlled trials that met the predefined inclusion criteria. The primary outcome was overall survival (OS); secondary outcomes were endometrial cancer–specific survival, locoregional recurrence, distant recurrence, and toxicity. Hazard ratios (HRs) were estimated and pooled if possible; otherwise, dichotomous data were extracted. All statistical tests were two-sided.

Results.—Of the eight included trials, seven trials (3628 women) compared external beam radiotherapy (EBRT) and no EBRT (or vaginal brachytherapy [VBT]), and one trial (645 women) compared VBT and no additional treatment. EBRT statistically significantly reduced locoregional recurrence compared with no EBRT (or VBT alone) (HR = 0.36, 95% confidence Interval [CI] = 0.25 to 0.52; $P < .001$), but this did not translate into an improvement in OS (HR = 0.99, 95% CI = 0.82 to 1.20; $P = .95$), endometrial cancer–specific survival (HR = 0.96, 95% CI = 0.72 to 1.28; $P = .80$), or distant recurrence rates (risk ratio = 1.04, 95% CI = 0.80 to 1.35; $P = .77$). EBRT was associated with an increased risk of severe acute toxicity, severe late toxicity, and reduced quality of life scores.

Conclusions.—EBRT reduces the risk of locoregional recurrence but has no statistically significant impact on cancer-related deaths or OS. However, EBRT is associated with clinically and statistically significant morbidity and a reduction in quality of life.

▶ The role of radiotherapy in the treatment of patients with endometrial carcinoma has come under increased scrutiny based on a Gynecologic Oncology Group study (GOG 122) that showed that chemotherapy was superior to abdomen-pelvic radiation after surgical bulk reduction for stage III to IV endometrial carcinoma. This meta-analysis of the value of radiation focuses on earlier disease (stage I) and seeks to determine, from the 8 randomized trials assessing the role of radiation in stage I disease, whether it is possible to identify an evidence-based role. The results of the meta-analysis show essentially that external beam radiation reduces the risk of locoregional recurrence with no discernible overall or cancer-specific survival advantage and clinically and statistically significant morbidity and decreased quality of life. Insufficient data were available to permit any comment on the role of vaginal brachytherapy. Based on current data, it would appear that surgical resection alone in earlier stage disease (stage I) and surgical resection followed by chemotherapy in more advanced disease (stages II—IVA) represent the current treatments of choice unless, of course, one believes that decreased local recurrence rate alone is adequate reason to subject the patient to greater toxicity and decreased quality of life.

J. T. Thigpen, MD

Adjuvant Therapy for High-Grade, Uterus-Limited Leiomyosarcoma: Results of a Phase 2 Trial (SARC 005)
Hensley ML, Wathen JK, Maki RG, et al (Memorial Sloan-Kettering Cancer Ctr, NY; Janssen Res and Development, Titusville, NJ; Mt Sinai Med Ctr, NY; et al)
Cancer 119:1555-1561, 2013

Background.—Between 30% and 50% of women who have high-grade uterine leiomyosarcoma (uLMS) limited to the uterus at diagnosis remain progression-free at 2 years. Adjuvant pelvic radiation does not improve outcome. The objective of the current study was to determine the 2-year and 3-year progression-free survival (PFS) among a prospective cohort of women who received adjuvant gemcitabine plus docetaxel followed by doxorubicin.

Methods.—Women with uterus-limited, high-grade uLMS and adequate organ function were eligible. Within 12 weeks of complete resection and after confirmation that they had no evidence of disease on computed tomography (CT) images, the patients received 4 cycles of fixed-dose-rate gemcitabine plus docetaxel. Those who were confirmed disease-free on CT scans after cycle 4 received 4 cycles of doxorubicin. CT imaging for recurrence was performed every 3 months for 2 years, then every 6 months for 3 years.

Results.—In total, 47 women were enrolled (46 evaluable) in 3 years. Characteristics included a median age of 53 years; 1988 International Federation of Gynecology and Obstetrics stage I disease in 81% of patients, stage II disease in 15%, and serosa-only stage IIIA disease in 4%; American Joint Committee on Cancer stage II disease in 13% of patients and stage III disease in 87%; a median tumor size of 8 cm (range, 2.5-30 cm); and a median mitotic rate of 18 mitoses per 10 high-power fields (range, 5-83 mitoses per 10 high-power fields). At a median follow-up of 39.8 months, 21 of 46 patients developed recurrent disease (45.7%). The median time to recurrence was 27.4 months (range, 3-40 months). Seventy-eight percent of patients (95% confidence interval, 67%-91%) were progression-free at 2 years, and 57% (95% confidence interval, 44%-74%) were progression-free at 3 years. The median PFS was not reached and exceeded 36 months.

Conclusions.—Among women with high-grade, uterus-limited uLMS who received treatment with adjuvant gemcitabine plus docetaxel followed by doxorubicin, 78% remained progression-free at 2 years, and 57% remained progression-free at 3 years. A randomized trial of adjuvant chemotherapy versus observation to determine whether adjuvant chemotherapy can improve survival in women with uterus-limited uLMS is underway.

▶ Uterine sarcomas constitute approximately 1000 cases of cancer per year in the United States. There are 2 major types: carcinosarcoma and leiomyosarcoma. A recent Gynecologic Oncology Group (GOG) study identified a high order of activity for the combination of gemcitabine plus docetaxel in advanced or recurrent leiomyosarcomas. At the same time, a European Organisation for the Research and Treatment of Cancer trial evaluating radiation vs observation after surgical resection of gross disease in patients with limited disease found a 50% recurrence in both arms. This article presents the results of a phase II trial evaluating the combination of gemcitabine plus docetaxel in patients with completely grossly resected uterine leiomyosarcomas. The purpose of the study was to ascertain whether there was sufficient evidence to justify a phase III trial of systemic therapy vs observation in patients with completely resected leiomyosarcoma of the uterus. The study yielded a higher percentage of patients progression free at 2 years than that previously reported and a substantially higher-than-expected percentage of patients progression free at 3 years. The study regimen was 4 cycles of gemcitabine plus docetaxel followed by 4 cycles of single-agent doxorubicin. These results led to the activation of GOG 277, which randomizes this study regimen against observation in patients with completely grossly resected uterine leiomyosarcoma. This trial is ongoing.

J. T. Thigpen, MD

Recurrence and Survival After Random Assignment to Laparoscopy Versus Laparotomy for Comprehensive Surgical Staging of Uterine Cancer: Gynecologic Oncology Group LAP2 Study
Walker JL, Piedmonte MR, Spirtos NM, et al (Univ of Oklahoma Health Sciences Ctr; Roswell Park Cancer Inst, Buffalo, NY; Women's Cancer Ctr of Nevada, Las Vegas; et al)
J Clin Oncol 30:695-700, 2012

Purpose.—The primary objective was to establish noninferiority of laparoscopy compared with laparotomy for recurrence after surgical staging of uterine cancer.

Patients and Methods.—Patients with clinical stages I to IIA disease were randomly allocated (two to one) to laparoscopy (n = 1,696) versus laparotomy (n = 920) for hysterectomy, salpingo-oophorectomy, pelvic cytology, and pelvic and para-aortic lymphadenectomy. The primary study end point was noninferiority of recurrence-free interval defined as no more than a 40% increase in the risk of recurrence with laparoscopy compared with laparotomy.

Results.—With a median follow-up time of 59 months for 2,181 patients still alive, there were 309 recurrences (210 laparoscopy; 99 laparotomy) and 350 deaths (229 laparoscopy; 121 laparotomy). The estimated hazard ratio for laparoscopy relative to laparotomy was 1.14 (90% lower bound, 0.92; 95% upper bound, 1.46), falling short of the protocol-specified definition of noninferiority. However, the actual recurrence rates were substantially lower than anticipated, resulting in an estimated 3-year recurrence rate of 11.4% with laparoscopy and 10.2% with laparotomy, or a difference of 1.14% (90% lower bound, −1.28; 95% upper bound, 4.0). The estimated 5-year overall survival was almost identical in both arms at 89.8%.

Conclusion.—This study previously reported that laparoscopic surgical management of uterine cancer is superior for short-term safety and length-of-stay end points. The potential for increased risk of cancer recurrence with laparoscopy versus laparotomy was quantified and found to be small, providing accurate information for decision making for women with uterine cancer.

▶ The use of minimally invasive surgery via the laparoscope has been touted and advertised to be a superior form of surgery over standard open procedures for a number of malignancies. Yet for the majority, the science to prove this is lacking. Even more unusual are head-to-head trials comparing open vs laparoscopic approaches for many cancers.

Congratulations need to go to the Gynecologic Oncology Group (GOG) for assessing these 2 forms of surgery for patients with uterine cancer. Not only did the GOG run this randomized trial to assess outcomes of cancer recurrence and overall survival, they also addressed quality-of-life issues. Their results suggest a benefit to the laparoscopic approach in terms of quality-of-life issues, such as a decrease in the number of complications and a shorter hospital stay without a decrease in recurrence rates or survival.

This approach to the evaluation of new techniques and technologies needs to be reproduced in a plethora of other cancers where adoption of new techniques and technologies has occurred without such scientific evaluation.

C. Lawton, MD

Ovarian

Long-Term Ovarian Cancer Survival Associated With Mutation in BRCA1 or BRCA2

McLaughlin JR, Rosen B, Moody J, et al (Mount Sinai Hosp, Toronto, Canada; Univ of Toronto, Ontario, Canada; et al)
J Natl Cancer Inst 105:141-148, 2013

Background.—Studies have suggested that the 5-year survival of women with ovarian cancer and a BRCA1 or BRCA2 mutation is better than expected. We sought to evaluate the impact of carrying a BRCA1 or BRCA2 mutation on long-term survival of women after a diagnosis of invasive ovarian cancer.

Methods.—One thousand six hundred twenty-six unselected women diagnosed with invasive ovarian cancer in Ontario, Canada, or in Tampa,

Florida, between 1995 and 2004 were followed for a mean of 6.9 years (range = 0.3 to 15.7 years). Mutation screening for BRCA1 and BRCA2 revealed mutations in 218 women (13.4%). Left-truncated survival analysis was conducted to estimate ovarian cancer-specific survival at various time points after diagnosis for women with and without mutations.

Results.—In the 3-year period after diagnosis, the presence of a BRCA1 or BRCA2 mutation was associated with a better prognosis (adjusted hazard ratio = 0.68, 95% confidence interval [CI] = 0.48 to 0.98; $P = .03$), but at 10 years after diagnosis, the hazard ratio was 1.00 (95% CI = 0.83 to 1.22; $P = .90$). Among women with serous ovarian cancers, 27.4% of women who were BRCA1 mutation carriers, 27.7% of women who were BRCA2 carriers, and 27.1% of women who were noncarriers were alive at 12 years past diagnosis.

Conclusion.—For women with invasive ovarian cancer, the short-term survival advantage of carrying a BRCA1 or BRCA2 mutation does not lead to a long-term survival benefit.

▶ Approximately 10% to 15% of women with ovarian cancer have a familial syndrome associated with ovarian cancer. Most of these (about 90%) will have mutations in *BRCA1* or *BRCA2*. Most studies of patients with these mutations suggest that they have a survival advantage compared with the more common sporadic form of high-grade serous ovarian carcinoma, but these studies have followed up with these patients for relatively short periods of time. This study looked at 1626 patients and found 218 with *BRCA1* or *BRCA2* mutations. Over the first 3 years after diagnosis, the group with *BRCA* mutations exhibited an improved survival rate compared with the other patients in the population (hazard ratio [HR] = 0.68). At 10 years, however, the survival advantage had been lost (HR = 1.0). One other observation of note in the trial was that, of the 309 women who survived more than 12 years, only one subsequent death from ovarian cancer has been seen. Survival disease free to 12 years may, therefore, be a reasonable surrogate for cure.

J. T. Thigpen, MD

Patient reported outcomes of a randomized, placebo-controlled trial of bevacizumab in the front-line treatment of ovarian cancer: A Gynecologic Oncology Group Study
Monk BJ, Huang HQ, Burger RA, et al (Creighton Univ School of Medicine at St. Joseph's Hosp and Med Ctr, Phoenix, AZ; Roswell Park Cancer Inst, Buffalo, NY; Fox Chase Cancer Ctr, Philadelphia, PA; et al)
Gynecol Oncol 128:573-578, 2013

Purpose.—To analyze quality of life (QOL) in a randomized, placebo-controlled phase III trial concluding that the addition of concurrent and maintenance bevacizumab (Arm 3) to carboplatin and paclitaxel prolongs progression-free survival in front-line treatment of advanced ovarian cancer compared to chemotherapy alone (Arm 1) or chemotherapy with bevacizumab in cycles 2—6 only (Arm 2).

Patients and Methods.—The Trial Outcome Index of the Functional Assessment of Cancer Therapy-Ovary (FACT-O TOI) was used to assess QOL before cycles 1, 4, 7, 13, and 21; and 6 months after completing study therapy. Differences in QOL scores were assessed using a linear mixed model, adjusting for baseline score, and age. The significance level was set at 0.0167 to account for multiple comparisons.

Results.—1693 patients were queried. Arm 2 ($p < 0.001$) and Arm 3 ($p < 0.001$) reported lower QOL scores than those in Arm 1. The treatment differences were observed mainly at cycle 4, when the patients receiving bevacizumab (Arm 2 and Arm 3) reported 2.72 points (98.3% CI: 0.88—4.57; effect size = 0.18) and 2.96 points (98.3% CI: 1.13—4.78; effect size = 0.20) lower QOL respectively, than those in Arm 1. The difference in QOL scores between Arm 1 and Arm 3 remained statistically significant up to cycle 7. The percentage of patients who reported abdominal discomfort dropped over time, without significant differences among study arms.

Conclusion.—The small QOL difference observed during chemotherapy did not persist during maintenance bevacizumab.

▶ Two years ago, 2 large, phase III trials of chemotherapy with bevacizumab in the management of chemo-naive advanced ovarian carcinoma found a progression-free survival advantage for the addition of bevacizumab to carboplatin-based chemotherapy. Subsequently, additional phase III trials in platinum-sensitive (OCEANS) and platinum-resistant (AURELIA) ovarian carcinoma also found a significant prolongation of progression-free survival. Cumulatively, more than 4500 patients involved on these 4 trials now show the same thing: Adding bevacizumab to chemotherapy followed by maintenance bevacizumab in those who exhibit at least stable disease results in clear clinical benefit for the patients so treated. This study examines the quality-of-life component of one of the front-line trials described above: Gynecologic Oncology Group 218. The main concern was whether the addition of the third agent would adversely impact quality of life. The study showed that there was a small adverse impact on quality of life with the administration of bevacizumab in combination with chemotherapy but not with the maintenance phase of the trial when patients were receiving bevacizumab alone. These data tend to support the value of adding bevacizumab. The lack of an overall survival advantage almost certainly relates to the extensive postprogression therapy that essentially all ovarian cancer patients receive.

J. T. Thigpen, MD

Results of Annual Screening in Phase I of the United Kingdom Familial Ovarian Cancer Screening Study Highlight the Need for Strict Adherence to Screening Schedule

Rosenthal AN, Fraser L, Manchanda R, et al (Queen Mary Univ of London, UK; Univ College London, UK; et al)
J Clin Oncol 31:49-57, 2013

Purpose.—To establish the performance characteristics of annual transvaginal ultrasound and serum CA125 screening for women at high risk of ovarian/fallopian tube cancer (OC/FTC) and to investigate the impact of delayed screening interval and surgical intervention.

Patients and Methods.—Between May 6, 2002, and January 5, 2008, 3,563 women at an estimated ≥10% lifetime risk of OC/FTC were recruited and screened by 37 centers in the United Kingdom. Participants were observed prospectively by centers, questionnaire, and national cancer registries.

Results.—Sensitivity for detection of incident OC/FTC at 1 year after last annual screen was 81.3% (95% CI, 54.3% to 96.0%) if occult cancers were classified as false negatives and 87.5% (95% CI, 61.7% to 98.5%) if they were classified as true positives. Positive and negative predictive values of incident screening were 25.5% (95% CI, 14.3 to 40.0) and 99.9% (95% CI, 99.8 to 100) respectively. Four (30.8%) of 13 incident screen-detected OC/FTCs were stage I or II. Compared with women screened in the year before diagnosis, those not screened in the year before diagnosis were more likely to have ≥ stage IIIc disease (85.7% v 26.1%; *P* = .009). Screening interval was delayed by a median of 88 days before detection of incident OC/FTC. Median interval from detection screen to surgical intervention was 79 days in prevalent and incident OC/FTC.

Conclusion.—These results in the high-risk population highlight the need for strict adherence to screening schedule. Screening more frequently than annually with prompt surgical intervention seems to offer a better chance of early-stage detection.

▶ Investigators in the United Kingdom reported 4 years ago the results of a screening trial that involved more than 202 000 women. Half of the women were randomly assigned to no screening. The other half were randomly assigned to screening, half to be screened annually with transvaginal sonography and half with what the investigators called "multimodality screening." In the latter, patients had annual CA-125 samples analyzed by the risk of ovarian cancer algorithm, which then triggered the use of transvaginal sonography with color-flow Doppler. In the group assigned to multimodality screening, the positive predictive value was reported at 35%, an astounding result substantially better than anything reported to that date. This article looks at a high-risk population and suggests that delays in screening and surgical intervention may have reduced the efficacy of screening and caused cancers that were diagnosed to consist of mostly advanced disease. This prompted a further trial reported at American Society of Clinical Oncology 2013. Screening in this study was carried out at

4-month intervals instead of annually, and extra effort was devoted to eliminating delays in screening and intervention. The results, unfortunately, showed insignificant improvement in the percentage of cases diagnosed at stage I or II. On the positive side, the data did show a major reduction in delays and suggest that a higher percentage of the cases identified could be completely, grossly cytoreduced at surgery. The positive predictive value of the screening test, however, decreased from 35% to 13%. Until mortality data are in and show a reduced mortality rate, these approaches cannot be said to constitute a valid screening approach for ovarian cancer.

J. T. Thigpen, MD

Randomized, Open-Label, Phase III Study Comparing Patupilone (EPO906) With Pegylated Liposomal Doxorubicin in Platinum-Refractory or -Resistant Patients With Recurrent Epithelial Ovarian, Primary Fallopian Tube, or Primary Peritoneal Cancer

Colombo N, Kutarska E, Dimopoulos M, et al (Univ of Milan-Bicocca and European Inst of Oncology, Italy; Centrum Onkologii Ziemi Lubelskej, Lublin, Poland; Univ of Athens, Greece; et al)

J Clin Oncol 30:3841-3847, 2012

Purpose.—This study compared the efficacy and safety of patupilone with those of pegylated liposomal doxorubicin (PLD) in patients with platinum-refractory or -resistant epithelial ovarian, primary fallopian tube, or primary peritoneal cancer.

Patients and Methods.—Patients with three or fewer prior regimens were eligible if they had received first-line taxane/platinum-based combination chemotherapy and were platinum refractory or resistant. Patients were randomly assigned to receive patupilone (10 mg/m^2 intravenously every 3 weeks) or PLD (50 mg/m^2 intravenously every 4 weeks).

Results.—A total of 829 patients were randomly assigned (patupilone, n = 412; PLD, n = 417). There was no statistically significant difference in overall survival (OS), the primary end point, between the patupilone and PLD arms (P =.195; hazard ratio, 0.93; 95% CI, 0.79 to 1.09), with median OS rates of 13.2 and 12.7 months, respectively. Median progression-free survival was 3.7 months for both arms. The overall response rate (all partial responses) was higher in the patupilone arm than in the PLD arm (15.5% v 7.9%; odds ratio, 2.11; 95% CI, 1.36 to 3.29), although disease control rates were similar (59.5% v 56.3%, respectively). Frequently observed adverse events (AEs) of any grade included diarrhea (85.3%) and peripheral neuropathy (39.3%) in the patupilone arm and mucositis/stomatitis (43%) and hand-foot syndrome (41.8%) in the PLD arm.

Conclusion.—Patupilone did not demonstrate significant improvement in OS compared with the active control, PLD. No new or unexpected serious AEs were identified.

▶ At the start of the 1990s, there was a new paradigm for the treatment of patients with recurrent or persistent ovarian carcinoma after initial platinum-based therapy. Based on studies conducted independently by Markman[1] in the United States and Blackledge[2] in the United Kingdom, patients were classified into 2 categories based on their response to first-line, platinum-based therapies. Those who responded to first-line, platinum-based therapy and achieved a clinical complete response that lasted at least 6 months were categorized as potentially platinum sensitive, whereas those whose best response was stable disease or those who progressed through initial therapy or who responded with a duration of less than 6 months were categorized as clinically platinum resistant. Patients with platinum-sensitive disease were best treated with another platinum-based regimen, whereas those with platinum-resistant disease were best treated with nonplatinum single agents with demonstrated activity against ovarian carcinoma. This trial is a study in platinum-resistant patients and represents one of a relatively small number of randomized comparisons of one single agent with another. The experimental agent, patupilone, had shown evidence of activity in phase II studies. The control agent was pegylated liposomal doxorubicin, which was approved by the US Food and Drug Administration for use in recurrent or persistent ovarian carcinoma. Among 829 patients included in the trial, there was no evidence of a difference in efficacy between the 2 agents. The relatively low response rates reported on both arms illustrate the challenge posed by platinum-resistant ovarian carcinoma.

J. T. Thigpen, MD

References

1. Markman M, Rothman R, Hakes T, et al. Second-line platinum therapy in patients with ovarian cancer previously treated with cisplatin. *J Clin Oncol.* 1991;9:389-393.
2. Blackledge G, Lawton F, Redman C, et al. Response of patients in phase II studies of chemotherapy in ovarian cancer: implications for patient treatment and the design of phase II trials. *Br J Cancer.* 1989;59:650-653.

Abagovomab As Maintenance Therapy in Patients With Epithelial Ovarian Cancer: A Phase III Trial of the AGO OVAR, COGI, GINECO, and GEICO—The MIMOSA Study
Sabbatini P, Harter P, Scambia G, et al (Memorial Sloan-Kettering Cancer Ctr, NY; Universitaetsklinikum Essen, Germany; Universitá Cattolica Sacro Cuore, Italy; et al)
J Clin Oncol 31:1554-1561, 2013

Purpose.—To determine whether abagovomab maintenance therapy prolongs recurrence-free (RFS) and overall survival (OS) in patients with ovarian cancer in first clinical remission.

Patients and Methods.—Patients with International Federation of Gynecology and Obstetrics stage III to IV ovarian cancer in complete clinical remission after primary surgery and platinum- and taxane-based chemotherapy were randomly assigned at a ratio of 2:1 in a phase III, double-blind, placebo-controlled, multicenter study. Abagovomab 2 mg or placebo was administered as 1-mL suspension once every 2 weeks for 6 weeks (induction phase) and then once every 4 weeks (maintenance phase) until recurrence or up to 21 months after random assignment of the last patient. The primary end point was RFS; secondary end points were OS and immunologic response.

Results.—Characteristics of the 888 patients included: mean age, 56.3 years; Eastern Cooperative Oncology Group performance status, ≤1 in >99% of patients; serous papillary subtype, 81.5%; stage III, 85.9%; and cancer antigen 125 ≤ 35U/mL after third cycle, 80.9%. Mean exposure to study treatment (± standard deviation) was 449.7 ± 333.08 days. Hazard ratio (HR) of RFS for the treatment group using tumor size categorization (≤1 cm, >1 cm) was 1.099 (95% CI, 0.919 to 1.315; $P = .301$). HR of OS using tumor size categorization (≤1 cm, >1 cm) was 1.150 (95% CI, 0.872 to 1.518; $P = .322$). The most frequently reported type of adverse event was an injection site reaction in 445 patients (50.2%), followed by injection site erythema and fatigue in 227 (25.6%) and 212 patients (23.9%), respectively. By the final visit, median anti-anti-idiotypic antibody level was 493,000.0 ng/mL, indicating a robust response.

Conclusion.—Abagovomab administered as repeated monthly injections is safe and induces a measurable immune response. Administration as maintenance therapy for patients with ovarian cancer in first remission does not prolong RFS or OS.

▶ Advanced ovarian cancer, contrary to some belief, is actually a very sensitive disease process to the effects of front-line systemic therapy. Up to 75% of patients with stage III to IV epithelial ovarian cancer will complete initial chemotherapy with paclitaxel/carboplatin in a clinical complete remission. A number of approaches to consolidating or maintaining the remission have been studied through the last 3 decades. To date, 4 agents have shown, in randomized trials, the ability to prolong progression-free survival in patients who have demonstrated at least stable disease to initial chemotherapy: paclitaxel (one phase III trial), bevacizumab (2 phase III trials), pazopanib (one phase III trial), and olaparib (one randomized, phase II trial in platinum-sensitive patients). None of these trials showed an overall survival advantage, but one must remember that patients, when they progressed in the study, received multiple additional lines of therapy, which serve to make the interpretation of the survival endpoint difficult. In the case of the trial of abagovomab, there is no indication that abagovomab produced any clinically significant improvement. Even the trends were in favor of the control. The positives were that the agent was safe and that a measurable immune response was induced. Based on these data, abagovomab does not appear to be an active approach to maintaining remission in ovarian cancer.

J. T. Thigpen, MD

A phase II trial of docetaxel and bevacizumab in recurrent ovarian cancer within 12 months of prior platinum-based chemotherapy

Wenham RM, Lapolla J, Lin H-Y, et al al (H. Lee Moffitt Cancer Ctr and Res Inst, Tampa, FL; Women's Cancer Associates, St Petersburg, FL; et al)
Gynecol Oncol 130:19-24, 2013

Objectives.—The efficacy and safety of bevacizumab and docetaxel were evaluated in women who developed recurrent epithelial ovarian, fallopian, or peritoneal cancer within 12 months of platinum-based therapy.

Methods.—Patients received docetaxel (40 mg/m^2) on days 1 and 8 and bevacizumab (15 mg/kg) on day 1 of a 21-day cycle. Primary endpoint was 6-month progression-free survival (PFS).

Results.—Forty-one patients were evaluable for PFS and 38 for best response; 46% had platinum-free intervals (PFI) of <6 months and 54% between 6 and 12 months. The 6-month PFS was 43.9% (95% confidence interval $(CI_{95\%}) = 28.6-58.2\%$). Median PFS (months) was 5.2 $(CI_{95\%} = 4.4-7.2)$ for all patients, 6.2 $(CI_{95\%} = 4.1-7.4)$ for patients with PFI <6 months, and 5.1 $(CI_{95\%} = 3.0-7.2)$ for those with PFI ≥6 months. Twenty-two patients showed overall response (CR + PR) (57.9%; $CI_{95\%} = 40.8-73.7\%$), and 32 showed clinical benefit (CR + PR + SD) (84.2%; $CI_{95\%} = 68.8-94.0\%$). For those with complete or partial responses, median duration of response was 4.8 months (0.7−14.5). Median overall survival was 12.4 months ($CI_{95\%} = 10.0-21.9$). The most common grade 3/4 adverse events (AEs) were neutropenia (14.6% of patients), followed by leukopenia, fatigue, metabolic, and gastrointestinal, with 66% showing any grade 3/4 toxicity. Most common AEs of any grade were gastrointestinal (93%), fatigue (73%), and pain (73%). Four (10%) patients developed hypertension, 1 a gastrointestinal perforation, and another a colovesicular fistula.

Conclusions.—Bevacizumab and docetaxel administered in patients with recurrent ovarian cancer is an active regimen without new unanticipated toxicities. This combination should be an option for further study or clinical use in recurrent ovarian cancer.

▶ For recurrent ovarian cancer, several active agents have been identified. For patients who are considered platinum resistant based on response to initial platinum-based therapy, these agents are usually used as single agents because of the absence of evidence to support increased efficacy for combination regimens. The one exception to this appears to be the combination of cytotoxic agents with bevacizumab. In the AURELIA trial of chemotherapy with or without bevacizumab presented at the 2012 American Society of Clinical Oncology oral session on gynecologic cancers, chemotherapy (1 of 3 agents: weekly paclitaxel, pegylated liposomal doxorubicin, or weekly topotecan) with or without bevacizumab showed an advantage in terms of progression-free survival for the combination of one of these agents with bevacizumab. This phase II trial of docetaxel plus bevacizumab extends those observations to yet another combination. The regimen showed significant activity as assessed by percentage of patients who were progression free at 6 months (43.9%), response rate (57.9%), and median overall survival (12.4 months); all results were better than would be expected. Although this is not a randomized trial against docetaxel alone, it is reasonable to conclude that the doublet has activity similar to that seen in the AURELIA trial.

J. T. Thigpen, MD

Declining Second Primary Ovarian Cancer After First Primary Breast Cancer
Schonfeld SJ, de Gonzalez AB, Visvanathan K, et al (Natl Insts of Health (NIH), Bethesda, MD; Johns Hopkins Bloomberg School of Public Health, Baltimore, MD)
J Clin Oncol 31:738-743, 2013

Purpose.—Although ovarian cancer incidence rates have declined in the United States, less is known of ovarian cancer trends among survivors of breast cancer. Therefore, we examined second primary ovarian cancers after first primary breast cancer.

Methods.—Data were obtained from the Surveillance, Epidemiology, and End Results program (1973 to 2008). Standardized incidence ratios (SIRs) were calculated as the observed numbers of ovarian cancers among survivors of breast cancer compared with the expected numbers in the general population. Absolute rates were measured as the incidence rates for second primary ovarian cancer by year of diagnosis of the first primary breast cancer adjusted for age of breast cancer diagnosis and years since diagnosis.

Results.—SIRs for second primary ovarian cancer were elevated over the entire study period (SIR, 1.24; 95% CI, 1.2 to 1.3), whereas the absolute rates declined with an estimated annual percentage change near 1% (−1.34% to −0.09% per year). Secular trends for second ovarian cancers were similar after estrogen receptor (ER) —positive and ER-negative breast cancers, whereas the age-specific patterns varied significantly by ER expression (P for interaction < .001). The largest SIR was among women age less than 50 years with ER-negative breast cancer (SIR, 4.35; 95% CI, 3.5 to 5.4).

Conclusion.—Persistently elevated SIRs along with decreasing absolute rates over the entire study period suggest that ovarian cancers in both the general population and survivors of breast cancer are declining in parallel, possibly because of common risk factor exposures. Analytic studies are needed to further assess the parallel overall trends and the age-specific interaction by ER expression.

▶ In the United States, the overall incidence of ovarian cancer has been declining at an estimated overall rate of 1% per year over the last 30 + years. In survivors of breast cancer, the same phenomenon exists of a declining incidence of ovarian cancer at the same rate as in those who have not had breast cancer. In addition, throughout the period covered by the study, there is a consistent elevation of the risk for a second primary ovarian cancer of about 1.24 (24% increase in risk). The greatest risk of a second primary ovarian cancer in breast cancer survivors was in the younger patients, particularly those who incurred breast cancer at an age of less than 40. The reason for the overall declining risk for ovarian cancer over the period of the study is not clear. Some have speculated that this reflects a declining exposure to those things that increase risk, but this is not certain. The principal impact of these observations on practice is to identify those patients at the greatest risk for ovarian cancer. Unfortunately, in the absence of an effective screening test for ovarian cancer, intervention focuses on prevention by such approaches as bilateral risk-reducing salpingo-oophorectomy.

J. T. Thigpen, MD

8 Gastrointestinal

Colon: Advanced

Effect of Oxaliplatin, Fluorouracil, and Leucovorin With or Without Cetuximab on Survival Among Patients With Resected Stage III Colon Cancer: A Randomized Trial

Alberts SR, Sargent DJ, Nair S, et al (Mayo Clinic Rochester, MN; Lehigh Valley Hosp, Allentown, PA; et al)
JAMA 307:1383-1393, 2012

Context.—Leucovorin, fluorouracil, and oxaliplatin (FOLFOX) is the standard adjuvant therapy for resected stage III colon cancer. Adding cetuximab to FOLFOX benefits patients with metastatic wild-type *KRAS* but not mutated *KRAS* colon cancer.

Objective.—To assess the potential benefit of cetuximab added to the modified sixth version of the FOLFOX regimen (mFOLFOX6) in patients with resected stage III wild-type *KRAS* colon cancer.

Design, Setting, and Participants.—A randomized trial of 2686 patients aged 18 years or older at multiple institutions across North America enrolled following resection and informed consent between February 10, 2004, and November 25, 2009. The primary randomized comparison was 12 biweekly cycles of mFOLFOX6 with and without cetuximab. *KRAS* mutation status was centrally determined. The trial was halted after a planned interim analysis of 48% of predicted events (246/515) occurring in 1863 (of 2070 planned) patients with tumors having wild-type *KRAS*. A total of 717 patients with mutated *KRAS* and 106 with indeterminate *KRAS* were accrued. The 2070 patients with wild-type KRAS provided 90% power to detect a hazard ratio (HR) of 1.33 (2-sided $\alpha = .05$), with planned interim efficacy analyses after 25%, 50%, and 75% of expected relapses.

Main Outcome Measures.—Disease-free survival in patients with wild-type *KRAS* mutations. Secondary end points included overall survival and toxicity.

Results.—Median (range) follow-up was 28 (0-68) months. The trial demonstrated no benefit when adding cetuximab. Three-year disease-free survival for mFOLFOX6 alone was 74.6% vs 71.5% with the addition of cetuximab (HR, 1.21; 95% CI, 0.98-1.49; $P = .08$) in patients with wild-type *KRAS*, and 67.1% vs 65.0% (HR, 1.12; 95% CI, 0.86-1.46;

$P = .38$) in patients with mutated *KRAS*, with no significant benefit in any subgroups assessed. Among all patients, grade 3 or higher adverse events (72.5% vs 52.3%; odds ratio [OR], 2.4; 95% CI, 2.1-2.8; $P < .001$) and failure to complete 12 cycles (33% vs 23%; OR, 1.6; 95% CI, 1.4-1.9; $P < .001$) were significantly higher with cetuximab. Increased toxicity and greater detrimental differences in all outcomes were observed in patients aged 70 years or older.

Conclusion.—Among patients with stage III resected colon cancer, the use of cetuximab with adjuvant mFOLFOX6 compared with mFOLFOX6 alone did not result in improved disease-free survival.

Trial Registration.—clinicaltrials.gov Identifier: NCT00079274.

▶ Colon cancer is the third-leading cause of cancer death in the United States in men and women behind prostate and lung vs breast and lung, respectively. Those patients most at risk for death from this disease are those whose disease is more advanced and, in particular, those patients whose disease has spread beyond the colon to the lymph nodes or other organs.

Stage III patients, whose disease has not yet metastasized to other organs, represent a group of patients for whom cure is possible, but surgery alone is not enough. Postoperative chemotherapy in the form of leucovorin, fluorouracil, and oxaliplatin (FOLFOX) is the standard of care in these patients, many of whom also benefit from postoperative radiation.

Despite the benefits of these treatments, upward of 40% to 50% of these patients recur and, thus, trying to improve outcomes, as was done in this trial with cetuximab, is important. The trial does not support the use of cetuximab in addition to FOLFOX for these patients, but it is an important example of the continued need to scientifically assess new compounds and treatments to increase cure rates for these patients.

C. Lawton, MD

Colorectal Cancer

Randomized trial of short-course radiotherapy versus long-course chemoradiation comparing rates of local recurrence in patients with T3 rectal cancer: Trans-Tasman Radiation Oncology Group trial 01.04
Ngan SY, Burmeister B, Fisher RJ, et al (Peter MacCallum Cancer Centre, Melbourne, Victoria, Australia)
J Clin Oncol 30:3827-3833, 2012

Purpose.—To compare the local recurrence (LR) rate between short-course (SC) and long-course (LC) neoadjuvant radiotherapy for rectal cancer.

Patients and Methods.—Eligible patients had ultrasound- or magnetic resonance imaging-staged T3N0-2M0 rectal adenocarcinoma within 12 cm from anal verge. SC consisted of pelvic radiotherapy 5×5 Gy in 1 week, early surgery, and six courses of adjuvant chemotherapy. LC was 50.4 Gy, 1.8 Gy/fraction, in 5.5 weeks, with continuous infusional fluorouracil 225 mg/m^2 per day, surgery in 4 to 6 weeks, and four courses of chemotherapy.

Results.—Three hundred twenty-six patients were randomly assigned; 163 patients to SC and 163 to LC. Median potential follow-up time was 5.9 years (range, 3.0 to 7.8 years). Three-year LR rates (cumulative incidence) were 7.5% for SC and 4.4% for LC (difference, 3.1%; 95% CI, −2.1 to 8.3; $P = .24$). For distal tumors (<5 cm), six of 48 SC patients and one of 31 LC patients experienced local recurrence ($P = .21$). Five-year distant recurrence rates were 27% for SC and 30% for LC (log-rank $P = 0.92$; hazard ratio [HR] for LC:SC, 1.04; 95% CI, 0.69 to 1.56). Overall survival rates at 5 years were 74% for SC and 70% for LC (log-rank $P = 0.62$; HR, 1.12; 95% CI, 0.76 to 1.67). Late toxicity rates were not substantially different (Radiation Therapy Oncology Group/European Organisation for Research and Treatment of Cancer G3-4: SC, 5.8%; LC, 8.2%; $P = .53$).

Conclusion.—Three-year LR rates between SC and LC were not statistically significantly different; the CI for the difference is consistent with either no clinically important difference or differences in favor of LC. LC may be more effective in reducing LR for distal tumors. No differences in rates of distant recurrence, relapse-free survival, overall survival, or late toxicity were detected.

▶ The use of both radiation and chemotherapy in addition to surgery in patients with T3 rectal cancers has become the standard. Several trials have found a benefit to the use of preoperative chemotherapy and radiation therapy over postoperative treatment; therefore, preoperative treatment has become the standard. Yet, preoperative chemotherapy and radiation therapy has been done in many different ways. Essentially, the preoperative radiation can be divided into 2 groups: short course, in which the radiation is given in 1-2 weeks, and standard fractionation (long course) of 1.8 Gy per fraction to approximately 50.4 Gy over 5.5 weeks.

There have been components for both the short-course and the long-course options such that each has become a relative standard. Thus, this trial performed by the Trans-Tasmin RT Group is very important. These phase III trials represent the gold standard to evaluate these types of seemingly equally beneficial options. The reported median follow-up is 5.9 years, and at this point it appears as if long-course treatment is better for patients with distal tumors. Longer follow-up is clearly needed to verify this endpoint, and, if convenience is a significant factor, short-course radiation therapy remains an excellent option for these patients.

C. Lawton, MD

Preoperative versus postoperative chemoradiotherapy for locally advanced rectal cancer: results of the German CAO/ARO/AIO-94 randomized phase III trial after a median follow-up of 11 years
Sauer R, Liersch T, Merkel S, et al (Univ of Erlangen, Germany)
J Clin Oncol 30:1926-1933, 2012

Purpose.—Preoperative chemoradiotherapy (CRT) has been established as standard treatment for locally advanced rectal cancer after first results of the CAO/ARO/AIO-94 [Working Group of Surgical Oncology/Working Group of Radiation Oncology/Working Group of Medical Oncology of the Germany Cancer Society] trial, published in 2004, showed an improved local control rate. However, after a median follow-up of 46 months, no survival benefit could be shown. Here, we report long-term results with a median follow-up of 134 months.

Patients and Methods.—A total of 823 patients with stage II to III rectal cancer were randomly assigned to preoperative CRT with fluorouracil (FU), total mesorectal excision surgery, and adjuvant FU chemotherapy, or the same schedule of CRT used postoperatively. The study was designed to have 80% power to detect a difference of 10% in 5-year overall survival as the primary end point. Secondary end points included the cumulative incidence of local and distant relapses and disease-free survival.

Results.—Of 799 eligible patients, 404 were randomly assigned to preoperative and 395 to postoperative CRT. According to intention-to-treat analysis, overall survival at 10 years was 59.6% in the preoperative arm and 59.9% in the postoperative arm ($P =.85$). The 10-year cumulative incidence of local relapse was 7.1% and 10.1% in the pre- and postoperative arms, respectively ($P =.048$). No significant differences were detected for 10-year cumulative incidence of distant metastases (29.8% and 29.6%; $P =.9$) and disease-free survival.

Conclusion.—There is a persisting significant improvement of pre- versus postoperative CRT on local control; however, there was no effect on overall survival. Integrating more effective systemic treatment into the multimodal therapy has been adopted in the CAO/ARO/AIO-04 trial to possibly reduce distant metastases and improve survival.

▶ It is well understood that within many malignancies local control is imperative to improve overall survival. Data in breast cancer, prostate cancer, and lung cancer would support this tenet. So there is reason to assume that this is likely true in colorectal carcinoma as well.

Thus, when the results of this German preoperative vs postoperative chemoradiation phase III trial first reported a local control benefit, it was not unreasonable to assume that with increased follow-up a survival advantage might be reached. The median follow-up for the first report was 46 months (just shy of 4 years). The current report has a median follow-up of 11 years. It does not, unfortunately, show a difference in either overall survival or incidence of distant metastasis.

This certainly indicates that the control of systemic disease remains a serious problem in rectal cancer. It also indicates that the chemotherapy in this trial with fluorouracil is inadequate and improvements are urgently needed to lower the distance metastatic rate and, thus, improve survival. The take-home message still supports the use of preoperative chemotherapy and radiation, as increased local control is important. We simply need more trials with different or additional chemotherapy to improve the systemic endpoints.

C. Lawton, MD

Colorectal-Cancer Incidence and Mortality with Screening Flexible Sigmoidoscopy
Schoen RE, for the PLCO Project Team (Univ of Pittsburgh, PA; et al)
N Engl J Med 366:2345-2357, 2012

Background.—The benefits of endoscopic testing for colorectal-cancer screening are uncertain. We evaluated the effect of screening with flexible sigmoidoscopy on colorectal-cancer incidence and mortality.

Methods.—From 1993 through 2001, we randomly assigned 154,900 men and women 55 to 74 years of age either to screening with flexible sigmoidoscopy, with a repeat screening at 3 or 5 years, or to usual care. Cases of colorectal cancer and deaths from the disease were ascertained.

Results.—Of the 77,445 participants randomly assigned to screening (intervention group), 83.5% underwent baseline flexible sigmoidoscopy and 54.0% were screened at 3 or 5 years. The incidence of colorectal cancer after a median follow-up of 11.9 years was 11.9 cases per 10,000 person-years in the intervention group (1012 cases), as compared with 15.2 cases per 10,000 person-years in the usual-care group (1287 cases), which represents a 21% reduction (relative risk, 0.79; 95% confidence interval [CI], 0.72 to 0.85; $P < 0.001$). Significant reductions were observed in the incidence of both distal colorectal cancer (479 cases in the intervention group vs. 669 cases in the usual-care group; relative risk, 0.71; 95% CI, 0.64 to 0.80; $P < 0.001$) and proximal colorectal cancer (512 cases vs. 595 cases; relative risk, 0.86; 95% CI, 0.76 to 0.97; $P = 0.01$). There were 2.9 deaths from colorectal cancer per 10,000 person-years in the intervention group (252 deaths), as compared with 3.9 per 10,000 person-years in the usual-care group (341 deaths), which represents a 26% reduction (relative risk, 0.74; 95% CI, 0.63 to 0.87; $P < 0.001$). Mortality from distal colorectal cancer was reduced by 50% (87 deaths in the intervention group vs. 175 in the usual-care group; relative risk, 0.50; 95% CI, 0.38 to 0.64; $P < 0.001$); mortality from proximal colorectal cancer was unaffected (143 and 147 deaths, respectively; relative risk, 0.97; 95% CI, 0.77 to 1.22; $P = 0.81$).

Conclusions.—Screening with flexible sigmoidoscopy was associated with a significant decrease in colorectal-cancer incidence (in both the distal and proximal colon) and mortality (distal colon only). (Funded by the National Cancer Institute; PLCO ClinicalTrials.gov number, NCT00002540.)

▶ Screening for colorectal cancer via flexible sigmoidoscopy or colonoscopy has been the recommendation for patients beginning at age 50 and above for many years. It was well understood that the use of these screening procedures decreased the incidence of invasive colorectal cancer. The beauty of these screening procedures, unlike mammograms or prostate-specific antigen screening tools, is that with sigmoidoscopy or colonoscopy precancerous polyps can be detected and removed before carcinoma in situ is even found. Thus, these procedures not only potentially decrease the incidence of invasive colorectal cancer but could also have a large effect on mortality for this disease.

Large, randomized screening trials such as this study are needed to verify that, in fact, these screening procedures do just what we physicians think they do. These data confirmed the significant benefit of screening flexible sigmoidoscopy in decreasing the risk of colorectal cancer and also confirmed a mortality benefit. Interestingly, the mortality benefit is seen only in the distal colorectal cancers and not the proximal cancers, despite a decrease in the incidence of both. This begs the question whether colonoscopy is better than flexible sigmoidoscopy to address the entire colon. Important studies like this give us critical answers, but they always generate more questions.

C. Lawton, MD

Colonoscopic Polypectomy and Long-Term Prevention of Colorectal-Cancer Deaths

Zauber AG, Winawer SJ, O'Brien MJ, et al (Memorial Sloan-Kettering Cancer Ctr, NY; Boston Univ School of Medicine, MA; et al)
N Engl J Med 366:687-696, 2012

Background.—In the National Polyp Study (NPS), colorectal cancer was prevented by colonoscopic removal of adenomatous polyps. We evaluated the long-term effect of colonoscopic polypectomy in a study on mortality from colorectal cancer.

Methods.—We included in this analysis all patients prospectively referred for initial colonoscopy (between 1980 and 1990) at NPS clinical centers who had polyps (adenomas and nonadenomas). The National Death Index was used to identify deaths and to determine the cause of death; follow-up time was as long as 23 years. Mortality from colorectal cancer among patients with adenomas removed was compared with the expected incidence-based mortality from colorectal cancer in the general population, as estimated from the Surveillance Epidemiology and End Results (SEER) Program, and with the observed mortality from colorectal cancer among patients with nonadenomatous polyps (internal control group).

Results.—Among 2602 patients who had adenomas removed during participation in the study, after a median of 15.8 years, 1246 patients had died from any cause and 12 had died from colorectal cancer. Given an estimated 25.4 expected deaths from colorectal cancer in the general population, the standardized incidence-based mortality ratio was 0.47 (95% confidence interval [CI], 0.26 to 0.80) with colonoscopic polypectomy, suggesting a 53% reduction in mortality. Mortality from colorectal cancer was similar among patients with adenomas and those with nonadenomatous polyps during the first 10 years after polypectomy (relative risk, 1.2; 95% CI, 0.1 to 10.6).

Conclusions.—These findings support the hypothesis that colonoscopic removal of adenomatous polyps prevents death from colorectal cancer. (Funded by the National Cancer Institute and others.)

▶ The use of colonoscopy to find and remove (especially adenomatous) polyps before they turn malignant has been shown to decrease the incidence of invasive colon cancer. In addition, the use of colonoscopy to diagnose colon cancer at an earlier stage has been shown to decrease deaths from colon cancer in screening trials. But the question remains: Does removal of colonic polyps actually decrease the risk of death from colon cancer? In other words, are these polyps the ones likely to be responsible for the ultimate deaths from colon cancer?

We know that screening colonoscopies are expensive and that there remains some question as to their required frequency, especially when the initial one is negative for polyps. So are they truly worth the cost and patient discomfort?

These data give us the definitive answer. Screening colonoscopies with associated polypectomy, as needed, does decrease the risk of death from colon cancer. These data reinforce the need for screening colonoscopy and help the patient and physician understand the benefits of this screening tool, despite the cost and discomfort. Questions remain, however, as to the appropriate frequency of such screening.

C. Lawton, MD

Association of *KRAS* G13D Tumor Mutations With Outcome in Patients With Metastatic Colorectal Cancer Treated With First-Line Chemotherapy With or Without Cetuximab

Tejpar S, Celik I, Schlichting M, et al (Univ Hosp Gasthuisberg, Leuven, Belgium; Merck KGaA, Darmstadt, Germany; et al)
J Clin Oncol 30:3570-3577, 2012

Purpose.—We investigated in the first-line setting our previous finding that patients with chemorefractory *KRAS* G13D—mutated metastatic colorectal cancer (mCRC) benefit from cetuximab treatment.

Methods.—Associations between tumor *KRAS* mutation status (wild-type, G13D, G12V, or other mutations) and progression-free survival (PFS), survival, and response were investigated in pooled data from 1,378 evaluable patients from the CRYSTAL and OPUS studies. Multivariate analysis correcting for differences in baseline prognostic factors was performed.

Results.—Of 533 patients (39%) with *KRAS*-mutant tumors, 83 (16%) had G13D, 125 (23%) had G12V, and 325 (61%) had other mutations. Significant variations in treatment effects were found for tumor response ($P = .005$) and PFS ($P = .046$) in patients with G13D-mutant tumors versus all other mutations (including G12V). Within *KRAS* mutation subgroups, cetuximab plus chemotherapy versus chemotherapy alone significantly improved PFS (median, 7.4 *v* 6.0 months; hazard ratio [HR], 0.47; $P = .039$) and tumor response (40.5% *v* 22.0%; odds ratio, 3.38; $P = .042$) but not survival (median, 15.4 *v* 14.7 months; HR, 0.89; $P = .68$) in patients with G13D-mutant tumors. Patients with G12V and other mutations did not benefit from this treatment combination. Patients with *KRAS* G13D—mutated tumors receiving chemotherapy alone experienced worse outcomes (response, 22.0% *v* 43.2%; odds ratio, 0.40; $P = .032$) than those with other mutations. Effects were similar in the separate CRYSTAL and OPUS studies.

Conclusion.—The addition of cetuximab to first-line chemotherapy seems to benefit patients with *KRAS* G13D—mutant tumors. Relative treatment effects were similar to those in patients with *KRAS* wild-type tumors but with lower absolute values.

▶ It is well known that the epidermal growth factor receptor (EGFR)-blocking antibodies, cetuximab and panitumumab, are not recommended for metastatic colorectal cancer patients whose tumors harbor *KRAS* mutations. Tejpar et al report on the differential effect that the *KRAS* G13D mutation may have on the relative benefit from cetuximab with chemotherapy in the CRYSTAL and OPUS studies.

CRYSTAL compared FOLFIRI with or without cetuximab, and OPUS compared FOLFOX with or without cetuximab for first-line treatment of metastatic colorectal cancer.[1,2] Overall, a *KRAS* G13V mutation is expected to occur in only 8% of all metastatic colorectal cancer patients and mostly in tumors with defective DNA repair genes.

In the CRYSTAL study, clinical efficacy was superior for cetuximab and FOLFIRI vs FOLFIRI alone only in patients with *KRAS* wild-type disease.[3] As preclinical data and other pooled analyses of chemorefractory patients suggested potential benefit from cetuximab in patients with *KRAS* codon 13 mutations, this study intended to validate previous results.

Among 1535 patients treated in CRYSTAL and OPUS, 533 patients (39%) had *KRAS* mutant tumors, of which 83 patients (16%) had a G13D mutation. Specifically, significant benefit from the addition of cetuximab was noted with regard to progression-free survival (7.4 vs 6 months; hazard ratio [HR], 0.47; $P = .039$) and response rate (40.5% vs 22%; odds ratio, 3.38; $P = .042$) but not for overall survival (15.4 vs 14.7 months; HR, 0.89; $P = .68$) in this pooled analysis.

Although outcomes with cetuximab plus chemotherapy in patients with *KRAS* G13D mutations are still inferior to those noted in *KRAS* wild-type tumors, these data show that *KRAS* mutations are clearly distinct in their biological role on influencing anti-EGFR treatment effect.

Clinical trials with panitumumab and chemotherapy have not all been consistent with a relative benefit in *KRAS* G13D mutated colorectal cancer.[4] Therefore, the role of EGFR-targeted therapies in patients with *KRAS* G13D mutated colorectal cancer will need to be studied further in a prospective manner and possibly in conjunction with new molecular markers.

E. G. Chiorean, MD

References

1. Van Cutsem E, Köhne CH, Hitre E, et al. Cetuximab and chemotherapy as initial treatment for metastatic colorectal cancer. *N Engl J Med.* 2009;360:1408-1417.
2. Bokemeyer C, Bondarenko I, Makhson A, et al. Fluorouracil, leucovorin, and oxaliplatin with and without cetuximab in the first-line treatment of metastatic colorectal cancer. *J Clin Oncol.* 2009;27:663-671.
3. Van Cutsem E, Köhne CH, Láng I, et al. Cetuximab plus irinotecan, fluorouracil, and leucovorin as first-line treatment for metastatic colorectal cancer: updated analysis of overall survival according to tumor KRAS and BRAF mutation status. *J Clin Oncol.* 2011;29:2011-2019.
4. Peeters M, Douillard JY, Van Cutsem E, et al. Mutant KRAS codon 12 and 13 alleles in patients with metastatic colorectal cancer: assessment as prognostic and predictive biomarkers of response to panitumumab. *J Clin Oncol.* 2013;31:759-765.

Regorafenib monotherapy for previously treated metastatic colorectal cancer (CORRECT): an international, multicentre, randomised, placebo-controlled, phase 3 trial

Grothey A, for the CORRECT Study Group (Mayo Clinic, Rochester, MN; et al)

Lancet 381:303-312, 2013

Background.—No treatment options are available for patients with metastatic colorectal cancer that progresses after all approved standard therapies, but many patients maintain a good performance status and could be candidates for further therapy. An international phase 3 trial was done to assess the multikinase inhibitor regorafenib in these patients.

Methods.—We did this trial at 114 centres in 16 countries. Patients with documented metastatic colorectal cancer and progression during or within 3 months after the last standard therapy were randomised (in a 2:1 ratio; by computer-generated randomisation list and interactive voice response system; preallocated block design (block size six); stratified by previous treatment with VEGF-targeting drugs, time from diagnosis of metastatic disease, and geographical region) to receive best supportive care plus oral regorafenib 160 mg or placebo once daily, for the first 3 weeks of each 4 week cycle. The primary endpoint was overall survival. The study sponsor, participants, and investigators were masked to treatment assignment. Efficacy analyses were by intention to treat. This trial is registered at ClinicalTrials.gov, number NCT01103323.

Findings.—Between April 30, 2010, and March 22, 2011, 1052 patients were screened, 760 patients were randomised to receive regorafenib (n=505) or placebo (n=255), and 753 patients initiated treatment (regorafenib n=500; placebo n=253; population for safety analyses). The primary endpoint of overall survival was met at a preplanned interim analysis; data cutoff was on July 21, 2011. Median overall survival was 6·4 months in the regorafenib group versus 5·0 months in the placebo group (hazard ratio 0·77; 95% CI 0·64–0·94; one-sided $p=0·0052$). Treatment-related adverse events occurred in 465 (93%) patients assigned regorafenib and in 154 (61%) of those assigned placebo. The most common adverse events of grade three or higher related to regorafenib were hand-foot skin reaction (83 patients, 17%), fatigue (48, 10%), diarrhoea (36, 7%), hypertension (36, 7%), and rash or desquamation (29, 6%).

Interpretation.—Regorafenib is the first small-molecule multikinase inhibitor with survival benefits in metastatic colorectal cancer which has progressed after all standard therapies. The present study provides evidence for a continuing role of targeted treatment after disease progression, with regorafenib offering a potential new line of therapy in this treatment-refractory population.

▶ The treatment of colorectal cancer has changed dramatically over the last 15 years with the addition of new agents, such as irinotecan, oxaliplatin, bevacizumab, and cetuximab among others. This study focused on a new agent, regorafenib, which is a multikinase inhibitor with effects on angiogenesis, oncogenesis, and the tumor microenvironment. The patient population for the trial consisted of patients whose cancer had progressed despite all currently available therapies; hence, this was a very difficult population to treat. A total of 753 patients were treated with best supportive care plus or minus regorafenib. Those receiving regorafenib achieved a superior median overall survival (6.4 months vs 5.0 months, hazard ratio = 0.77). This adds yet another potential line of therapy for patients with metastatic colorectal cancer, a line that consists of targeted therapy. The ultimate role for this option will be determined by future trials looking at combination regimens and studies in patients with less prior therapy.

J. T. Thigpen, MD

Estrogen Plus Progestin and Colorectal Cancer Incidence and Mortality
Simon MS, Chlebowski RT, Wactawski-Wende J, et al (Wayne State Univ, Detroit, MI; Harbor-Univ of California at Los Angeles Med Ctr, Torrance; State Univ of New York at Buffalo; et al)
J Clin Oncol 30:3983-3990, 2012

Purpose.—During the intervention phase in the Women's Health Initiative (WHI) clinical trial, use of estrogen plus progestin reduced the colorectal cancer diagnosis rate, but the cancers were found at a substantially higher stage. To assess the clinical relevance of the findings, analyses of the influence of combined hormone therapy on colorectal cancer incidence and colorectal cancer mortality were conducted after extended follow-up.

Patients and Methods.—The WHI study was a randomized, double-blind, placebo-controlled clinical trial involving 16,608 postmenopausal women with an intact uterus who were randomly assigned to daily

0.625 mg conjugated equine estrogen plus 2.5 mg medroxyprogesterone acetate (n = 8,506) or matching placebo (n = 8,102). Colorectal cancer diagnosis rates and colorectal cancer mortality were assessed.

Results.—After a mean of 5.6 years (standard deviation [SD], 1.03 years) of intervention and 11.6 years (SD, 3.1 years) of total follow-up, fewer colorectal cancers were diagnosed in the combined hormone therapy group compared with the placebo group (diagnoses/year, 0.12% v 0.16%; hazard ratio [HR], 0.72; 95% CI, 0.56 to 0.94; P = .014). Bowel screening examinations were comparable between groups throughout. Cancers in the combined hormone therapy group more commonly had positive lymph nodes (50.5% v 28.6%; P < .001) and were at higher stage (regional or distant, 68.8% v 51.4%; P = .003). Although not statistically significant, there was a higher number of colorectal cancer deaths in the combined hormone therapy group (37 v 27 deaths; 0.04% v 0.03%; HR, 1.29; 95% CI, 0.78 to 2.11; P = .320).

Conclusion.—The findings, suggestive of diagnostic delay, do not support a clinically meaningful benefit for combined hormone therapy on colorectal cancer.

▶ The Women's Health Initiative study was a double-blind, placebo-controlled clinical trial involving 16 608 postmenopausal women with an intact uterus randomly assigned to estrogen/progestin or placebo who were initially reported to have an increased risk of breast cancer in the hormonal therapy arm. This led to an early closure of the trial and intense discussion of whether hormone replacement therapy should be used. Lost in all of the discussion of the breast cancer risk was an observation that use of hormone replacement therapy reduced the number of colorectal cancers diagnosed with a hazard ratio of 0.72 (28% reduction in the risk of getting colon cancer). This article reports on a longer follow-up of these data out to in excess of 11 years. These additional data show that women on hormone replacement therapy tended to have a greater frequency of positive lymph nodes and a higher-stage cancer. In the final analysis, there were more deaths in the hormone arm, a difference that was not statistically significant. Because of this trend to an increased mortality from colon cancer, one can no longer cite a beneficial effect of hormones on colon cancer risk as a potential benefit of the treatment.

J. T. Thigpen, MD

Aspirin Use, Tumor *PIK3CA* Mutation, and Colorectal-Cancer Survival
Liao X, Lochhead P, Nishihara R, et al (Dana-Farber Cancer Inst and Harvard Med School, Boston, MA; et al)
N Engl J Med 367:1596-1606, 2012

Background.—Regular use of aspirin after a diagnosis of colon cancer has been associated with a superior clinical outcome. Experimental evidence suggests that inhibition of prostaglandin-endoperoxide synthase 2 (PTGS2) (also known as cyclooxygenase-2) by aspirin down-regulates phosphatidylinositol 3-kinase (PI3 K) signaling activity. We hypothesized that the effect of aspirin on survival and prognosis in patients with cancers characterized by mutated *PIK3CA* (the phosphatidylinositol-4, 5-bisphosphonate 3-kinase, catalytic subunit alpha polypeptide gene) might differ from the effect among those with wild-type *PIK3CA* cancers.

Methods.—We obtained data on 964 patients with rectal or colon cancer from the Nurses' Health Study and the Health Professionals Follow-up Study, including data on aspirin use after diagnosis and the presence or absence of *PIK3CA* mutation. We used a Cox proportional-hazards model to compute the multivariate hazard ratio for death. We examined tumor markers, including PTGS2, phosphorylated AKT, *KRAS, BRAF,* microsatellite instability, CpG island methylator phenotype, and methylation of long interspersed nucleotide element 1.

Results.—Among patients with mutated-*PIK3CA* colorectal cancers, regular use of aspirin after diagnosis was associated with superior colorectal cancer–specific survival (multivariate hazard ratio for cancer-related death, 0.18; 95% confidence interval [CI], 0.06 to 0.61; $P < 0.001$ by the log-rank test) and overall survival (multivariate hazard ratio for death from any cause, 0.54; 95% CI, 0.31 to 0.94; $P = 0.01$ by the log-rank test). In contrast, among patients with wild-type *PIK3CA*, regular use of aspirin after diagnosis was not associated with colorectal cancer–specific survival (multivariate hazard ratio, 0.96; 95% CI, 0.69 to 1.32; $P = 0.76$ by the log-rank test; $P = 0.009$ for interaction between aspirin and *PIK3CA* variables) or overall survival (multivariate hazard ratio, 0.94; 95% CI, 0.75 to 1.17; $P = 0.96$ by the log-rank test; $P = 0.07$ for interaction).

Conclusions.—Regular use of aspirin after diagnosis was associated with longer survival among patients with mutated-*PIK3CA* colorectal cancer, but not among patients with wild-type *PIK3CA* cancer. The findings from this molecular pathological epidemiology study suggest that the *PIK3CA* mutation in colorectal cancer may serve as a predictive molecular biomarker for adjuvant aspirin therapy.

▶ Liao et al studied the effect of aspirin in patients with colorectal cancer to determine whether it confers a differential protective effect for survival, depending on the presence or absence of an activated phosphatidylinositol 3-kinase (PI3K) pathway, that is, activating *PIK3CA* mutations. Aspirin is known to affect the prostaglandin-endoperoxide synthase 2 (PTGS2, or cyclooxygenase-2), and is known to be, overall, beneficial for colorectal cancer survival,[1] particularly when PTGS2 is overactive.[2] Nevertheless, colorectal cancers are heterogenous, and certain mutations or epigenetic events may affect outcomes. An overactive PI3K pathway activates PTGS2, resulting in inhibition of apoptosis[3]; therefore, aspirin may be particularly useful in colorectal cancers harboring *PIK3CA* mutations. The authors used 964 participants with known *PIK3CA* mutational status from 2 large prospective cohort studies: the Nurses' Health Study and the Health Professionals Follow-up Study. This analysis demonstrates that, as hypothesized, patients with *PIK3CA*-mutated tumors derive significant survival benefit from regular aspirin use, particularly after colorectal cancer resection, whereas aspirin was not protective for patients with wild-type *PIK3CA*. Previous data noted survival benefit from aspirin in colorectal cancer patients whose tumors overexpressed PTGS2 by immunohistochemistry. Among the patients studied here, PTGS2 overexpression did not confer survival advantage when the *PIK3CA* status was wild type, whereas for *PIK3CA*-mutated cancers, the benefit appeared to be the strongest. Although patients' subsets were small, and data must be interpreted with caution, this landmark study suggests that regular aspirin use should be used as adjuvant treatment for colorectal cancer patients harboring *PIK3CA* mutations (approximately 10% to 17% of colorectal cancers).

E. G. Chiorean, MD

References

1. Chan AT, Ogino S, Fuchs CS. Aspirin use and survival after diagnosis of colorectal cancer. *JAMA*. 2009;302:649-658.
2. Chan AT, Ogino S, Fuchs CS. Aspirin and the risk of colorectal cancer in relation to the expression of COX-2. *N Engl J Med*. 2007;356:2131-2142.
3. Kaur J, Sanyal SN. PI3-kinase/Wnt association mediates COX-2/PGE(2) pathway to inhibit apoptosis in early stages of colon carcinogenesis: chemoprevention by diclofenac. *Tumour Biol*. 2010;31:623-631.

Pancreas

Open-Label, Multicenter, Randomized Phase III Trial of Adjuvant Chemoradiation Plus Interferon Alfa-2b Versus Fluorouracil and Folinic Acid for Patients With Resected Pancreatic Adenocarcinoma
Schmidt J, Abel U, Debus J, et al (Ruprecht-Karls-Univ, Heidelberg, Germany; et al)
J Clin Oncol 30:4077-4083, 2012

Purpose.—Adjuvant chemotherapy prolongs survival in patients with pancreatic cancer, but its benefit is limited. Long-term survival times of up to 44 months after adjuvant chemoradioimmunotherapy in phase II trials motivated the present study.

Patients and Methods.—Between 2004 and 2007, 132 R0/R1 resected patients received either fluorouracil (FU), cisplatin, and interferon alfa-2b (IFN α-2b) plus radiotherapy followed by two cycles of FU (arm A, n = 64) or six cycles of FU monotherapy (arm B, n = 68). One hundred ten patients (arm A, n = 53; arm B, n = 57) received at least one dose of the study medication, and these patients composed the per-protocol (PP) population. Biomarkers were analyzed longitudinally for their predictive value.

Results.—Median survival for all randomly assigned patients was 26.5 months (95% CI, 21.6 to 39.5 months) in arm A and 28.5 months (95% CI, 20.4 to 38.6 months) in arm B. The hazard ratio was 1.04 (arm A *v* arm B: 95% CI, 0.66 to 1.53; $P = .99$). Median survival for the PP population was 32.1 months (95% CI, 22.8 to 42.2 months) in arm A and 28.5 months (95% CI, 19.5 to 38.6 months) in arm B ($P = .49$).

Eighty-five percent of patients in arm A and 16% of patients in arm B experienced grade 3 or 4 toxicity. The quality of life was temporarily negatively affected in arm A.

Conclusion.—The FU, cisplatin, and IFN α-2b plus radiotherapy regimen did not improve the survival compared with FU monotherapy. Given the substantial adverse effects, this treatment can currently not be recommended. Nevertheless, the outcome in both arms represents the best survival, to our knowledge, ever reported for patients with resected pancreatic cancer in randomized controlled trials. Future studies will demonstrate whether immune response to IFN α-2b challenge has a predictive value.

▶ Patients with resected pancreatic adenocarcinoma have median overall survival of 24 months and a 5-year overall survival rate of 20% to 25% after surgery and adjuvant gemcitabine or fluoropyrimidine therapy (CONKO 001 study, ESPAC-1, and ESPAC-3 studies).[1-3] Investigators at Virginia Mason Cancer Institute reported a superior 5-year survival rate of 55% in a phase 2 single institution trial, with a combined chemoimmunotherapy plus radiotherapy regimen,[4] and a single-arm phase 2 ACOSOG Z05031 trial using this therapy observed median survival of 27 months, albeit with significant toxicity requiring study termination.[5] Preclinical data indicate that interferon-α2b (IFN-α2b) may have chemotherapy and radiotherapy potentiating effects as well as provide antitumor immunologic efficacy.[6]

To further assess the efficacy and safety of cisplatin and IFN-α2b plus 5-fluorouracil (5-FU)- based chemoradioimmunotherapy after surgical resection, this study randomly assigned 130 patients to receive adjuvant chemoradioimmunotherapy vs standard 5-FU and leucovorin. The study aimed to observe a 2-year survival rate of 60% in the investigational arm.

With a median follow-up of 43 months in the intent-to-treat population, there was no difference in median overall survival (OS) between the investigational and standard arm: 26.5 vs 28.5 months, respectively. Among patients who received at least one dose of treatment (per protocol population), the median OS rates were not statistically different: 32.1 vs 28.5 months ($P = .49$) in favor of the investigational arm. The median disease-free survival was 15.2 vs 11.5 months in favor of the investigational arm (not significant).

Chemoradioimmunotherapy was associated with significant and prohibitive toxicity compared with standard chemotherapy (85% vs 16% grade 3–4 adverse events) and worsening quality of life during treatment.

In this study, patients treated with standard 5-FU/folinic acid had 2-year OS of 54%, higher than the historical 35% 2-year survival rates. This could be explained by improved patient selection, by proper radiologic staging, and possibly by improved supportive care.

It is nevertheless clear that the chemoradioimmunotherapy regimen with cisplatin, 5-FU, and IFN-α2b, while significantly more toxic, did not provide a meaningful increase in overall survival and is not justified in the adjuvant setting of resected pancreatic adenocarcinoma.

E. G. Chiorean, MD

References

1. Oettle H, Post S, Neuhaus P, et al. Adjuvant chemotherapy with gemcitabine vs observation in patients undergoing curative-intent resection of pancreatic cancer: a randomized controlled trial. *JAMA.* 2007;297:267-277.
2. Neoptolemos J, Stocken D, Friess H, et al; European Study Group for Pancreatic Cancer. A randomized trial of chemoradiotherapy and chemotherapy after resection of pancreatic cancer. *N Engl J Med.* 2004;350:1200-1210.
3. Picozzi VJ, Kozarek RA, Traverso LW. Interferon-based adjuvant chemoradiation therapy after pancreaticoduodenectomy for pancreatic adenocarcinoma. *Am J Surg.* 2003;185:476-480.
4. Picozzi J, Abrams R, Traverso L, et al. ACOSOG Z05031: report on a multicenter, phase II trial for adjuvant therapy of resected pancreatic cancer using cisplatin, 5-FU, and alpha-interferon. *J Clin Oncol.* 2008;26:214s.
5. Schmidt J, Patrut EM, Ma J, et al. Immunomodulatory impact of interferon-alpha in combination with chemoradiation of pancreatic adenocarcinoma (CapRI). *Cancer Immunol Immunother.* 2006;55:1396-1405.
6. Holsti LR, Mattson K, Niiranen A, et al. Enhancement of radiation effects by alpha interferon in the treatment of small cell carcinoma of the lung. *Int J Radiat Oncol Biol Phys.* 1987;13:1161-1166.

Carbohydrate Antigen 19-9 is a Prognostic and Predictive Biomarker in Patients With Advanced Pancreatic Cancer Who Receive Gemcitabine-Containing Chemotherapy: A Pooled Analysis of 6 Prospective Trials

Bauer TM, El-Rayes BF, Li X, et al (The Ohio State Univ Comprehensive Cancer Ctr, Columbus; Emory Univ, Atlanta, GA; The Ohio State Univ, Columbus; et al)
Cancer 119:285-292, 2013

Background.—Carbohydrate antigen 19-9 (CA19-9) is a widely used biomarker in pancreatic cancer. There is no consensus on the interpretation of the change in CA19-9 serum levels and its role in the clinical management of patients with pancreatic cancer.

Methods.—Individual patient data from 6 prospective trials evaluating gemcitabine-containing regimens from 3 different institutions were pooled. CA19-9 values were obtained at baseline and after successive cycles of treatment. The objective of this study was to correlate a decline in CA19-9 with outcomes while undergoing treatment.

Results.—A total of 212 patients with locally advanced (n = 50) or metastatic (n = 162) adenocarcinoma of the pancreas were included. Median baseline CA19-9 level was 1077 ng/mL (range, 15-492,241 ng/mL). Groups were divided into those levels below (low) or above (high) the median. Median overall survival (mOS) was 8.7 versus 5.2 months ($P = .0018$) and median time to progression (mTTP) was 5.8 versus 3.7 months ($P = .082$) in the low versus high groups, respectively. After 2 cycles of chemotherapy, up to a 5% increase versus ≥5% increase in CA19-9 levels conferred an improved mOS (10.3 vs 5.1 months, $P = .0022$) and mTTP (7.5 vs 3.5 months, $P = 0.0005$).

Conclusions.—In patients who have advanced pancreatic cancer treated with gemcitabine-containing regimens baseline CA19-9 is prognostic for outcome. A decline in CA19-9 after the second cycle of chemotherapy is not predictive of improved mOS or mTTP; thus, CA19-9 decline is not a useful surrogate endpoint in clinical trials. Clinically, a ≥5% rise in CA19-9 after 2 cycles of chemotherapy serves as a negative predictive marker.

▶ Pancreatic cancer continues to be an exceptionally lethal cancer for which chemotherapy offers relatively limited benefits. Median survival times for all but those cases of very limited extent of the disease uniformly are less than a year and in many instances substantially less than a year. The most common regimens used focus on gemcitabine as a central part of the treatment regimen. For purposes of following the course of response to treatment, physicians have often used the biomarker carbohydrate antigen 19-9 (CA 19-9). The study presents a pooled analysis of 6 prospective trials to assess the value of CA 19-9 as a prognostic and predictive marker of treatment success or failure. A total of 212 patients with locally advanced or metastatic pancreatic cancer with a median baseline CA 19-9 level of 1077 were included in the analysis. Key observations included the following: First, the baseline CA 19-9 was a prognostic marker. Patients with a baseline CA 19-9 level above the median exhibited a significantly poorer median overall survival (5.2 vs 8.7 months) and median time to progression (3.7 vs 5.8 months). In certain other cancers, the rate of decrease of the biomarker level over the first 2 cycles of therapy is predictive of outcome with more rapid rates suggestive of a better response to therapy (eg, ovarian cancer and CA-125). This was not the case with CA 19-9 and pancreatic cancer. Instead, there was a difference between any decline in the CA 19-9 level vs no decline in the level after 2 cycles (overall survival, 10.3 months vs 5.2 months, and time to progression, 7.6 months vs 3.9 months) and between a less than 5% increase in CA 19-9 level vs greater increase (overall survival, 10.3 months vs 5.1 months). The authors' overall conclusion is that CA 19-9 changes cannot serve as surrogate markers because of a low positive predictive value, but these changes can be useful as a general guide to what therapy is accomplishing.

J. T. Thigpen, MD

EGFR pathway biomarkers in erlotinib-treated patients with advanced pancreatic cancer: translational results from the randomised, crossover phase 3 trial AIO-PK0104
Boeck S, Jung A, Laubender RP, et al (Ludwig-Maximilians-Univ of Munich, Germany; et al)
Br J Cancer 108:469-476, 2013

Background.—We aimed to identify molecular epidermal growth factor receptor (EGFR) tissue biomarkers in pancreatic cancer (PC) patients treated with the anti-EGFR agent erlotinib within the phase 3 randomised AIO-PK0104 study.

Methods.—AIO-PK0104 was a multicenter trial comparing gemcitabine/erlotinib followed by capecitabine with capecitabine/erlotinib followed by gemcitabine in advanced PC; primary study end point was the time-to-treatment failure after first- and second-line therapy (TTF2). Translational analyses were performed for KRAS exon 2 mutations, EGFR expression, PTEN expression, the EGFR intron 1 and exon 13 R497K polymorphism (PM). Biomarker data were correlated with TTF, overall survival (OS) and skin rash.

Results.—Archival tumour tissue was available from 208 (74%) of the randomised patients. The KRAS mutations were found in 70% (121 out of 173) of patients and exclusively occurred in codon 12. The EGFR over-expression was detected in 89 out of 181 patients (49%) by immunohisto-chemistry (IHC), and 77 out of 166 patients (46%) had an *EGFR* gene amplification by fluorescence *in-situ* hybridisation (FISH); 30 out of 171 patients (18%) had a loss of PTEN expression, which was associated with an inferior TTF1 (first-line therapy; HR 0.61, $P = 0.02$) and TTF2 (HR 0.66, $P = 0.04$). The KRAS wild-type status was associated with improved OS (HR 1.68, $P = 0.005$); no significant OS correlation was found for EGFR-IHC (HR 0.96), EGFR-FISH (HR 1.22), PTEN-IHC (HR 0.77), intron 1 (HR 0.91) or exon 13 R497K PM (HR 0.83). None of the six biomarkers correlated with the occurrence of skin rash.

Conclusion.—The KRAS wild-type was associated with an improved OS in erlotinib-treated PC patients in this phase 3 study; it remains to be defined whether this association is prognostic or predictive.

▶ Erlotinib, an anti—epidermal growth factor receptor (EGFR) inhibitor, has shown modest survival benefit when added to gemcitabine compared with gemcitabine alone in a large, randomized, phase 3 study (6.2 vs 5.9 months overall survival, respectively, hazard ratio, 0.82; $P = .038$),[1] leading to its approval for treatment of advanced pancreatic cancer. Patients with grade 2 or higher rash were noted to derive higher survival benefit (median overall survival > 10 months) but no other biological markers, including EGFR copy number or *KRAS* mutational status, have correlated with improved response or survival in the PA.3 study.[2]

Given the potential survival benefit noted with second-line fluoropyrimidine-based therapy after gemcitabine failure in phase 2 studies,[3] the AIO-PK0104 phase 3 trial was designed to study the efficacy of sequential treatment of gemcitabine plus erlotinib followed by capecitabine upon progression vs capecitabine plus erlotinib followed by gemcitabine upon progression, and compared time to first and second treatment failure and overall survival between groups.[4] Overall, median survival rates were similar with both regimens (6.2 vs 6.9 months). In a preplanned analysis of KRAS exon 2 mutational status, KRAS wild-type pancreatic cancers (30%) were associated with improved overall survival compared with KRAS-mutated tumors, (7.9 vs 5.7 months, $P = .005$), but it could not be determined whether KRAS was a prognostic or predictive factor for benefit from erlotinib-based therapy.[4] As previously documented with erlotinib, skin rash grade 2 or higher remained significantly associated with survival (9.6 months vs 3.4 months for patients without skin rash).[4] Because no definitive biomarkers have been predictors of benefit from erlotinib-based therapy, the investigators further collected tumor specimens for biological correlative studies.

Boeck et al report on the translational EGFR pathway—related biomarkers from the AIO-PK0104 study. Among 281 patients randomly chosen, archival tumor tissue was obtained retrospectively from 208 patients. EGFR expression by immunohistochemistry (IHC), EGFR gene copy number by fluorescence in situ hybridization, EGFR gene polymorphisms (intron 1 and exon 13), *PTEN* expression by IHC, and *KRAS* mutational status were correlated with survival as well as time-to-treatment failure and occurrence of rash.

Although no marker correlated with response to treatment or the incidence of skin rash, lack of *PTEN* loss seemed to correlate with favorable time-to-treatment failure from first-line (2.4 vs 2 months, $P = .02$) and second-line therapy (4.1 vs 3 months, $P = .04$) and a trend for improved survival (6.8 vs 4.5 months, $P = .22$). As previously described above,[4] *KRAS* wild-type status conferred superior overall survival but did not correlate with time-to-progression failure (4.2 vs 4 months) or response to therapy.

Overall, *KRAS* and *PTEN* status should be explored prospectively as prognostic or predictive biomarkers in larger therapeutic clinical trials in pancreatic cancer to further define their role. With the evolution of treatment options in pancreatic cancer, defining biomarkers to predict clinical benefit is urgently needed.

E. G. Chiorean, MD

References

1. Moore MJ, Goldstein D, Hamm J, et al. Erlotinib plus gemcitabine compared with gemcitabine alone in patients with advanced pancreatic cancer: a phase III trial of the National Cancer Institute of Canada Clinical Trials Group. *J Clin Oncol.* 2007;25:1960-1966.
2. da Cunha Santos G, Dhani N, Tu D, et al. Molecular predictors of outcome in a phase 3 study of gemcitabine and erlotinib therapy in patients with advanced pancreatic cancer: National Cancer Institute of Canada Clinical Trials Group Study PA.3. *Cancer.* 2010;116:5599-5607.
3. Kulke MH, Blaszkowsky LS, Ryan DR, et al. Capecitabine plus erlotinib in gemcitabine-refractory advanced pancreatic cancer. *J Clin Oncol.* 2007;25: 4787-4792.
4. Heinemann V, Vehling-Kaiser U, Waldschmidt D, et al. Gemcitabine plus erlotinib followed by capecitabine versus capecitabine plus erlotinib followed by gemcitabine in advanced pancreatic cancer: final results of a randomised phase 3 trial of the 'Arbeitsgemeinschaft Internistische Onkologie' (AIO-PK0104). *Gut.* 2013; 62:751-759.

Re-resection for Isolated Local Recurrence of Pancreatic Cancer is Feasible, Safe, and Associated with Encouraging Survival
Strobel O, Hartwig W, Hackert T, et al (Univ Hosp Heidelberg, Germany)
Ann Surg Oncol 20:964-972, 2013

Background.—Local recurrence of pancreatic cancer occurs in 80 % of patients within 2 years after potentially curative resections. Around 30 % of patients have isolated local recurrence (ILR) without evidence of metastases. In spite of localized disease these patients usually only receive palliative chemotherapy and have a short survival.

Purpose.—To evaluate the outcome of surgery as part of a multimodal treatment for ILR of pancreatic cancer.

Methods.—All consecutive operations performed for suspected ILR in our institution between October 2001 and October 2009 were identified from a prospective database. Perioperative outcome, survival, and prognostic parameters were assessed.

Results.—Of 97 patients with histologically proven recurrence, 57 (59 %) had ILR. In 40 (41 %) patients surgical exploration revealed metastases distant to the local recurrence. Resection was performed in 41 (72 %) patients with ILR, while 16 (28 %) ILR were locally unresectable. Morbidity and mortality were 25 and 1.8 % after resections and 10 and 0 % after explorations, respectively. Median postoperative survival was 16.4 months in ILR versus 9.4 months in metastatic disease ($p < 0.0001$). In ILR median survival was significantly longer after resection (26.0 months) compared with exploration without resection (10.8 months, $p = 0.0104$). R0 resection was achieved in 18 patients and resulted in 30.5 months median survival. Presence of metastases, incomplete resection, and high preoperative CA 19-9 serum values were associated with lesser survival.

Conclusions.—Resection for isolated local recurrence of pancreatic cancer is feasible, safe, and associated with favorable survival outcome. This concept warrants further evaluation in other institutions and in randomized controlled trials.

▶ Resectable pancreatic cancer is associated with median overall survival of 24 months and a 5-year survival rate of 20% after surgery and adjuvant chemotherapy.[1] Although metastatic disease recurrence predominates, occasionally the disease recurs locally only (20%–30% isolated local recurrence [ILR]) and may thus be amenable to either combined chemoradiotherapy or systemic chemotherapy alone. Median survival with medical therapy after recurrence ranges from 10 to 17 months.[2]

Redo surgery has been reported in small series' but had variable results.[3] With increasing staging accuracy by pancreas-protocol computed tomography scans and magnetic resonance imaging, it may be possible to better select patients who are candidates for aggressive multidisciplinary approaches, including reresection of ILR.

Strobel et al report on the feasibility and outcomes of surgical resection of ILR, including local pancreatic and retroperitoneal local recurrence, in 105 patients selected by radiologic criteria based on no evidence of systemic recurrence. Encasement of the celiac artery or the superior mesenteric artery was criterion for unresectability. All patients with ILR, if operable, were to be treated with surgery preceded (neoadjuvant) or followed (adjuvant) by additional chemotherapy or chemoradiotherapy.

Among the 105 initial patients with suspected local recurrence, 97 had histologically confirmed pancreatic cancer, and, among them, 40 (41%) were found to have distant metastases intraoperatively. Thus, only 57 patients (59%) were deemed to have ILR, and, among them, 41 were operable per resectability criteria. Intraoperative radiation was used in 22 patients.

Overall survival after reoperation in patients with ILR vs those found intraoperatively to have metastases was 16.4 vs 9.4 months, respectively, reflecting the natural biology of the disease.

In patients with ILR, those able to undergo resection achieved a significantly better survival compared with those who did not and were only treated with local intraoperative or postoperative radiotherapy and systemic chemotherapy (median overall survival, 26 months and 5-year survival, 20% from reoperation vs 10.8 months median survival and 2-year survival of 15% for patients with localized inoperable disease). Intraoperative radiotherapy for resected ILR did not convey better survival rates, but it seemed beneficial for patients with inoperable cancer.

R2 resection (24%) and preoperative serum CA19-9 levels at or above 400 ng/mL were prognostic for worse survival.

This large, nonrandomized observational study does not compare outcomes of local resection combined with systemic chemotherapy vs systemic therapy combined with local radiotherapy for locoregional recurrence of pancreatic cancer but raises the important issue of a potentially aggressive, multidisciplinary approach that could benefit select patients.

It may be difficult to definitively prove the role of reresection for ILR in pancreatic cancer without a randomized trial, but this modality appears safe and feasible and should be encouraged in large specialized centers. This approach may further affect guidelines for relapse surveillance after primary pancreatic cancer surgery to detect potentially resectable local recurrences early.

E. G. Chiorean, MD

References

1. Neoptolemos JP, Stocken DD, Bassi C, et al. Adjuvant chemotherapy with fluorouracil plus folinic acid vs gemcitabine following pancreatic cancer resection: a randomized controlled trial. *JAMA*. 2010;304:1073-1081.
2. Wilkowski R, Thoma M, Bruns C, Duhmke E, Heinemann V. Combined chemoradiotherapy for isolated local recurrence after primary resection of pancreatic cancer. *JOP*. 2006;7:34-40.
3. Kleeff J, Reiser C, Hinz U, et al. Surgery for recurrent pancreatic ductal adenocarcinoma. *Ann Surg*. 2007;245:566-572.

Miscellaneous

Long-Term Update of US GI Intergroup RTOG 98-11 Phase III Trial for Anal Carcinoma: Survival, Relapse, and Colostomy Failure With Concurrent Chemoradiation Involving Fluorouracil/Mitomycin Versus Fluorouracil/Cisplatin

Gunderson LL, Winter KA, Ajani JA, et al (Mayo Clinic Arizona, Scottsdale; Radiation Therapy Oncology Group Statistical Ctr, Philadelphia, PA; MD Anderson Cancer Ctr, Houston, TX; et al)
J Clin Oncol 30:4344-4351, 2012

Purpose.—On initial publication of GI Intergroup Radiation Therapy Oncology Group (RTOG) 98-11 [A Phase III Randomized Study of 5-Fluorouracil (5-FU), Mitomycin, and Radiotherapy Versus 5-Fluorouracil, Cisplatin and Radiotherapy in Carcinoma of the Anal Canal], concurrent chemoradiation (CCR) with fluorouracil (FU) plus mitomycin (MMC) decreased colostomy failure (CF) when compared with induction plus concurrent FU plus cisplatin (CDDP), but did not significantly impact disease-free survival (DFS) or overall survival (OS) for anal canal carcinoma. The intent of the updated analysis was to determine the long-term impact of treatment on survival (DFS, OS, colostomy-free survival [CFS]), CF, and relapse (locoregional failure [LRF], distant metastasis) in this patient group.

Patients and Methods.—Stratification factors included sex, clinical node status, and primary size. DFS and OS were estimated univariately by the Kaplan-Meier method, and treatment arms were compared by log-rank test. Time to relapse and CF were estimated by the cumulative incidence method and treatment arms were compared by using Gray's test. Multivariate analyses used Cox proportional hazard models to test for treatment differences after adjusting for stratification factors.

Results.—Of 682 patients accrued, 649 were analyzable for outcomes. DFS and OS were statistically better for RT + FU/MMC versus RT + FU/CDDP (5-year DFS, 67.8% v 57.8%; P =.006; 5-year OS, 78.3% v 70.7%; P =.026). There was a trend toward statistical significance for CFS (P =.05), LRF (P =.087), and CF (P =.074). Multivariate analysis was statistically significant for treatment and clinical node status for both DFS and OS, for tumor diameter for DFS, and for sex for OS.

Conclusion.—CCR with FU/MMC has a statistically significant, clinically meaningful impact on DFS and OS versus induction plus concurrent FU/CDDP, and it has borderline significance for CFS, CF, and LRF. Therefore, RT + FU/MMC remains the preferred standard of care.

▶ The Radiation Therapy Oncology Group 98-11 phase III trial in anal cancer patients compared concurrent chemoradiotherapy with 5-fluorouracil (5FU) and mitomycin C, vs 5FU and cisplatin. The initial results of the study were published in 2008 and showed superior local control and lower colostomy rates (10% vs 19%) for patients treated with 5FU/mitomycin C[1] but with no improvement in disease-free survival (DFS) or overall survival (OS). Subsequent subgroup analyses showed that tumor size greater than 5 cm and node-positive disease impacted DFS and OS.[2] The primary endpoint of the study was to observe an increase in DFS from 63% with 5FU/mitomycin C plus radiotherapy (RT) to 73% with 5FU/cisplatin plus RT. Secondary endpoints were OS, colostomy failure, and relapse (local and metastatic).

This analysis reports long-term outcomes in both treatment arms. Eligibility criteria included T2-T4 and any anal canal cancers. Patients assigned to 5FU/mitomycin C were treated up front with chemoradiotherapy, whereas patients assigned to 5FU/cisplatin received an induction phase with chemotherapy alone followed by chemoradiotherapy. A total of 682 patients were randomly selected and 649 patients are evaluable for long-term outcomes analysis.

Five-year DFS was significantly higher with 5FU/mitomycin C/RT vs 5FU/cisplatin/RT: 68% vs 58% (hazard ratio [HR] 1.39, $P = .006$), and the 5-year OS was similarly higher: 78% vs 71% (HR 1.39, $P = .026$).

Five-year colostomy-free survival rates were 72% vs 65% ($P = .05$), 5-year locoregional failure rates were 20% vs 26% ($P = .087$), 5-year colostomy failure rates were 12% vs 17% ($P = .074$), and 5-year distant metastases rates were 13% vs 18% ($P = .12$), respectively, for 5FU/mitomycin C/RT and 5FU/cisplatin/RT.

This study clearly indicated that 5FU/mitomycin C/RT is the standard regimen for squamous carcinoma of the anus. Nevertheless, the study has its own design drawbacks, namely, the delay in chemoradiotherapy in the 5FU/cisplatin arm[3] and the fact that cisplatin induction therapy may have contributed to radioresistance by inducing DNA repair and preventing radiation-induced cytotoxicity,[4] thus confounding a direct comparison.

E. G. Chiorean, MD

References

1. Ajani JA, Winter KA, Gunderson LL, et al. Fluorouracil, mitomycin, and radiotherapy vs fluorouracil, cisplatin, and radiotherapy for carcinoma of the anal canal: a randomized controlled trial. *JAMA*. 2008;299:1914-1921.
2. Ajani JA, Winter KA, Gunderson LL, et al. Prognostic factors derived from a prospective database dictate clinical biology of anal cancer: the intergroup trial (RTOG 98-11). *Cancer*. 2010;116:4007-4013.
3. Ben-Josef E, Moughan J, Ajani JA, et al. Impact of overall treatment time on survival and local control in patients with anal cancer: a pooled data analysis of Radiation Therapy Oncology Group trials 87-04 and 98-11. *J Clin Oncol*. 2010; 28:5061-5066.
4. Glynne-Jones R, Hoskin P. Neoadjuvant cisplatin chemotherapy before chemoradiation: a flawed paradigm? *J Clin Oncol*. 2007;25:5281-5286.

9 Hematologic Malignancies

Leukemia and Myelodysplastic Syndrome

Secondary genetic lesions in acute myeloid leukemia with inv(16) or t(16;16): a study of the German-Austrian AML Study Group (AMLSG)
Paschka P, Du J, Schlenk RF, et al (Universitätsklinikum Ulm, Germany)
Blood 121:170-177, 2013

In this study, we evaluated the impact of secondary genetic lesions in acute myeloid leukemia (AML) with inv(16)(p13.1q22) or t(16;16)(p13.1;q22); CBFB-MYH11. We studied 176 patients, all enrolled on prospective treatment trials, for secondary chromosomal aberrations and mutations in N-/KRAS, KIT, FLT3, and JAK2 (V617F) genes. Most frequent chromosomal aberrations were trisomy 22 (18%) and trisomy 8 (16%). Overall, 84% of patients harbored at least 1 gene mutation, with RAS being affected in 53% (45% NRAS; 13% KRAS) of the cases, followed by KIT (37%) and FLT3 (17%; FLT3-TKD [14%], FLT3-ITD [5%]). None of the secondary genetic lesions influenced achievement of complete remission. In multivariable analyses, KIT mutation hazard ratio [HR] = 1.67; $P = .04$], log(10)(WBC) (HR = 1.33; $P = .02$), and trisomy 22 (HR = 0.54; $P = .08$) were relevant factors for relapse-free survival; for overall survival, FLT3 mutation (HR = 2.56; $P = .006$), trisomy 22 (HR = 0.45; $P = .07$), trisomy 8 (HR = 2.26; $P = .02$), age (difference of 10 years, HR = 1.46; $P = .01$), and therapy-related AML (HR = 2.13; $P = .14$) revealed as prognostic factors. The adverse effects of KIT and FLT3 mutations were mainly attributed to exon 8 and tyrosine kinase domain mutations, respectively. Our large study emphasizes the impact of both secondary chromosomal aberrations as well as gene mutations for outcome in AML with inv(16)/t (16;16).

▶ As different cancer types get genomically sliced and diced, their increasing heterogeneity becomes almost unthinkable in terms of how to best apply molecularly targeted therapy. But the "groupers" have a trick up their sleeve that the "splitters" did not necessarily anticipate. That trick is pathway analysis and pathway-directed therapy. The report by Paschka et al covers both aspects of the process by diving deep into the secondary genetic lesions associated with the inv(16) or t(16;16) subtype of acute myeloid leukemia. They define multiple combinations of mutant genes plus additional chromosome abnormalities showing 41 sub-subtypes with only 8.4% of cases having no additional genetic lesions noted. However, all the subtypes could be broken down into essentially 3 major pathways or groups that included *RAS*, *KIT*, and *FLT3*. Clearly, even these have extensive overlap. Thus, although it might be assumed that genetic heterogeneity can be simplified in terms of targeted pathway-directed therapy, rigorous studies linking extensive genomic and functional studies to clinical responses to determine the contextual nature of response or no response will be needed to determine whether this approach will truly improve the lives of patients.

R. J. Arceci, MD, PhD

Sequential gain of mutations in severe congenital neutropenia progressing to acute myeloid leukemia
Beekman R, Valkhof MG, Sanders MA, et al (Erasmus Univ Med Ctr, Rotterdam, The Netherlands; et al)
Blood 119:5071-5077, 2012

Severe congenital neutropenia (SCN) is a BM failure syndrome with a high risk of progression to acute myeloid leukemia (AML). The underlying genetic changes involved in SCN evolution to AML are largely unknown. We obtained serial hematopoietic samples from an SCN patient who developed AML 17 years after the initiation of G-CSF treatment. Next-generation sequencing was performed to identify mutations during disease progression. In the AML phase, we found 12 acquired nonsynonymous mutations. Three of these, in *CSF3R*, *LLGL2*, and *ZC3H18*, co-occurred in a subpopulation of progenitor cells already in the early SCN phase. This population expanded over time, whereas clones harboring only CSF3R mutations disappeared from the BM. The other 9 mutations were only apparent in the AML cells and affected known AML-associated genes (*RUNX1* and *ASXL1*) and chromatin remodelers (*SUZ12* and *EP300*). In addition, a novel *CSF3R* mutation that conferred autonomous proliferation to myeloid progenitors was found. We conclude that progression from SCN to AML is a multistep process, with distinct mutations arising early during the SCN phase and others later in AML development. The sequential gain of 2 *CSF3R* mutations implicates abnormal G-CSF signaling as a driver of leukemic transformation in this case of SCN.

▶ Rare diseases continue to inform us about the basic biology of cancer. In the case of severe congenital neutropenia (SCN), also called *Kostmann syndrome*, there has been a known increased risk of acute myeloid leukemia (AML) development over time. Several inherited gene mutations have been associated with and are thought to be the cause of SCN, including the *ELANE* gene, which this patient had. Whether the use of granulocyte colony-stimulating factor (G-CSF) in such patients increases the incidence of the conversion to AML has been controversial but clinically important in terms of reducing the risk of infection.

Beekman et al now present genome-wide studies at different time points in a single patient with SCN. They observed early mutations, some of which were activating, of the CSF3R receptor, AC3H18, and LLGL2. Of particular interest was the observation that not all of the CSF3R receptor clones emerged but only one that subsequently developed a series of mutations in genes character-istic of AML. Although this patient required high doses of G-CSF, the case of one patient cannot answer that question of causality. Murine experiments with transgenic models have not been able to definitively link G-CSF exposure to the progression to leukemia. Nevertheless, this single-patient report should pave the way for similar analyses and hopefully a shared, worldwide database. Such a database will collect sufficient information that may provide clues to how best to follow up with such patients and their risk of leukemia based on identification of specific mutational events.

R. J. Arceci, MD, PhD

DNA methylation changes are a late event in acute promyelocytic leukemia and coincide with loss of transcription factor binding
Schoofs T, Rohde C, Hebestreit K, et al (Univ of Münster, Germany; et al)
Blood 121:178-187, 2013

The origin of aberrant DNA methylation in cancer remains largely unknown. In the present study, we elucidated the DNA methylome in primary acute promyelocytic leukemia (APL) and the role of promyelocytic leukemia—retinoic acid receptor α (PML-RARα) in establishing these patterns. Cells from APL patients showed increased genome-wide DNA methylation with higher variability than healthy CD34$^+$ cells, promyelo-cytes, and remission BM cells. A core set of differentially methylated regions in APL was identified. Age at diagnosis, Sanz score, and Flt3-mutation status characterized methylation subtypes. Transcription factor-binding sites (eg, the c-myc—binding sites) were associated with low methylation. However, SUZ12- and REST-binding sites identified in embryonic stem cells were pref-erentially DNA hypermethylated in APL cells. Unexpectedly, PML-RAR-α—binding sites were also protected from aberrant DNA methylation in APL cells. Consistent with this, myeloid cells from preleukemic PML-RARα knock-in mice did not show altered DNA methylation and the expression of PML-RARα in hematopoietic progenitor cells prevented differentiation without affecting DNA methylation. Treatment of APL blasts with all-*trans* retinoic acid also did not result in immediate DNA methylation changes. The results of the present study suggest that aberrant DNA methylation is associated with leukemia phenotype but is not required for PML-RARα—mediated initiation of leukemogenesis.

▶ The role of DNA methylation in cancer development has seen its ups and downs. Some reports have shown that altered methylation is a mechanism by which a second allele of a mutated tumor suppressor gene could be inactivated. Other reports have suggested that altered DNA methylation patterns are a secondary consequence of gene mutations and chromosomal translocation-generated fusion proteins. The report by Schoofs et al is one of the few that tries to provide a chronology to DNA methylation and function. They studied a series of patient samples of acute promyelocytic leukemia (APL). Altered DNA methylation patterns were able to be identified in key genes. These patterns, which include decreased methylation of transcription binding sites such as c-MYC, but also key embryonic stem cell genes, like SUZ12, showed increased methylation. However, induced differentiation of APL cells with all-trans retinoic acid did not show altered genomic methylation patterns. In addition, the initiation of APL by promyelocytic leukemia—retinoic acid receptor α in the murine APL model was also not associated with measurable genomic methylation changes. Although it is possible key methylation changes were not detected by the methods utilized, the results suggest that changes in DNA methylation patterns in APL are a later phenomenon and not required for the initiation of the leukemia. The therapeutic consequences of these observations are that histone—and not DNA methylatione—modifying drugs may provide a more rational approach to treatment in such cancers.

R. J. Arceci, MD, PhD

Dexamethasone exposure and asparaginase antibodies affect relapse risk in acute lymphoblastic leukemia

Kawedia JD, Liu C, Pei D, et al (St Jude Children's Res Hosp, Memphis, TN; et al)

Blood 119:1658-1664, 2012

We have previously hypothesized that higher systemic exposure to asparaginase may cause increased exposure to dexamethasone, both critical chemotherapeutic agents for acute lymphoblastic leukemia. Whether inter-patient pharmaco-kinetic differences in dexamethasone contribute to relapse risk has never been studied. The impact of plasma clearance of dexamethasone and anti—asparaginase antibody levels on risk of relapse was assessed in 410 children who were treated on a front-line clinical trial for acute lymphoblastic leukemia and were evaluable for all pharmacologic measures, using multivariate analyses, adjusting for standard clinical and biologic prognostic factors. Dexamethasone clearance (mean ± SD) was higher $(P = 3 \times 10^{-8})$ in patients whose sera was positive $(17.7 \pm 18.6$ L/h per m$^2)$ versus negative $(10.6 \pm 5.99$ L/h per m$^2)$ for anti—asparaginase antibodies. In multivariate analyses, higher dexamethasone clearance was associated with a higher risk of any relapse $(P = .01)$ and of central nervous system relapse $(P = .014)$. Central nervous system relapse was also more common in patients with anti-asparaginase antibodies $(P = .019)$. In conclusion, systemic clearance of dexamethasone is higher in patients with anti–asparaginase antibodies. Lower exposure to both drugs was associated with an increased risk of relapse.

▶ Predictive response biomarkers in leukemia continue to be an important area of investigation. Although molecular biomarkers have taken up a great deal of attention, less attention has been partitioned to pharmacologic markers. Kawedia et al report on the pharmacologic clearance of dexamethasone in children with acute lymphoblastic leukemia (ALL) who have or do not have antibodies against L-asparaginase. The observation was made previously by this group that those children with L-asparaginase antibodies had higher dexamethasone clearance, although it remains completely unclear in terms of mechanism and, thus, a persisting and simple association. However, in this report the authors show that increased clearance of dexamethasone is associated with an increased frequency of ALL relapse. Because there is such a tight association with dexamethasone clearance and L-asparaginase antibodies, it is less clear what the critical characteristic is, whether it be dexamethasone clearance or L-asparaginase antibodies. It should be noted that the analysis also did not attempt to utilize balanced learning and test cohorts. Nevertheless, finding approaches to identify and correct dexamethasone clearance would be important. The role of L-asparaginase antibodies in this remains elusive.

R. J. Arceci, MD, PhD

The genetic basis of early T-cell precursor acute lymphoblastic leukaemia
Zhang J, Ding L, Holmfeldt L, et al (St Jude Children's Res Hosp, Memphis, TN; The Genome Inst at Washington Univ, St Louis, MO; et al)
Nature 481:157-163, 2012

Early T-cell precursor acute lymphoblastic leukaemia (ETP ALL) is an aggressive malignancy of unknown genetic basis. We performed whole-genome sequencing of 12 ETP ALL cases and assessed the frequency of the identified somatic mutations in 94 T-cell acute lymphoblastic leukaemia cases. ETP ALL was characterized by activating mutations in genes regulating cytokine receptor and RAS signalling (67% of cases; *NRAS*, *KRAS*, *FLT3*, *IL7R*, *JAK3*, *JAK1*, *SH2B3* and *BRAF*), inactivating lesions disrupting haematopoietic development (58%; *GATA3*, *ETV6*, *RUNX1*, *IKZF1* and *EP300*) and histone-modifying genes (48%; *EZH2*, *EED*, *SUZ12*, *SETD2* and *EP300*). We also identified new targets of recurrent mutation including *DNM2*, *ECT2L* and *RELN*. The mutational spectrum is similar to myeloid tumours, and moreover, the global transcriptional profile of ETP ALL was similar to that of normal and myeloid leukaemia haematopoietic stem cells. These findings suggest that addition of myeloid-directed therapies might improve the poor outcome of ETP ALL.

▶ The molecular analysis of leukemia has helped to define an increasing number of distinct subtypes. Thymic-derived lymphoid leukemias and lymphomas have been known for many years to represent distinct immunophenotypes and clinical behavior. Zhang et al report on an extensive molecular analysis of what they now term *ETP ALL*, which is short for early T-cell precursor acute lymphoblastic leukemia (ALL). The gene mutation and ribonucleic acid expression patterns appeared to be more similar to that of acute myeloid leukemia (AML) and hematopoietic myeloid precursors, or as the authors state, closer to a myeloid stem cell leukemia. The results present a number of possible clinically actionable new targets for this subtype of ALL, which has quite a poor outcome. The suggestion of using cytarabine-based, AML-directed therapies may, however, have stretched the interpretation of the data to a thin breaking point, as even AML therapy has not been overwhelmingly effective in early stem cell disease. Nevertheless, this type of study is a superb example of providing the basis for further experimental work and ultimately clinical testing of new approaches.

R. J. Arceci, MD, PhD

---

inv(16)/t(16;16) acute myeloid leukemia with non−type A *CBFB-MYH11* fusions associate with distinct clinical and genetic features and lack *KIT* mutations

Schwind S, on behalf of the Alliance for Clinical Trials in Oncology (The Ohio State Univ Comprehensive Cancer Ctr, Columbus; et al)
Blood 121:385-391, 2013

The inv(16)(p13q22)/t(16;16)(p13;q22) in acute myeloid leukemia results in multiple *CBFB-MYH11* fusion transcripts, with type A being most frequent. The biologic and prognostic implications of different fusions are unclear. We analyzed *CBFB-MYH11* fusion types in 208 inv(16)/t(16;16) patients with de novo disease, and compared clinical and cytogenetic features and the *KIT* mutation status between type A ($n = 182$; 87%) and non−type A ($n = 26$; 13%) patients. At diagnosis, non−type A patients had lower white blood counts ($P = .007$), and more often trisomies of chromosomes 8 ($P = .01$) and 21 ($P < .001$) and less often trisomy 22 ($P = .02$). No patient with non−type A fusion carried a *KIT* mutation, whereas 27% of type A patients did ($P = .002$). Among the latter, *KIT* mutations conferred adverse prognosis; clinical outcomes of non−type A and type A patients with wild-type *KIT* were similar. We also derived a fusion-type-associated global gene-expression profile. Gene Ontology analysis of the differentially expressed genes revealed—among others—an enrichment of up-regulated genes involved in activation of caspase activity, cell differentiation and cell cycle control in non−type A patients. We conclude that non−type A fusions associate with distinct clinical and genetic features, including lack of *KIT* mutations, and a unique gene-expression profile.

▶ The inv(16)/t(16;16) subtype of acute myeloid leukemia (AML) has been known for decades and confers a favorable prognosis. Nevertheless, a subset of patients with this subtype is not cured, suggesting inherent differences associated with the good vs poor prognostic groups within this category of AML. Schwind et al examine 2 different types of inv(16) AML based on a type A vs non—type A *CBFB-MYH11* fusion. They show that not only did AML with a non—type A fusion not show mutations of *KIT*, but that the type A AML with *KIT* mutations had an inferior outcome. The presence of the *KIT* mutation was the distinguishing prognostic factor. Further, those with non—type A fusions showed a distinctive gene expression profile. So although the type of the *CBFB-MYH11* fusion can be partitioned with or without *KIT* mutations, it is unclear whether these observations are mechanistically linked or just an association. Regardless, the role of *KIT* in this subtype of AML remains a key prognostic factor.

R. J. Arceci, MD, PhD

Prognostic Relevance of Integrated Genetic Profiling in Acute Myeloid Leukemia
Patel JP, Gönen M, Figueroa ME, et al (Memorial Sloan-Kettering Cancer Ctr, NY; Weill Cornell Med College, NY; et al)
N Engl J Med 366:1079-1089, 2012

Background.—Acute myeloid leukemia (AML) is a heterogeneous disease with respect to presentation and clinical outcome. The prognostic value of recently identified somatic mutations has not been systematically evaluated in a phase 3 trial of treatment for AML.

Methods.—We performed a mutational analysis of 18 genes in 398 patients younger than 60 years of age who had AML and who were randomly assigned to receive induction therapy with high-dose or standard-dose daunorubicin. We validated our prognostic findings in an independent set of 104 patients.

Results.—We identified at least one somatic alteration in 97.3% of the patients. We found that internal tandem duplication in *FLT3 (FLT3-*ITD*)*, partial tandem duplication in *MLL (MLL*-PTD), and mutations in ASXL1 and PHF6 were associated with reduced overall survival ($P = 0.001$ for *FLT3*-ITD, $P = 0.009$ for *MLL*-PTD, $P = 0.05$ for *ASXL1*, and $P = 0.006$ for PHF6); *CEBPA* and *IDH2* mutations were associated with improved overall survival ($P = 0.05$ for *CEBPA* and $P = 0.01$ for *IDH2*). The favorable effect of NPM1 mutations was restricted to patients with co-occurring *NPM1* and *IDH1* or *IDH2* mutations. We identified genetic predictors of outcome that improved risk stratification among patients with AML, independently of age, white-cell count, induction dose, and post-remission therapy, and validated the significance of these predictors in an independent cohort. High-dose daunorubicin, as compared with standard-dose daunorubicin, improved the rate of survival among patients with *DNMT3A* or *NPM1* mutations or *MLL* translocations ($P = 0.001$) but not among patients with wild-type *DNMT3A*, *NPM1*, and *MLL* ($P = 0.67$).

Conclusions.—We found that *DNMT3A* and *NPM1* mutations and *MLL* translocations predicted an improved outcome with high-dose induction chemotherapy in patients with AML. These findings suggest that mutational profiling could potentially be used for risk stratification and to inform prognostic and therapeutic decisions regarding patients with AML. (Funded by the National Cancer Institute and others).

▶ Predicting the outcome for patients with leukemia to conventional chemotherapy remains a major challenge in oncology. Integrated analyses of mutational data from patients with acute myeloid leukemia (AML) have been studied, but the Patel et al analysis linked an in-depth study of 18 genes in a relatively select group of patients all older than 60 years of age. Nearly 100% of patient AML samples showed at least one somatic mutation in the group of genes studied. A subset of mutated genes, including some known players such as *FLT3-ITD* or partial duplications of *MLL*, and mutations of *ASX1* and *PHF6*, were all correlated with a reduced overall survival. Others, again mostly those correlated with good outcomes in a variety of studies, included mutations of *CEBPA*, *NPM1*, and IDH1/2. Of note, however, was the observation that the favorable impact of *NPM1* mutations occurred when present in conjunction with IDH1/2 mutations. In addition, a higher dose of daunorubicin appeared to improve the survival selectively in patients with AML characterized by mutations in *DMT3A*, *NPM1*, and *MLL* translocations. This held true regardless of other factors, including transplantation. So where does this leave us? Although interesting, without prospective analysis of a uniformly treated patient population, such information may not change practice. However, the data do point to the possibility of using such approaches to predict more accurately the responses to targeted agents in a clinically actionable timeframe. That would be real progress.

R. J. Arceci, MD, PhD

Retinoic Acid and Arsenic Trioxide for Acute Promyelocytic Leukemia
Lo-Coco F, for Gruppo Italiano Malattie Ematologiche dell'Adulto, the German—Austrian Acute Myeloid Leukemia Study Group, and Study Alliance Leukemia (Università Tor Vergata, Rome, Italy; et al)
N Engl J Med 369:111-121, 2013

Background.—All-*trans* retinoic acid (ATRA) with chemotherapy is the standard of care for acute promyelocytic leukemia (APL), resulting in cure rates exceeding 80%. Pilot studies of treatment with arsenic trioxide with or without ATRA have shown high efficacy and reduced hematologic toxicity.

Methods.—We conducted a phase 3, multicenter trial comparing ATRA plus chemotherapy with ATRA plus arsenic trioxide in patients with APL classified as low-to-intermediate risk (white-cell count, $\leq 10 \times 10^9$ per liter). Patients were randomly assigned to receive either ATRA plus arsenic trioxide for induction and consolidation therapy or standard ATRA—idarubicin induction therapy followed by three cycles of consolidation therapy with ATRA plus chemotherapy and maintenance therapy with low-dose chemotherapy and ATRA. The study was designed as a noninferiority trial to show that the difference between the rates of event-free survival at 2 years in the two groups was not greater than 5%.

Results.—Complete remission was achieved in all 77 patients in the ATRA—arsenic trioxide group who could be evaluated (100%) and in 75 of 79 patients in the ATRA—chemotherapy group (95%) (*P* = 0.12). The median follow-up was 34.4 months. Two-year event-free survival rates were 97% in the ATRA—arsenic trioxide group and 86% in the ATRA-chemotherapy group (95% confidence interval for the difference, 2 to 22 percentage points; *P* < 0.001 for noninferiority and *P* = 0.02 for superiority of ATRA—arsenic trioxide). Overall survival was also better with ATRA—arsenic trioxide (*P* = 0.02). As compared with ATRA—chemotherapy, ATRA—arsenic trioxide was associated with less hematologic toxicity and fewer infections but with more hepatic toxicity.

Conclusions.—ATRA plus arsenic trioxide is at least not inferior and may be superior to ATRA plus chemotherapy in the treatment of patients with low-to-intermediate-risk APL. (Funded by Associazione Italiana contro le Leucemie and others; ClinicalTrials.gov number, NCT00482833.)

▶ The introduction of targeted therapies for patients with acute promyelocytic leukemia (APL) has completely changed the former dismal outcomes for patients to some of the best overall survival in those with acute myeloid leukemias. Now the combination of such targeted therapies is continuing this approach with equally impressive findings. Lo-Coco et al report on a large, randomized trial for patients with low-/intermediate-risk APL to test whether the combination of retinoic acid and arsenic trioxide is at least as efficacious (designed as a noninferiority trial) as conventional therapy with retinoic acid plus chemotherapy followed by 2 years of retinoic acid and low-dose chemotherapy maintenance. The results clearly show that the retinoic acid plus arsenic combination is as efficacious as, and likely more effective than, the retinoic acid plus chemotherapy regimen. Toxicity was also less prevalent. This is a landmark study for sure. A remaining question is what the outcome for patients with high-risk disease will be.

R. J. Arceci, MD, PhD

The level of residual disease based on mutant *NPM1* is an independent prognostic factor for relapse and survival in AML
Shayegi N, on behalf of the Study Alliance Leukemia (SAL) (Universitätsklinikum Carl Gustav Carus der Technischen Universität, Dresden, Germany; et al)
Blood 122:83-92, 2013

Mutations of the *NPM1* gene (*NPM1^{mut}*) are among the most common genetic alterations in acute myeloid leukemia and are suitable for minimal residual disease detection. We retrospectively investigated the prognostic impact of $NPM1^{mut}$-based minimal residual disease detection from bone marrow for development of relapse by using a newly developed real-time polymerase chain reaction based on locked nucleic acid—containing primers in 174 patients, 155 of whom were treated within prospective protocols. The prognostic value of 5 cutoff values after completion of treatment or after allogeneic transplantation was studied by using cause-specific hazard models. Subsequent validation using cross-validated partial likelihood analysis revealed that an increase of more than 1% $NPM1^{mut}/ABL1$ was most prognostic for relapse after chemotherapy, whereas an increase of more than 10% $NPM1^{mut}/ABL1$ was most prognostic for relapse after allogeneic transplantation. Univariate and multivariate analysis of disease-free survival and overall survival revealed a significantly worse outcome in patients with >1% $NPM1^{mut}/ABL1$ and >10% $NPM1^{mut}ABL1$, respectively, which remained significant after adjustment for $FLT3$—internal tandem duplication status. Our results in a large data set define and optimize cutoff values for early diagnosis of molecular relapse. These results may be especially important for defining triggers for early therapeutic intervention.

▶ The ability to determine minimal residual disease (MRD) in patients with leukemia using several flow cytometric or molecular methods has become an essential aspect of risk stratifying patients. However, several issues have partly compromised the use of MRD, including the loss of some markers, the lack of a stable marker across all of the different subtypes, and the varying sensitivity of the detection method. In addition, most MRD markers are based on sampling the bone marrow. While mutant $NPM1$ is found in up to about 60% of adult patients with normal karyotype acute myeloid leukemia (AML), it is found in about one-third of all adult AML. The report by Shayegi et al shows that detection of $NPM1$ mutation in morphologic remission bone marrow is able to predict the chance of relapse. Of interest, greater than 1% and greater than 10% mutant $NPM1$ to ABL (used to normalize values) are the optimal for bone marrow after chemotherapy only and bone marrow transplantation, respectively. An explanation for this difference is uncertain, but a possibility is that an antileukemia allogeneic immune response may be able to omit lower levels of MRD. Using peripheral blood proved less sensitive than using bone marrow MRD measurement. Thus, detection of $NPM1$ mutations appears to be another tool in the MRD toolbox. The stability of the marker suggests that it represents a leukemia driver mutation. Nevertheless, the Holy Grail of finding a pan-leukemia subtype MRD marker that predicts relapse 100% of the time remains elusive.

R. J. Arceci, MD, PhD

Clonal evolution in relapsed *NPM1*-mutated acute myeloid leukemia

Krönke J, Bullinger L, Teleanu V, et al (Univ of Ulm, Germany; et al)
Blood 122:100-108, 2013

Mutations in the nucleophosmin 1 (*NPM1*) gene are considered a founder event in the pathogenesis of acute myeloid leukemia (AML). To address the role of clonal evolution in relapsed *NPM1*-mutated (*NPM1^{mut}*) AML, we applied high-resolution, genome-wide, single-nucleotide polymorphism array profiling to detect copy number alterations (CNAs) and uniparental disomies (UPDs) and performed comprehensive gene mutation screening in 53 paired bone marrow/peripheral blood samples obtained at diagnosis and relapse. At diagnosis, 15 aberrations (CNAs, n = 10; UPDs, n = 5) were identified in 13 patients (25%), whereas at relapse, 56 genomic alterations (CNAs, n = 46; UPDs, n = 10) were detected in 29 patients (55%) indicating an increase in genomic complexity. Recurrent aberrations acquired at relapse included deletions affecting tumor suppressor genes (*ETV6* [n = 3], *TP53* [n = 2], *NF1* [n = 2], *WT1* [n = 3], *FHIT* [n = 2]) and homozygous *FLT3* mutations acquired via UPD13q (n = 7). *DNMT3A* mutations (*DNMT3A^{mut}*) showed the highest stability (97%). Persistence of *DNMT3A^{mut}* in 5 patients who lost *NPM1^{mut}* at relapse suggests that *DNMT3A^{mut}* may precede *NPM1^{mut}* in AML pathogenesis. Of note, all relapse samples shared at least 1 genetic aberration with the matched primary AML sample, implying common ancestral clones. In conclusion, our study reveals novel insights into clonal evolution in *NPM1^{mut}* AML.

▶ The molecular heterogeneity of cancer has become more evident with the application of genomic sequencing and gene copy number arrays to the problem. The implications of such heterogeneity are that various clones with different drug sensitivities may be present at the initiation of treatment and then be selected for by the treatment or that new clones with varying drug sensitivities may arise during treatment. In either case, the eradication of such clones would appear key to providing effective curative therapies. Krönke et al analyze in considerable depth a cohort of patient acute myeloid leukemia (AML) samples to examine this question. They observe that the most stable mutations (ie, at diagnosis and relapse) include mutations in *DNMT3a* followed by *NPM1* and *IDH2*. Other genes that are more likely to acquire mutations or alternations include *NRAS*, *FLT3*, and *IDH1* along with changes in copy number of selected genomic regions. They conclude from these results that *DNMT3a* is possibly one of, if not the, earliest mutational events in this subset of AML. It is somewhat unclear, however, if the stability of *DNMT3a* is simply more critical to the leukemia survival. This is even more interesting if one assumes, backed by some experimental evidence, that many of the epigenetic patterns established by alterations of DNA methyl transferases are stable over many generations. Thus, once the epigenetic pattern is established, why does the *DNMT3a* mutation need to be so stable over time? It might be of some interest to examine the stability of such downstream epigenetic changes in experimental systems as well as in patient samples.

R. J. Arceci, MD, PhD

Epigenetic silencing of *microRNA-193a* contributes to leukemogenesis in t(8;21) acute myeloid leukemia by activating the *PTEN*/PI3K signal pathway

Li Y, Gao L, Luo X, et al (Chinese PLA General Hosp, Beijing, China; et al)
Blood 121:499-509, 2013

---

t(8;21) is one of the most frequent chromosomal translocations occurring in acute myeloid leukemia (AML) and is considered the leukemia-initiating event. The biologic and clinical significance of microRNA dysregulation associated with AML1/ETO expressed in t(8;21) AML is unknown. Here, we show that AML1/ETO triggers the heterochromatic silencing of *microRNA-193a* (*miR-193a*) by binding at AML1-binding sites and recruiting chromatin-remodeling enzymes. Suppression of *miR-193a* expands the oncogenic activity of the fusion protein AML-ETO, because *miR-193a* represses the expression of multiple target genes, such as *AML1/ETO, DNMT3a, HDAC3, KIT, CCND1*, and *MDM2* directly, and increases *PTEN* indirectly. Enhanced *miR-193a* levels induce G_1 arrest, apoptosis, and restore leukemic cell differentiation. Our study identifies *miR-193a* and *PTEN* as targets for AML1/ETO and provides evidence that links the epigenetic silencing of tumor suppressor genes *miR-193a* and *PTEN* to differentiation block of myeloid precursors. Our results indicated a feedback circuitry involving *miR-193a* and *AML1/ETO/DNMTs/HDACs*, cooperating with the *PTEN*/PI3K signaling pathway and contributing to leukemogenesis in vitro and in vivo, which can be successfully targeted by pharmacologic disruption of the *AML1/ETO/DNMTs/HDACs* complex or enhancement of *miR-193a* in t(8;21)—leukemias.

▶ The role of microRNAs in cancer has mostly been a result of suggested function based on altered expression patterns. Few functional pathways have shown a clear role for microRNAs in cancer, but the Li et al report is an exception. The study shows first that microRNA 193a (miR-193a) is a direct target of the AML1/ETO fusion protein generated from the classic driver translocation t(8;21). The epigenetic silencing of miR-193a results in enhanced expression of the fusion itself, *DNMT3a, HDAC3, KIT, CCND1*, and *MDM2* as well as the AML1/ETO silencing of the PTEN promoter. The overall results indicate upregulation of the cytokine driven *c-KIT* receptor and activation of PI3K signaling. Reintroduction of miR-193a by transduction of the RNA into a leukemia cell line induced some degree of differentiation antigen expression, decreased growth, and increased apoptosis. The study shows important targets of AML1/ETO targeting that have direct impact as drivers of this subtype of acute myeloid leukemia and further provides some specific targets for epigenetic re-engineering.

R. J. Arceci, MD, PhD

A phase 3 study of gemtuzumab ozogamicin during induction and postconsolidation therapy in younger patients with acute myeloid leukemia

Petersdorf SH, Kopecky KJ, Slovak M, et al (Fred Hutchinson Cancer Res Ctr, Seattle, WA)

Blood 121:4854-4860, 2013

This randomized phase 3 clinical trial evaluated the potential benefit of the addition of gemtuzumab ozogamicin (GO) to standard induction and postconsolidation therapy in patients with acute myeloid leukemia. Patients were randomly assigned to receive daunorubicin (45 mg/m(2) per day on days 1, 2, and 3), cytarabine (100 mg/m(2) per day by continuous infusion on days 1-7), and GO (6 mg/m(2) on day 4; DA+GO) vs standard induction therapy with daunorubicin (60 mg/m(2) per day on days 1, 2, and 3) and cytarabine alone (DA). Patients who achieved complete remission (CR) received 3 courses of high-dose cytarabine. Those remaining in CR after consolidation were randomly assigned to receive either no additional therapy or 3 doses of GO (5 mg/m(2) every 28 days). From August 2004 until August 2009, 637 patients were registered for induction. The CR rate was 69% for DA+GO and 70% for DA ($P =.59$). Among those who achieved a CR, the 5-year relapse-free survival rate was 43% in the DA+GO group and 42% in the DA group ($P =.40$). The 5-year overall survival rate was 46% in the DA+GO group and 50% in the DA group ($P =.85$). One hundred seventy-four patients in CR after consolidation underwent the postconsolidation randomization. Disease-free survival was not improved with postconsolidation GO (HR, 1.48; $P =.97$). In this study, the addition of GO to induction or postconsolidation therapy failed to show improvement in CR rate, disease-free survival, or overall survival. This trial is registered with www.clinicaltrials.gov as #NCT00085709.

▶ The introduction of new, effective agents that do not show similar toxicity profiles to chemotherapy for patients with acute myeloid leukemia (AML) has been particularly challenging. The introduction of gemtuzumab ozogamicin (GO), a toxin-conjugated monoclonal antibody directed against CD33, a myeloid differentiation antigen, showed efficacy in phase I and II trials of adult and pediatric patients with relapsed/refractory disease. Although toxicities were noted, especially relating to liver and bone marrow, the antibody was well tolerated overall and, thus, likely to satisfy the requirements of added efficacy without significantly increased toxicity. The randomized phase III study by Petersdorf et al unfortunately was not able to find added benefit in the cohort of patients receiving GO, but the rate of fatal nonhematologic induction toxicity was significantly higher in the group that received GO. These results stand in contrast to reports from the United Kingdom and Europe that have shown significant overall survival and relapse-free benefit in randomized studies for patients allocated to receive GO. So what, if anything, went wrong with the Petersdorf et al study? First, it is unfortunate that the study reduced daunorubicin from 60 mg/m^2 in the standard arm to 45 mg/m^2 in the GO arm. From one point of view, the study could conclude that GO allowed the reduction of anthracycline exposure. But then the significant increase in induction mortality in the GO cohort needs to be recognized. Was this a statistical aberration? Regardless of one's interpretation, the results were not compelling enough to stop the US Food and Drug Administration from nixing the further approval of GO. In the United Kingdom and Europe, the use of GO, at least in some patients with selective subtypes of AML, is accepted as a standard of care now. Clearly, much needs to be learned. Perhaps the randomized pediatric trial testing GO will provide further insight into what was once a promising drug for AML and may still have a heartbeat worth resuscitating.

R. J. Arceci, MD, PhD

10 Thoracic Cancer

Biology

Lung Cancer That Harbors a *HER2* Mutation: Epidemiologic Characteristics and Therapeutic Perspectives
Mazières J, Peters S, Lepage B, et al (Hôpital Larrey, Toulouse, France; Centre Hospitalier Universitaire Vaudois, Lausanne, Switzerland; Centre Hospitalier Universitaire Toulouse, France; et al)
J Clin Oncol 2013 [Epub ahead of print]

Purpose.—*HER2* mutations are identified in approximately 2% of non–small-cell lung cancers (NSCLC). There are few data available that describe the clinical course of patients with *HER2*-mutated NSCLC.

Patients and Methods.—We retrospectively identified 65 NSCLC, diagnosed with a *HER2* in-frame insertion in exon 20. We collected clinicopathologic characteristics, patients' outcomes, and treatments.

Results.—*HER2* mutation was identified in 65 (1.7%) of 3,800 patients tested and was almost an exclusive driver, except for one single case with a concomitant *KRAS* mutation. Our population presented with a median age of 60 years (range, 31 to 86 years), a high proportion of women (45 women v 20 men; 69%), and a high proportion of never-smokers (n = 34; 52.3%). All tumors were adenocarcinomas and 50% were stage IV at diagnosis. For these latter cases, 22 anti–human epidermal growth factor receptor 2 (HER2) treatments were administered after conventional chemotherapy in 16 patients. Subsequently, four patients experienced progressive disease, seven experienced disease stabilizations, and 11 experienced partial responses (overall response rate, 50%; disease control rate [DCR], 82%). Specifically, we observed a DCR of 93% for trastuzumab-based therapies (n = 15) and a DCR of 100% for afatinib (n = 3) but no response to other HER2-targeted drugs (n = 3). Progression-free survival for patients with HER2 therapies was 5.1 months. Median survival was of 89.6 and 22.9 months for early-stage and stage IV patients, respectively.

Conclusion.—This study, the largest to date dedicated to *HER2*-mutated NSCLC, reinforces the importance of screening for *HER2* mutations in lung adenocarcinomas and suggests the potential efficacy of HER2-targeted drugs in this population.

▶ In the era of genomic sequencing, subgroups of patients are emerging with unique gene mutations or amplifications that are potentially targetable with novel agents. The authors reported on the largest series of *HER2*-mutated patients (in frame exon 20 insertion) and showed significant clinical benefit with the use of *HER2*-targeted agents (trastuzumab and afatinib).

This study is important for the lung cancer field because earlier trials using *HER2*-directed therapies (ie, trastuzumab) were resoundingly negative in non–small cell lung cancer patients with HER2 protein overexpression (by immunohistochemistry) or *HER2* gene amplification (by fluorescence in situ hybridization). This was in contrast to the breast cancer literature, and enthusiasm for *HER2*-directed therapies in lung cancer waned. This study reopens the issue by identifying a population of patients with a specific mutation in the *HER2* gene (which occurs in 1.7%-2% of all lung cancer patients). This initial report indicates that these *HER2* mutants are more likely to be women, never-smokers, and adenocarcinomas (some lepidic pattern). These patients have a response to *HER2*-directed therapies (trastuzumab or afatinib), and this study provides support that *HER2* exon 20 insertion mutations should be included in the lung cancer genomic profile analysis. Ongoing trials with pertuzumab (unselected) and trastuzumab (*HER2* mutation selected) will hopefully provide more definitive results in the near future.

A. S. Tsao, MD

Effect of crizotinib on overall survival in patients with advanced non-small-cell lung cancer harbouring *ALK* gene rearrangement: a retrospective analysis
Shaw AT, Yeap BY, Solomon BJ, et al (Massachusetts General Hosp Cancer Ctr, Boston; Peter MacCallum Cancer Centre, Melbourne, Victoria, Australia; et al)
Lancet Oncol 12:1004-1012, 2011

Background.—*ALK* gene rearrangement defines a new molecular subtype of non-small-cell lung cancer (NSCLC). In a recent phase 1 clinical trial, the ALK tyrosine-kinase inhibitor (TKI) crizotinib showed marked antitumour activity in patients with advanced, ALK-positive NSCLC. To assess whether crizotinib affects overall survival in these patients, we did a retrospective study comparing survival outcomes in crizotinib-treated patients in the trial and crizotinib-naive controls screened during the same time period.

Methods.—We examined overall survival in patients with advanced, ALK-positive NSCLC who enrolled in the phase 1 clinical trial of crizotinib, focusing on the cohort of 82 patients who had enrolled through Feb 10, 2010. For comparators, we identified 36 ALK-positive patients from trial sites who were not given crizotinib (ALK-positive controls), 67 patients without *ALK* rearrangement but positive for *EGFR* mutation, and 253 wild-type patients lacking either *ALK* rearrangement or *EGFR* mutation. To assess differences in overall survival, we assessed subsets of clinically comparable ALK-positive and ALK-negative patients.

Findings.—Among 82 ALK-positive patients who were given crizotinib, median overall survival from initiation of crizotinib has not been reached (95% CI 17 months to not reached); 1-year overall survival was 74% (95% CI 63—82), and 2-year overall survival was 54% (40—66). Overall survival did not differ based on age, sex, smoking history, or ethnic origin. Survival in 30 ALK-positive patients who were given crizotinib in the second-line or third-line setting was significantly longer than in 23 ALK-positive controls given any second-line therapy (median overall survival not reached [95% CI 14 months to not reached] *vs* 6 months [4—17], 1-year overall survival 70% [95% CI 50—83] *vs* 44% [23—64], and 2-year overall survival 55% [33—72] *vs* 12% [2—30]; hazard ratio 0·36, 95% CI 0·17—0·75; $p = 0·004$). Survival in 56 crizotinib-treated, ALK-positive patients was similar to that in 63 ALK-negative, EGFR-positive patients given EGFR TKI therapy (median overall survival not reached [95% CI 17 months to not reached] *vs* 24 months [15—34], 1-year overall survival 71% [95% CI 58—81] *vs* 74% [61—83], and 2-year overall survival 57% [40—71] *vs* 52% [38—65]; $p = 0·786$), whereas survival in 36 crizotinib-naive, ALK-positive controls was similar to that in 253 wild-type controls (median overall survival 20 months [95% CI 13—26] *vs* 15 months [13—17]; $p = 0·244$).

Interpretation.—In patients with advanced, ALK-positive NSCLC, crizotinib therapy is associated with improved survival compared with that of crizotinib-naive controls. *ALK* rearrangement is not a favourable prognostic factor in advanced NSCLC.

▶ This is a retrospective study comparing different cohorts of patients who were either screened for a phase I crizotinib trial or were identified via genetic screening at participating sites. Despite its inherent limitations, this is an important study for 2 reasons. First, it clearly demonstrates that echinoderm microtubule-associated protein-like 4 anaplastic lymphoma kinase (ALK) is a negative prognostic factor, and standard noncrizotinib salvage therapies are not as effective in this population of patients. Second, it is vital to identify these patients as early as possible and give them crizotinib treatment.

In this study, there were only 6 patients (11%) who received frontline crizotinib therapy and the numbers were too small to analyze. But the authors proceeded to do a comparative analysis focused on patients from the second-line and third-line setting and showed that ALK-positive patients who received crizotinib had a much longer overall survival rate than those ALK-positive patients treated only with chemotherapy. One can extrapolate that getting the right drug to the mutated patient earlier will ultimately improve his or her clinical outcome. The US Food and Drug Administration (FDA) agreed with this concept, because crizotinib is now an FDA-approved agent for all lines of therapy, although there has only been a salvage trial completed demonstrating overall survival benefit. Currently, it is highly recommended to identify ALK-mutated patients early on and treat them as soon as possible with crizotinib. It is becoming standard practice to screen all adenocarcinomas for genetic mutations, but as described in other studies, the ALK-positive patients are younger (median age 51 years) than the epidermal growth factor receptor (*EGFR*) mutation and *EGFR* wild-type ALK-negative control non—small cell lung cancer patients, and they tended to have adenocarcinomas with never less than 10 pack-year smoking histories.

A. S. Tsao, MD

Natural History and Molecular Characteristics of Lung Cancers Harboring *EGFR* Exon 20 Insertions
Oxnard GR, Lo PC, Nishino M, et al (Dana-Farber Cancer Inst, Boston, MA; Dana-Farber Cancer Inst and Brigham and Women's Hosp, Boston, MA)
J Thorac Oncol 8:179-184, 2013

Introduction.—Exon 20 insertions are the third most common family of epidermal growth factor receptor (*EGFR*) mutations found in non—small-cell lung cancer (NSCLC). Little is known about cancers harboring these mutations aside from their lack of response to *EGFR* tyrosine kinase inhibitors, impairing the development of effective targeted therapies.

Methods.—NSCLC patients with *EGFR* genotyping were studied using a mechanism approved by the Institutional Review Board. Cancers with exon 20 insertions were indentified, sequences were characterized, and effectiveness of different treatment regimens was reviewed retrospectively. Clinical characteristics and survival were compared with cancers harboring common *EGFR* mutations and cancers with wild-type *EGFR*.

Results.—One thousand eighty-six patients underwent *EGFR* genotyping from 2004 to 2012. Twenty seven (2.5%) harbored exon 20 insertions, making up 9.2% of all cancers with documented *EGFR* mutations. Compared with wild-type cancers, those with exon 20 insertions were more commonly found in never-smokers and Asian patients. Insertion sequences were highly variable, with the most common variant (V769_D770insASV) making up only 22% of cases. Median survival of patients with exon 20 insertions was 16 months, similar to the survival of wild-type cancers and shorter than the survival of cancers with common *EGFR* mutations.

Conclusions.—Patients with *EGFR* exon 20 insertions have similar clinical characteristics to those with common *EGFR* mutations but a poorer prognosis. The prevalence of this subset of NSCLC is similar to that of other genotype-defined subsets of lung adenocarcinoma (e.g. those with *BRAF* mutations, *HER2* insertions, *ROS1* rearrangements) and is a population of interest for trials of new targeted therapies.

▶ There are 3 epidermal growth factor receptor (*EGFR*) mutations that dominate the field: the 2 sensitive mutations (deletion exon 19 and exon 21 L858) and the resistance mutation T790M (mostly acquired resistance mutation in exon 20). These 3 mutations comprise over 85% of all the de novo *EGFR* mutations that are seen in non—small cell lung cancer. However, the rarer *EGFR* mutations often make an appearance, and it is unknown what the optimal therapy is for these patients.

These authors reported on 27 exon 20 insertion patients and their clinical outcomes. This is one of the largest series collected on this group of patients, and it shows that the insertion sequences were highly variable and survival rate was not as high as those seen with sensitive *EGFR* mutations. In preclinical models, exon 20 insertions have been found to be resistant to EGFR tyrosine kinase inhibitors, but few clinical trials have been able to discern the actual response and survival outcomes for this group of patients. In this study (which was partly retrospective), there were 8 exon 20 insertion patients who received erlotinib therapy. Their median time to treatment failure was 2.4 months, and in the 5 patients with available radiographic images, there were no radiographic responses. It remains to be seen whether the irreversible EGFR tyrosine kinase inhibitors will be more beneficial for this group of patients or whether Hsp90 inhibitors will be useful. Hsp90 inhibitors have shown preliminary benefit against oncogene-addicted tumors refractory to initial tyrosine kinase inhibition.

A. S. Tsao, MD

Mechanisms of Acquired Crizotinib Resistance in ALK-Rearranged Lung Cancers

Katayama R, Shaw AT, Khan TM, et al (Massachusetts General Hosp Cancer Ctr, Boston; et al)
Sci Transl Med 4:120ra17, 2012

Most anaplastic lymphoma kinase (*ALK*)−positive non−small cell lung cancers (NSCLCs) are highly responsive to treatment with ALK tyrosine kinase inhibitors (TKIs). However, patients with these cancers invariably relapse, typically within 1 year, because of the development of drug resistance. Herein, we report findings from a series of lung cancer patients ($n = 18$) with acquired resistance to the ALK TKI crizotinib. In about one-fourth of patients, we identified a diverse array of secondary mutations distributed throughout the *ALK* TK domain, including new resistance mutations located in the solvent-exposed region of the adenosine triphosphate−binding pocket, as well as amplification of the *ALK* fusion gene. Next-generation ALK inhibitors, developed to overcome crizotinib resistance, had differing potencies against specific resistance mutations. In addition to secondary *ALK* mutations and *ALK* gene amplification, we also identified aberrant activation of other kinases including marked amplification of *KIT* and increased autophosphorylation of epidermal growth factor receptor in drug-resistant tumors from patients. In a subset of patients, we found evidence of multiple resistance mechanisms developing simultaneously. These results highlight the unique features of TKI resistance in *ALK*-positive NSCLCs and provide the rationale for pursuing combinatorial therapeutics that are tailored to the precise resistance mechanisms identified in patients who relapse on crizotinib treatment.

▶ The identification of echinoderm microtubule-associated protein-like 4 (EML4) anaplastic lymphoma kinase (ALK) mutations and the beneficial effect of crizotinib have revolutionized lung cancer therapy. Unfortunately, the significant clinical benefits are not sustainable, and ALK patients on crizotinib will often progress with disease at 10 months.

This study is a critical step in advancing the field in resistance mechanisms for EML4 ALK patients. The subsequent biopsies from the 18 patients refractory to crizotinib demonstrated that 22% had secondary ALK mutations in the tyrosine kinase domain (3 new mutations and on ALK fusion gene amplification) and 50% had a bypass or alternate pathway activation (epidermal growth factor receptor and KIT, including *KIT* gene amplification). This study emphasizes the vital need to rebiopsy patients at the time of disease progression because, ultimately, different therapies will likely be needed based on the resistance mechanism. Even in crizotinib-refractory ALK patients who have secondary mutations in the *ALK* gene, there have been differential responses to the second-generation ALK inhibitors. Mutations in G1202R and 1151Tins both have high resistance to crizotinib and to the second-generation ALK inhibitors in preclinical models. These patients may be more likely to benefit from Hsp90 inhibitors. Patients with alternate bypass pathway activation will likely require dual inhibition, yet the sequence of treatment and dosing is unknown. Currently, the exact and optimal therapeutic options for these crizotinib-refractory EML4 ALK patients have yet to be elucidated, and this study demonstrates how complicated this process will be.

A. S. Tsao, MD

Genotypic and Histological Evolution of Lung Cancers Acquiring Resistance to EGFR Inhibitors
Sequist LV, Waltman BA, Dias-Santagata D, et al (Massachusetts General Hosp Cancer Ctr, Boston; Harvard Med School, Boston, MA; et al)
Sci Transl Med 3:75ra26, 2011

Lung cancers harboring mutations in the epidermal growth factor receptor (*EGFR*) respond to EGFR tyrosine kinase inhibitors, but drug resistance invariably emerges. To elucidate mechanisms of acquired drug resistance, we performed systematic genetic and histological analyses of tumor biopsies from 37 patients with drug-resistant non–small cell lung cancers (NSCLCs) carrying *EGFR* mutations. All drug-resistant tumors retained their original activating *EGFR* mutations, and some acquired known mechanisms of resistance including the *EGFR* T790M mutation or *MET* gene amplification. Some resistant cancers showed unexpected genetic changes including EGFR amplification and mutations in the *PIK3CA* gene, whereas others underwent a pronounced epithelial-to-mesenchymal transition. Surprisingly, five resistant tumors (14%) transformed from NSCLC into small cell lung cancer (SCLC) and were sensitive to standard SCLC treatments. In three patients, serial biopsies revealed that genetic mechanisms of resistance were lost in the absence of the continued selective pressure of EGFR inhibitor treatment, and such cancers were sensitive to a second round of treatment with EGFR inhibitors. Collectively, these results deepen our understanding of resistance to EGFR inhibitors and underscore the importance of repeatedly assessing cancers throughout the course of the disease.

▶ This article is a critical initiative that emphasizes the importance of rebiopsying after development of disease resistance. Sequist et al assessed 37 patients with non–small cell lung cancer who had activating epidermal growth factor receptor (*EGFR*) mutations, were on EGFR tyrosine kinase inhibitors (TKIs), and developed disease resistance. The rebiopsy specimen results showed a surprising range of mechanisms of resistance, including transformation to small cell lung cancer (SCLC), accumulation of second point mutations in *EGFR* T790M or PI3KCA, and *MET* or *EGFR* gene amplifications (Fig 1 in the original article). Patients who have activating *EGFR* gene mutations (del exon 19, L858) can usually remain on EGFR TKI for years with intermittent chemotherapy challenges. The optimal treatment (ie, remain on EGFR TKI or not) has not been established, and we now realize this is largely because the mechanisms of resistance have clearly varied with each individual patient. Additional reports have noted that some patients with T790M acquired resistance benefit with irreversible EGFR inhibitors, such as afatinib or the combination of afatinib with cetuximab. Other patients whose disease transforms to SCLC are treated with platinum-etoposide and revert back to having sensitivity to EGFR TKIs. This article clearly defines the necessary role of rebiopsying our *EGFR* mutation patients once resistance to EGFR TKI develops, as the salvage therapies can be optimized to their respective disease. Eventually, the *EGFR* mutation patients will continue to be treated with sequential targeted agents or chemotherapy based on their individual tumor genetic profile that evolves over time.

A. S. Tsao, MD

Fibroblast Growth Factor Receptor 1 Gene Amplification Is Associated With Poor Survival and Cigarette Smoking Dosage in Patients With Resected Squamous Cell Lung Cancer

Kim HR, Kim DJ, Kang DR, et al (Yonsei Univ College of Medicine, Seoul, Republic of Korea; et al)
J Clin Oncol 31:731-737, 2013

Purpose.—To investigate the frequency and the prognostic role of fibroblast growth factor receptor 1 (*FGFR1*) amplification in patients with surgically resected squamous cell carcinoma of the lung (SCCL) and the association between smoking and *FGFR1* amplification.

Patients and Methods.—Gene copy number of *FGFR1* was investigated in microarrayed tumors from 262 patients with SCCL who had tumor tissue as well as smoking and survival data available. Gene copy number was evaluated by fluorescent in situ hybridization, and an *FGFR1*-amplified tumor (*FGFR1* amp⁺) was prespecified as a tumor with nine or more copies of *FGFR1*.

Results.—Among 262 patients, the frequency of *FGFR1* amp⁺ was 13.0%. Patients with *FGFR1* amp⁺ had significantly shorter disease-free survival (DFS; 26.9 *v* 94.6 months; $P < .001$) as well as shorter overall survival (OS; 51.2 *v* 115.0 months; $P = .002$) than those without *FGFR1* amp⁺. Multivariate modeling confirmed that patients with *FGFR1* amp⁺ had a significantly greater risk of recurrence and death than those without *FGFR1* amp⁺ after adjusting for sex, smoking status, pathologic stage, and adjuvant chemotherapy (DFS: adjusted hazard ratio [AHR], 2.24; 95% CI, 1.45 to 3.45; $P < .001$; OS: AHR, 1.83; 95% CI, 1.15 to 2.89; $P = .01$). The frequency of *FGFR1* amp⁺ was significantly higher in current smokers than in former smokers and never-smokers (28.9% *v* 2.5% *v* 0%; $P_{trend} < .001$). As the smoking dosage increased, so did the incidence of *FGFR1* amp⁺ ($P_{trend} = .002$).

Conclusion.—*FGFR1* amplification is an independent negative prognostic factor in surgically resected SCCL and is associated with cigarette smoking in a dose-dependent manner. *FGFR1* amplification is a relevant therapeutic target in Asian patients with SCCL.

▶ Fibroblast growth factor receptor 1 (*FGFR1*) amplification in squamous cell carcinoma (SCC) of the lung has come under significant scrutiny after several articles showed the incidence of *FGFR1* amplification to be close to 20% in SCC.[1,2] The preclinical models of *FGFR1*-amplified cancer cells indicate that these cells are reliant on the *FGFR1* signaling pathway and are, therefore, potentially actionable with a targeted agent.

The Korean authors of this article reported a 13% incidence of *FGFR* amplification in 262 SCC patients (stages I to IIIB between the years 1998 and 2009) who underwent resections at their institution. This was a heterogeneous group of patients with differing stages and only half receiving adjuvant chemotherapy (starting after 2004). The authors reasonably concluded that *FGFR1* gene amplification was associated with higher smoking rates and worse clinical outcomes (shorter disease-free survival and overall survival). However, there were a few surprising findings in this article.

First, the authors reported 8 epidermal growth factor receptor-mutated and 2 *KRAS*-mutated SCC patients among 262 total patients. Because these mutations are more typically seen in adenocarcinomas, one should be concerned about the rigor of the pathologic histology review. Did some mixed histologies enter the study? Second, the authors reported in the multivariate analysis that adjuvant chemotherapy did not prolong overall survival except in stage II patients. They also reported that the 118 patients with no *FGFR* gene amplification had no benefit to adjuvant chemotherapy, whereas the 19 *FGFR1* gene amplified patients who received adjuvant chemotherapy did. This is not what one would expect given the literature and phase III clinical trial data, and it lends some concern to the overall analysis reported by the authors.

So, in a nutshell, *FGFR1* gene amplification is seen in SCC of the lung and may be a valuable target. The gene amplification appears to vary by geographic location: 20% Western Caucasian, 13% Korean, and 41% in the Japanese group (using polymerase chain reaction instead of florescence in situ hybridization as in the other groups). Most of these studies have been performed on retrospective tissue banks, and the true incidence will need to be identified with larger datasets and prospective collection of data. I think this study has merit with the correlation of higher smoking rates to the *FGFR1* gene amplification; however, the adjuvant chemotherapy effects remain unexplained and run contrary to the literature, and these data should not be used to make treatment decisions.

A. S. Tsao, MD

References

1. Dutt A, Ramos AH, Hammerman PS, et al. Inhibitor-sensitive FGFR1 amplification in human non-small cell lung cancer. *PLoS One.* 2011;6:e20351.
2. Weiss J, Sos ML, Seidel D, et al. Frequent and focal FGFR1 amplification associates with therapeutically tractable FGFR1 dependency in squamous cell lung cancer. *Sci Transl Med.* 2010;2:62ra93.

First Line Metastatic Non–Small-Cell Lung Cancer

Randomized Phase II Study of Ixabepilone or Paclitaxel Plus Carboplatin in Patients With Non–Small-Cell Lung Cancer Prospectively Stratified by Beta-3 Tubulin Status

Edelman MJ, Schneider C-P, Tsai C-M, et al (Univ of Maryland Greenebaum Cancer Ctr, Baltimore, MD; Zentralklinik Bad Berka, Germany; Taipei Veterans General Hosp, Taiwan; et al)
J Clin Oncol 2013 [Epub ahead of print]

Purpose.—Retrospective studies have reported that tumor expression of the beta-3 tubulin (β3T) isoform is an unfavorable prognostic factor in non–small-cell lung cancer (NSCLC) treated with tubulininhibiting chemotherapy. Ixabepilone is a tubulin-inhibiting agent with low susceptibility to multiple resistance mechanisms including β3T isoform expression in several tumor models. This randomized phase II study evaluated ixabepilone-based chemotherapy in stage IIIb/IV NSCLC, compared with paclitaxel-based chemotherapy. Tumor specimens were prospectively evaluated for β3T expression.

Patients and Methods.—Patients were stratified by β3T status (positive *v* negative) and randomly assigned at a ratio of 1:1 to receive ixabepilone (32 mg/m^2) and carboplatin (area under concentration-time curve [AUC], 6) or paclitaxel (200 mg/m^2) and carboplatin (AUC, 6) for up to six cycles. The primary end point was progression-free survival (PFS) in the β3T-positive subgroup.

Results.—Ninety-five patients (β3T positive, 52; β3T negative, 43) received ixabepilone plus carboplatin; 96 patients (β3T positive, 49; β3T negative, 47) received paclitaxel plus carboplatin. No significant differences in median PFS were observed between arms for either subgroup (β3T positive, 4.3 months in both arms; β3T negative, 5.8 v 5.3 months). Ixabepilone did not significantly improve overall survival (OS) for the β3T-positive subset or the overall population. Adverse events were similar between the two arms and comparable with those in previous studies.

Conclusion.—There was no predictive value of β3T in differentiating clinical activity of ixabepilone- or paclitaxel-containing regimens. Ixabepilone did not improve PFS or OS in patients with β3Tpositive tumors. β3T-positive patients had worse PFS relative to β3T-negative patients, regardless of treatment; hence, β3T expression seems to be a negative prognostic factor, but not a predictive factor, in advanced NSCLC treated with either ixabepilone or paclitaxel platinum-based doublets.

▶ Unfortunately, this trial placed yet another promising predictive biomarker into the ground. Beta-3 tubulin tumor expression was long considered to be a negative predictive biomarker for tubulin-inhibiting therapy. Ixabepilone (epothilone B analogue) was seen in preclinical models to have efficacy, despite high beta-3 tubulin expression and resilience against the multidrug resistance transporter. Because it was US Food and Drug Administration approved in taxane refractory breast cancer, there was a good rationale to move it into trials in lung cancer.

This trial was well designed and thoughtful with the integration of the biomarker in the stratification factors prior to randomization to carbo-ixabepilone (epothilone B analogue) vs carbo-paclitaxel. The lack of survival difference between the 2 arms for the intent-to-treat population was not unexpected. However, the complete lack of difference in the beta-3 tubulin positive and negative groups with treatment (especially the ixabepilone arm) was disheartening. The authors rightly conclude that beta-3 tubulin is likely a negative prognostic factor but has no predictive capability. Profiling companies that use beta-3 tubulin to declare what chemotherapeutic treatment to give patients should cease. To date, there are no predictive biomarkers for chemotherapeutic agents that are reliable enough to decide treatment options for patients. It is unlikely that ixabepilone will be developed further in non—small cell lung cancer.

A. S. Tsao, MD

Erlotinib versus standard chemotherapy as first-line treatment for European patients with advanced EGFR mutation-positive non-small-cell lung cancer (EURTAC): a multicentre, open-label, randomised phase 3 trial
Rosell R, on behalf of the Spanish Lung Cancer Group in collaboration with the Groupe Français de Pneumo-Cancérologie and the Associazione Italiana Oncologia Toracica (Catalan Inst of Oncology, Badalona, Spain; et al)
Lancet Oncol 13:239-246, 2012

Background.—Erlotinib has been shown to improve progression-free survival compared with chemotherapy when given as first-line treatment for Asian patients with non-small-cell lung cancer (NSCLC) with activating EGFR mutations. We aimed to assess the safety and efficacy of erlotinib compared with standard chemo therapy for first-line treatment of European patients with advanced EGFR-mutation positive NSCLC.

Methods.—We undertook the open-label, randomised phase 3 EURTAC trial at 42 hospitals in France, Italy, and Spain. Eligible participants were adults (>18 years) with NSCLC and EGFR mutations (exon 19 deletion or L858R mutation in exon 21) with no history of chemotherapy for metastatic disease (neoadjuvant or adjuvant chemotherapy ending $\geq$ 6 months before study entry was allowed). We randomly allocated participants (1:1) according to a computer-generated allocation schedule to receive oral erlotinib 150 mg per day or 3 week cycles of standard intravenous chemotherapy of cisplatin 75 mg/m^2 on day 1 plus docetaxel (75 mg/m^2 on day 1) or gemcitabine (1250 mg/m^2 on days 1 and 8). Carboplatin (AUC 6 with docetaxel 75 mg/m^2 or AUC 5 with gemcitabine 1000 mg/m^2) was allowed in patients unable to have cisplatin. Patients were stratified by EGFR mutation type and Eastern Cooperative Oncology Group performance status (0 *vs* 1 *vs* 2). The primary endpoint was progression-free survival (PFS) in the intention-to-treat population. We assessed safety in all patients who received study drug ($\geq$ 1 dose). This study is registered with ClinicalTrials.gov, number NCT00446225.

Findings.—Between Feb 15, 2007, and Jan 4, 2011, 174 patients with EGFR mutations were enrolled. One patient received treatment before randomisation and was thus withdrawn from the study; of the remaining patients, 86 were randomly assigned to receive erlotinib and 87 to receive standard chemotherapy. The preplanned interim analysis showed that the study met its primary endpoint; enrolment was halted, and full evaluation of the results was recommended. At data cutoff (Jan 26, 2011), median PFS was 9·7 months (95% CI 8·4−12·3) in the erlotinib group, compared with 5·2 months (4·5−5·8) in the standard chemotherapy group (hazard ratio 0·37, 95% CI 0·25−0·54; $p < 0·0001$). Main grade 3 or 4 toxicities were rash (11 [13%] of 84 patients given erlotinib *vs* none of 82 patients in the chemotherapy group), neutropenia (none *vs* 18 [22%]), anaemia (one [1%] *vs* three [4%]), and increased aminotransferase concentrations (two [2%] *vs* 0). Five (6%) patients on erlotinib had treatment-related severe adverse events compared with 16 patients (20%) on chemotherapy. One patient in the erlotinib group and two in the standard chemotherapy group died from treatment-related causes.

Interpretation.—Our findings strengthen the rationale for routine baseline tissue-based assessment of EGFR mutations in patients with NSCLC and for treatment of mutation-positive patients with EGFR tyrosine-kinase inhibitors.

▶ This phase III European trial was the counterpart to the IPASS Asian trial by Mok et al.[1] However, this study had a better scientific design, as it only enrolled non—small cell lung cancer patients with sensitive epidermal growth factor receptor (*EGFR*) mutations to receive either erlotinib or chemotherapy. This trial basically joins a long list of frontline Asian EGFR tyrosine kinase inhibitor (TKI) studies (IPASS, OPTIMAL, Japan WJTOG3405) that have consistently shown progression-free survival (PFS) superiority of EGFR TKIs over front-line platinum-doublet chemotherapy for *EGFR* mutation patients. The EURTAC trial is the first European (ie, Caucasian) study and, thus, shows that mutation genetic profiles are what ultimately matters for treatment outcomes and that ethnic differences do not matter if there is a driver mutation for the cancer. This trial was very specific and only enrolled chemo-naïve sensitive *EGFR* mutation patients (del exon 19, L858). The patients with deletion exon 19 mutations appeared to have a greater magnitude of PFS benefit from erlotinib than the L858 mutation patients. This would be consistent with preclinical data suggesting the deletion exon 19 *EGFR* mutants are more sensitive to the reversible EGFR TKIs. There were no new safety signals from the trial. Based off of the EURTAC trial and the others listed above, it is now standard of care to screen front-line chemo-naïve metastatic adenocarcinoma patients for the *EGFR* mutation before treating them with an EGFR TKI.

A. S. Tsao, MD

Reference

1. Mok TS, Wu YL, Thongprasert S, et al. Gefitinib or carboplatin-paclitaxel in pulmonary adenocarcinoma. *N Engl J Med*. 2009;361:947-957.

Second Line Metastatic Non—Small-Cell Lung Cancer

Randomized Phase II Study of Dacomitinib (PF-00299804), an Irreversible Pan—Human Epidermal Growth Factor Receptor Inhibitor, Versus Erlotinib in Patients With Advanced Non—Small-Cell Lung Cancer
Ramalingam SS, Blackhall F, Krzakowski M, et al (Winship Cancer Inst of Emory Univ, Atlanta, GA; Christie Natl Health Service Foundation Trust, Manchester, UK; The Maria Sklodowska-Curie Inst of Oncology, Warsaw, Poland; et al)
J Clin Oncol 30:3337-3344, 2012

Purpose.—This randomized, open-label trial compared dacomitinib (PF-00299804), an irreversible inhibitor of human epidermal growth factor receptors (EGFR)/HER1, HER2, and HER4, with erlotinib, a reversible EGFR inhibitor, in patients with advanced non—small-cell lung cancer (NSCLC).

Patients and Methods.—Patients with NSCLC, Eastern Cooperative Oncology Group performance status 0 to 2, no prior HER-directed therapy, and one/two prior chemotherapy regimens received dacomitinib 45 mg or erlotinib 150 mg once daily.

Results.—One hundred eighty-eight patients were randomly assigned. Treatment arms were balanced for most clinical and molecular characteristics. Median progression-free survival (PFS; primary end point) was 2.86 months for patients treated with dacomitinib and 1.91 months for patients treated with erlotinib (hazard ratio [HR] = 0.66; 95% CI, 0.47 to 0.91; two-sided *P* =.012); in patients with *KRAS* wild-type tumors, median PFS was 3.71 months for patients treated with dacomitinib and

1.91 months for patients treated with erlotinib (HR = 0.55; 95% CI, 0.35 to 0.85; two-sided *P* =.006); and in patients with *KRAS* wild-type/*EGFR* wild-type tumors, median PFS was 2.21 months for patients treated with dacomitinib and 1.84 months for patients treated with erlotinib (HR = 0.61; 95% CI, 0.37 to 0.99; two-sided *P* =.043). Median overall survival was 9.53 months for patients treated with dacomitinib and 7.44 months for patients treated with erlotinib (HR = 0.80; 95% CI, 0.56 to 1.13; two-sided *P* =.205). Adverse event-related discontinuations were uncommon in both arms. Common treatment-related adverse events were dermatologic and gastrointestinal, predominantly grade 1 to 2, and more frequent with dacomitinib.

Conclusion.—Dacomitinib demonstrated significantly improved PFS versus erlotinib, with acceptable toxicity. PFS benefit was observed in most clinical and molecular subsets, notably *KRAS* wild-type/*EGFR* any status, *KRAS* wild-type/*EGFR* wild-type, and *EGFR* mutants.

▶ Dacomitinib, an irreversible pan-*HER* family tyrosine kinase inhibitor, is one of the second-generation epidermal growth factor receptors (EGFR) family inhibitors and is presumed to have significant promise in the evolving field of targeted therapies in non—small cell lung cancer (NSCLC). In this phase II trial comparing salvage dacomitinib to salvage erlotinib (standard of care), the progression-free survival (PFS) was prolonged with statistical significance across most clinical and molecular subgroups. However, the overall survival benefit did not reach statistical significance and the side effects (gastrointestinal, skin toxicity) were higher in the dacomitinib arm. A phase III trial with a similar randomization of erlotinib vs dacomitinib is under way to establish dacomitinib's role in salvage NSCLC. The second-generation irreversible EGFR/EGFR family inhibitors have reached the phase III level and will likely soon be approved for use. It will initially be uncertain how the first-generation reversible and the second-generation irreversible inhibitors should be used in the course of a patient's therapy, especially if the patient has an *EGFR* mutation. Despite dacomitinib having prolonged PFS over erlotinib, the median PFS for an *EGFR* wild-type patient was still only 2.86 months and is by no means a home run. For the mutated *EGFR* patients, there were only 19 who received dacomitinib and 11 who received erlotinib. The hazard ratio was 0.46, favoring dacomitinib for the *EGFR* mutants. Therefore, it remains to be seen whether the irreversible quality of these second-generation agents will provide more optimal or just different clinical benefit over older agents. As a reminder, afatinib (irreversible EGFR tyrosine kinase inhibitor) is also on the horizon to be a potential front-line option for *EGFR* mutation patients.

A. S. Tsao, MD

Aflibercept and Docetaxel Versus Docetaxel Alone After Platinum Failure in Patients With Advanced or Metastatic Non–Small-Cell Lung Cancer: A Randomized, Controlled Phase III Trial

Ramlau R, Gorbunova V, Ciuleanu TE, et al (Poznań Univ of Med Sciences, Poland; N.N. Blokhin Russian Cancer Res Ctr, Moscow, Russia; Inst of Oncology, Cluj-Napoca, Romania; et al)
J Clin Oncol 30:3640-3647, 2012

Purpose.—To compare the efficacy of aflibercept (ziv-aflibercept), a recombinant human fusion protein targeting the vascular endothelial growth factor (VEGF) pathway, with or without docetaxel in platinum-pretreated patients with advanced or metastatic nonsquamous non–small-cell lung cancer.

Patients and Methods.—In this international, double-blind, placebo-controlled phase III trial, 913 patients were randomly assigned to (ziv-)aflibercept 6 mg/kg intravenous (IV; n = 456) or IV placebo (n = 457), both administered every 3 weeks and in combination with docetaxel 75 mg/m^2. The primary end point was overall survival (OS). Other efficacy outcomes, safety, and immunogenicity were also assessed.

Results.—Patient characteristics were balanced between arms; 12.3% of patients had received prior bevacizumab. (Ziv-)Aflibercept did not improve OS (hazard ratio [HR], 1.01; 95% CI, 0.87 to 1.17; stratified log-rank $P = .90$). The median OS was 10.1 months (95% CI, 9.2 to 11.6 months) for (ziv-)aflibercept and 10.4 months (95% CI, 9.2 to 11.9 months) for placebo. In exploratory analyses, median progression-free survival was 5.2 months (95% CI, 4.4 to 5.6 months) for (ziv-)aflibercept versus 4.1 months (95% CI, 3.5 to 4.3 months) for placebo (HR, 0.82; 95% CI, 0.72 to 0.94; $P = .0035$); overall response rate was 23.3% of evaluable patients (95% CI, 19.1% to 27.4%) in the (ziv-)aflibercept arm versus 8.9% (95% CI, 6.1% to 11.6%; $P < .001$) in the placebo arm. Grade ≥ 3 adverse events occurring more frequently in the (ziv-)aflibercept arm versus the placebo arm were neutropenia (28.0% v 21.1%, respectively), fatigue (11.1% v 4.2%, respectively), stomatitis (8.8% v 0.7%, respectively), and hypertension (7.3% v 0.9%, respectively).

Conclusion.—The addition of (ziv-)aflibercept to standard docetaxel therapy did not improve OS. In exploratory analyses, secondary efficacy end points did seem to be improved in the (ziv-) aflibercept arm. The study regimen was associated with increased toxicities, consistent with known anti-VEGF and chemotherapy-induced events.

▶ Aflibercept, a recombinant human fusion protein, has high affinity for ligand vascular endothelial growth factor (VEGF)-A and VEGF-B and placental growth factors-1 and -2. The international phase III VITAL trial conducted a randomized comparison of ziv-aflibercept with docetaxel vs docetaxel alone in second-line metastatic non–squamous cell carcinoma patients. As with most other antiangiogenic tyrosine kinase inhibitors when combined with salvage docetaxel, there were better response rates and progression-free survival rates with the combination. Also, consistent with the rest of the antiangiogenic literature, there was no difference in quality of life nor overall survival, and a higher rate of grade 3 adverse events was seen with ziv-aflibercept plus docetaxel (71.5% vs 49.7%). There was a higher rate of neutropenic complications leading to death in the combination arm. Unfortunately, we remain stuck in the same situation as before, in which a targeted antiangiogenic agent with no predictive biomarker helps the response/progression-free survival rates but adds side effects and no overall survival benefit. This trial goes into the heap of other failed antiangiogenic salvage studies. Future efforts need to focus on identifying a predictive biomarker for the antiangiogenic agents and ensuring that translational studies are incorporated into the trial. It is impossible to learn anything from this trial about whether placental growth factor inhibition adds anything to VEGF inhibition, as there were no reported translational studies.

A. S. Tsao, MD

Pemetrexed Versus Pemetrexed and Carboplatin As Second-Line Chemotherapy in Advanced Non–Small-Cell Lung Cancer: Results of the GOIRC 02-2006 Randomized Phase II Study and Pooled Analysis With the NVALT7 Trial

Ardizzoni A, Tiseo M, Boni L, et al (Azienda Ospedaliero-Universitaria, Parma, Italy; Azienda Ospedaliero-Universitaria Careggi, Firenze, Italy; et al)
J Clin Oncol 30:4501-4507, 2012

Purpose.—To compare efficacy of pemetrexed versus pemetrexed plus carboplatin in pretreated patients with advanced non-small-cell lung cancer (NSCLC).

Patients and Methods.—Patients with advanced NSCLC, in progression during or after first-line platinum-based chemotherapy, were randomly assigned to receive pemetrexed (arm A) or pemetrexed plus carboplatin (arm B). Primary end point was progression-free survival (PFS). A preplanned pooled analysis of the results of this study with those of the NVALT7 study was carried out to assess the impact of carboplatin added to pemetrexed in terms of overall survival (OS).

Results.—From July 2007 to October 2009, 239 patients (arm A, n = 120; arm B, n = 119) were enrolled. Median PFS was 3.6 months for arm A versus 3.5 months for arm B (hazard ratio [HR], 1.05; 95% CI, 0.81 to 1.36; $P = .706$). No statistically significant differences in response rate, OS, or toxicity were observed. A total of 479 patients were included in the pooled analysis. OS was not improved by the addition of carboplatin to pemetrexed (HR, 90; 95% CI, 0.74 to 1.10; $P = .316$; P heterogeneity = .495). In the subgroup analyses, the addition of carboplatin to pemetrexed in patients with squamous tumors led to a statistically significant improvement in OS from 5.4 to 9 months (adjusted HR, 0.58; 95% CI, 0.37 to 0.91; P interaction test = .039).

Conclusion.—Second-line treatment of advanced NSCLC with pemetrexed plus carboplatin does not improve survival outcomes as compared with single-agent pemetrexed. The benefit observed with carboplatin addition in squamous tumors may warrant further investigation.

▶ In ovarian cancer, the dominant paradigm in the management of recurrent disease is to categorize patients based on how they responded to front-line platinum-based therapy. Those who respond and have a response that lasts at least 6 months benefit most from retreatment with a platinum-based regimen, whereas those who do not respond or whose response lasts less than 6 months do better with alternative treatment. This article explores to some extent the same paradigm in lung cancer. Unfortunately, not enough information is given to allow a proper assessment of those with treatment-free intervals of greater than 6 months. The overall conclusion that the addition of platinum to pemetrexed does not offer greater benefit than pemetrexed alone thus does not provide a clear determination as to whether those with a treatment-free interval of greater than 6 months might actually benefit from carboplatin. Given the results in ovarian cancer, it is probably worthwhile to explore this further in additional studies focusing on those with treatment-free intervals of greater than 6 months. The caveat to this is that the level of efficacy of the platinum agents in lung cancer is nowhere near the level of efficacy seen for the platinum agents in ovarian cancer; hence, the enhanced efficacy may be so small as to be difficult to detect.

J. T. Thigpen, MD

Non—Small-Cell: Early Stage and Adjuvant Therapy

Incorporating Bevacizumab and Erlotinib in the Combined-Modality Treatment of Stage III Non—Small-Cell Lung Cancer: Results of a Phase I/II Trial
Socinski MA, Stinchcombe TE, Moore DT, et al (Univ of North Carolina, Chapel Hill; et al)
J Clin Oncol 30:3953-3959, 2012

Purpose.—Bevacizumab and erlotinib have been shown to improve survival in stage IV non—small-cell lung cancer (NSCLC). This phase I/II trial was designed to incorporate these agents with induction and concurrent chemoradiotherapy in stage III NSCLC.

Patients and Methods.—Patients received induction chemotherapy (carboplatin area under the curve [AUC] 6, paclitaxel 225 mg/m^2, and bevacizumab 15 mg/kg on days 1 and 22) followed by concurrent chemotherapy (carboplatin AUC 2 and paclitaxel 45 mg/m^2 weekly with bevacizumab 10 mg/kg every other week for four doses) and thoracic conformal radiation therapy (TCRT) to 74 Gy. In the phase I portion, cohort 1 received no erlotinib, whereas cohorts 2 and 3 received erlotinib at 100 and 150 mg, respectively, Tuesday through Friday, during TCRT. Consolidation therapy with erlotinib (150 mg daily) and bevacizumab (15 mg/kg every 3 weeks) was planned 3 to 6 weeks later for six cycles.

Results.—Forty-five eligible patients were enrolled. The objective response rates to induction and overall treatment were 39% (95% CI,

24% to 55%) and 60% (95% CI, 44% to 75%), respectively. The median progression-free and overall survival times were 10.2 months (95% CI, 8.4 to 18.3 months) and 18.4 months (95% CI, 13.4 to 31.7 months), respectively. The principal toxicity was esophagitis (29% grade 3 or 4 esophagitis, with one patient with grade 3 tracheoesophageal fistula), which was often prolonged. Consolidation therapy with bevacizumab and erlotinib was not feasible.

Conclusion.—The use of bevacizumab and erlotinib as administered in this trial is not recommended given the lack of an efficacy signal and the substantial risk of esophageal toxicity.

▶ This ambitious trial teaches us that more is not better, and that we can seriously harm patients with novel targeted agents if they are not appropriately used. This study was well intentioned with the goal of improving overall survival outcomes for stage III patients, who routinely have a 15% to 35% 5-year overall survival rate with multimodality therapy. The biggest problem with this trial was in the study regimen, which attempted to throw everything at the patient: induction chemotherapy and antiangiogenic agents, followed by chemoradiation with 2 targeted agents, followed by 2 targeted agents for maintenance therapy.

We now know from additional bevacizumab chemoradiation studies that bevacizumab chemoradiation has high toxicity rates with potentially fatal tracheal–esophageal fistulas. The patients in this trial could not tolerate the full aggressive treatment largely because of esophageal toxicity. Also, in the patients who did receive this aggressive regimen, there was no benefit to progression-free survival, a disturbing thought that confirms that trials with novel agents should be designed with a selected population of patients. Broad use of these agents in unselected patients is unlikely to demonstrate significant clinical benefit and just adds toxicity to the patients.

There were 2 additional problems with this clinical trial: (1) the inclusion of squamous cell carcinoma patients and (2) the dose of thoracic radiation to 74 Gy. The initial squamous cell carcinoma patients enrolled to the trial had a risk for delayed hemoptysis after the neoadjuvant chemoradiation bevacizumab and concurrent chemoradiation bevacizumab chemoradiotherapy. The trial was amended to exclude these squamous cell carcinoma patients after 2 episodes of grade 5 hemoptysis in the initial 12 patients and 1 grade 3 episode. The total dose of thoracic radiation was high—the RTOG-0617 trial had to close its high-dose (74 Gy) arms because of excessive early deaths. It is unknown whether this contributed to the poor outcomes in this trial, but it is definitely a factor that contributed to the high esophagitis rates. For our stage III, non–small cell lung cancer patients who are treated with multimodality therapy, future studies need to focus on genetic profiling, identifying prognostic and predictive biomarkers, and incorporating less toxic novel agents into the treatment strategies.

A. S. Tsao, MD

Advanced Diseases

Phase II Trial of Erlotinib Plus Concurrent Whole-Brain Radiation Therapy for Patients With Brain Metastases From Non–Small-Cell Lung Cancer
Welsh JW, Komaki R, Amini A, et al (The Univ of Texas MD Anderson Cancer Ctr, Houston; et al)
J Clin Oncol 31:895-902, 2013

Purpose.—Brain metastasis (BM) is a leading cause of death from non–small-cell lung cancer (NSCLC). Reasoning that activation of the epidermal growth factor receptor (EGFR) contributes to radiation resistance, we undertook a phase II trial of the EGFR inhibitor erlotinib with whole-brain radiation therapy (WBRT) in an attempt to extend survival time for patients with BM from NSCLC. Additional end points were radiologic response and safety.

Patients and Methods.—Eligible patients had BM from NSCLC, regardless of EGFR status. Erlotinib was given at 150 mg orally once per day for 1 week, then concurrently with WBRT (2.5 Gy per day 5 days per week, to 35 Gy), followed by maintenance. *EGFR* mutation status was tested by DNA sequencing at an accredited core facility.

Results.—Forty patients were enrolled and completed erlotinib plus WBRT (median age, 59 years; median diagnosis-specific graded prognostic assessment score, 1.5). The overall response rate was 86% (n = 36). No increase in neurotoxicity was detected, and no patient experienced grade ≥ 4 toxicity, but three patients required dose reduction for grade 3 rash. At a median follow-up of 28.5 months (for living patients), median survival time was 11.8 months (95% CI, 7.4 to 19.1 months). Of 17 patients with known *EGFR* status, median survival time was 9.3 months for those with wild-type *EGFR* and 19.1 months for those with *EGFR* mutations.

Conclusion.—Erlotinib was well tolerated in combination with WBRT, with a favorable objective response rate. The higher-than-expected rate of *EGFR* mutations in these unselected patients raises the possibility that *EGFR*-mutated tumors are prone to brain dissemination.

▶ This trial (N = 40) was important because it addresses an issue that plagues the treating oncologist—whether to give whole-brain radiation with erlotinib concurrently if the patient is already taking erlotinib or is starting it.

In this trial, there were no grade 4 or 5 acute treatment-related toxicities, and there was no evidence of worsening rash with the addition of radiation to erlotinib in the radiation portal site. Of the 40 patients, only 2 had possible long-term toxicity, with dementia in a 74-year-old and radiation necrosis in a patient with recurrent brain disease who had received a stereotactic radiosurgery boost. In terms of efficacy, the 3-month central nervous system response rate was 89% for epidermal growth factor receptor (*EGFR*) mutants and 63% for *EGFR* wild-type patients. The authors reported that the median overall survival in the intent-to-treat population was 11.8 months and, thus, markedly higher than the anticipated 3.9 months (per historical control).

This finding is perhaps not as dramatic as claimed. First, current median overall survival times for patients with brain metastases is higher than 3.9 months, given the new radiation technologies and supportive therapies. Also, this significant overall survival benefit is impacted by the high number of *EGFR* mutation patients included in the trial. This trial was open to all comers and did not select for *EGFR* mutation. Yet, in the subsequent analysis of 17 patients with available adequate tumor tissue, 9 were found to have *EGFR* mutations and 7 of these 9 patients had sensitive *EGFR* mutations (del exon 19, L858). *EGFR* mutation patients obviously had better outcomes on this trial because they were treated with erlotinib. This is clearly seen in the trial's median overall survival for *EGFR* mutants compared with *EGFR* wild-type—19.1 months vs 9.3 months, respectively. Although this study does demonstrate limited acute toxicity with the combination of whole-brain radiation and erlotinib, it remains unclear whether it is necessary to give erlotinib concurrently or whether it could be held for the 2 weeks and resumed after the whole-brain radiation is completed. Does the erlotinib heighten the effect of the radiation and cause long-term cognitive dysfunction or damage? Only a larger randomized trial of whole-brain radiation with or without erlotinib would answer this issue. In general as a standard practice, most patients on erlotinib who have a focal area of progression in the body or a painful refractory bone metastasis will continue the erlotinib and receive radiation to the focal area. It is still unclear whether it is necessary to give concurrent therapy to the brain and risk long-term cognitive deficits.

A. S. Tsao, MD

11 Head and Neck

Induction chemotherapy followed by concurrent chemoradiotherapy (sequential chemoradiotherapy) versus concurrent chemoradiotherapy alone in locally advanced head and neck cancer (PARADIGM): a randomized phase 3 trial

Haddad R, O'Neill A, Rabinowits G, et al (Harvard Med School, Boston, MA; Dana-Farber Cancer Inst, Boston, MA; et al)

Lancet Oncol 14:257-264, 2013

Background.—The relative efficacy of the addition of induction chemotherapy to chemoradiotherapy compared with chemoradiotherapy alone for patients with head and neck cancer is unclear. The PARADIGM study is a multicentre open-label phase 3 study comparing the use of docetaxel, cisplatin, and fluorouracil (TPF) induction chemotherapy followed by concurrent chemoradiotherapy with cisplatin-based concurrent chemoradiotherapy alone in patients with locally advanced head and neck cancer.

Methods.—Adult patients with previously untreated, non-metastatic, newly diagnosed head and neck cancer were eligible. Patients were eligible if their tumour was either unresectable or of low surgical curability on the basis of advanced tumour stage (3 or 4) or regional-node stage (2 or 3, except T1N2), or if they were a candidate for organ preservation. Patients were randomly assigned (in a 1:1 ratio) to receive either induction chemotherapy with three cycles of TPF followed by concurrent chemoradiotherapy with either docetaxel or carboplatin or concurrent chemoradiotherapy alone with two cycles of bolus cisplatin. A computer-generated randomisation schedule using minimisation was prepared and the treatment assignment was done centrally at one of the study sites. Patients, study staff, and investigators were not masked to group assignment. Stratification factors were WHO performance status, primary disease site, and stage. The primary endpoint was overall survival. Analysis was by intention to treat. Patient accrual was terminated in December, 2008, because of slow enrolment. The trial is registered with ClinicalTrials.gov, number NCT00095875.

Findings.—Between Aug 24, 2004, and Dec 29, 2008, we enrolled 145 patients across 16 sites. After a median follow-up of 49 months (IQR 39–63), 41 patients had died—20 in the induction chemotherapy followed by chemoradiotherapy group and 21 in the chemoradiotherapy alone group. 3-year overall survival was 73% (95% CI 60–82) in the induction therapy followed by chemoradiotherapy group and 78% (66–86) in the chemoradiotherapy alone group (hazard ratio 1·09, 95% CI 0·59–2·03;

$p=0\cdot77$). More patients had febrile neutropenia in the induction chemotherapy followed by chemoradiotherapy group (16 patients) than in the chemoradiotherapy alone group (one patient).

Interpretation.—Although survival results were good in both groups there was no difference noted between those patients treated with induction chemotherapy followed by chemoradiotherapy and those who received chemoradiotherapy alone. We cannot rule out the possibility of a difference in survival going undetected due to early termination of the trial. Clinicians should still use their best judgment, based on the available data, in the decision of how to best treat patients. The addition of induction chemotherapy remains an appropriate approach for advanced disease with high risk for local or distant failure.

▶ The PARADIGM trial attempted to address the role of induction therapy in high-risk patients with locally advanced squamous carcinoma of the head and neck. The study did not find any difference in overall survival between the 2 treatment arms; however, there are 2 significant issues with the study design and implementation. First, the study was designed before the impact of human papillomavirus (HPV)-associated oropharyngeal cancers on overall survival was clearly recognized. It is now known that HPV-associated cancers have a much better prognosis than cancers associated with smoking and alcohol use. In this study, 80% of patients had oropharyngeal primary tumors. Although HPV status was not assessed, the high rate of oropharyngeal cancers created the potential that a high percentage of patients in the study were low risk. This is borne out by the high overall survival for both treatment arms. The study was designed to detect an improvement in overall survival rate from 55% to 70% with the addition of induction chemotherapy. The overall survival rate was approximately 70% in both arms, indicating that the study did not enroll the targeted high-risk population. Second, the study was closed early after recruiting less than half of the expected number of patients because of poor accrual. Based on these flaws, the data from this study cannot be used to support or refute the role of induction chemotherapy in high-risk patients. It does, however, underscore the changing epidemiology of head and neck cancer within the United States and the need to incorporate HPV status into study design.

B. A. Murphy, MD

Phase III Randomized, Placebo-Controlled Trial of Docetaxel With or Without Gefitinib in Recurrent or Metastatic Head and Neck Cancer: An Eastern Cooperative Oncology Group Trial
Argiris A, Ghebremichael M, Gilbert J, et al (The Univ of Texas Health Science Ctr at San Antonio; Massachusetts General Hosp, Boston; Vanderbilt Univ, Nashville, TN; et al)
J Clin Oncol 31:1405-1414, 2013

Purpose.—We hypothesized that the addition of gefitinib, an epidermal growth factor receptor (EGFR) tyrosine kinase inhibitor, to docetaxel would enhance therapeutic efficacy in squamous cell carcinoma of the head and neck (SCCHN).

Patients and Methods.—Patients with recurrent or metastatic SCCHN with Eastern Cooperative Oncology Group (ECOG) performance status of 2, or patients with ECOG performance status of 0 to 2 but were previously treated with chemotherapy, were randomly assigned to receive weekly docetaxel plus either placebo (arm A) or gefitinib 250 mg/d, orally (arm B) until disease progression. At the time of progression, patients in the placebo arm could receive single-agent gefitinib. EGFR, c-MET, and KRAS mutations and polymorphisms in drug metabolizing enzymes and transporters were evaluated by pyrosequencing.

Results.—Two hundred seventy patients were enrolled before the study was closed early at interim analysis (arm A, n = 136; arm B, n = 134). Median overall survival was 6.0 months in arm A versus 7.3 months in arm B (hazard ratio, 0.93; 95% CI, 0.72 to 1.21; $P = .60$). An unplanned subset analysis showed that gefitinib improved survival in patients younger than 65 years (median 7.6 v 5.2 months; $P = .04$). Also, there was a trend for improved survival in patients with c-MET wild-type (5.7 v 3.6 months; $P = .09$) regardless of treatment. Grade 3/4 toxicities were comparable between the two arms except that grade 3/4 diarrhea was more common with docetaxel/gefitinib. Of 18 eligible patients who received gefitinib after disease progression in arm A, one patient had a partial response.

Conclusion.—The addition of gefitinib to docetaxel was well tolerated but did not improve outcomes in poor prognosis but otherwise unselected patients with SCCHN.

▶ Cetuximab has been found to improve overall survival when added to systemic chemotherapy for treatment of patients with recurrent or metastatic head and neck cancer. Thus, investigators are interested in determining the efficacy of other agents targeting the epidermal growth factor receptor pathway. Gefitinib is an orally administered tyrosine kinase inhibitor that has been studied previously in head and neck cancer patients. In a randomized phase III trial, 2 doses of gefitinib (500 mg and 250 mg) were compared with single-agent methotrexate as first-line therapy for patients with metastatic or recurrent squamous cell carcinoma of the head and neck. In this setting, gefitinib failed to demonstrate superiority to weekly single-agent methotrexate. Despite the disappointing results, preclinical data supporting the efficacy of gefitinib plus docetaxel prompted investigators to conduct a trial of the 2-drug combination compared with docetaxel as a single agent in patients who did not respond to first-line chemotherapy for metastatic or recurrent disease. No difference was noted in the overall survival between the 2 treatment arms. Of interest, in the subset of patients who were younger than 65, there was a significant survival advantage for patients receiving combination therapy vs single-agent treatment (7.6 months vs 5.2 months, $P = .04$). Although this difference may not be clinically robust, it does beg the question whether combination therapy for second-line treatment of fit younger patients with recurrent or metastatic head and neck cancer may be worth pushing.

B. A. Murphy, MD

Deintensification Candidate Subgroups in Human Papillomavirus–Related Oropharyngeal Cancer According to Minimal Risk of Distant Metastasis

O'Sullivan B, Huang SH, Siu LL, et al (Princess Margaret Hosp/Univ of Toronto, Ontario, Canada; et al)
J Clin Oncol 31:543-550, 2013

Purpose.—To define human papillomavirus (HPV) —positive oropharyngeal cancers (OPC) suitable for treatment deintensification according to low risk of distant metastasis (DM).

Patients and Methods.—OPC treated with radiotherapy (RT) or chemoradiotherapy (CRT) from 2001 to 2009 were included. Outcomes were compared for HPV-positive versus HPV-negative patients. Univariate and multivariate analyses identified outcome predictors. Recursive partitioning analysis (RPA) stratified the DM risk.

Results.—HPV status was ascertained in 505 (56%) of 899 consecutive OPCs. Median follow-up was 3.9 years. HPV-positive patients (n = 382), compared with HPV-negative patients (n = 123), had higher local (94% v 80%, respectively, at 3 years; $P < .01$) and regional control (95% v 82%, respectively; $P < .01$) but similar distant control (DC; 90% v 86%, respectively; $P = .53$). Multivariate analysis identified that HPV negativity (hazard ratio [HR], 2.9; 95% CI, 2.0 to 5.0), N2b-N3 (HR, 2.9; 95% CI, 1.8 to 4.9), T4 (HR, 1.8; 95% CI, 1.2 to 2.9), and RT alone (HR, 1.8; 95% CI, 1.1 to 2.5) predicted a lower recurrence-free survival (RFS; all $P < .01$). Smoking pack-years >10 reduced overall survival (HR, 1.72; 95% CI, 1.1 to 2.7; $P = .03$) but did not impact RFS (HR, 1.1; 95% CI, 0.7 to 1.9; $P = .65$). RPA segregated HPV-positive patients into low (T1-3N0-2c; DC, 93%) and high DM risk (N3 or T4; DC, 76%) groups and HPV-negative patients into different low (T1-2N0-2c; DC, 93%) and high DM risk (T3-4N3; DC, 72%) groups. The DC rates for HPV-positive, low-risk N0-2a or less than 10 pack-year N2b patients were similar for RT alone and CRT, but the rate was lower in the N2c subset managed by RT alone (73% v 92% for CRT; $P = .02$).

Conclusion.—HPV-positive T1-3N0-2c patients have a low DM risk, but N2c patients from this group have a reduced DC when treated with RT alone and seem less suited for deintensification strategies that omit chemotherapy.

▶ Over the last decade, there has been a dramatic shift in the epidemiology of head and neck cancer. The number of patients with human papillomavirus (HPV)-associated oropharyngeal cancers has increased dramatically. This cohort of patients receives diagnosis at an earlier age, is less likely to have a history of heavy smoking, and generally has a good outcome with regard to locoregional control and overall survival. That being said, sufficient data pertaining to recurrence patterns and outcome for patients with recurrent disease are just now becoming available. Data would indicate that locoregional recurrence is uncommon, and most patients have recurrence with distant metastases. Based on these observations, researchers are considering 2 potential treatment paradigms: (1) deintensification of locoregional therapy to minimize acute and late toxicities and (2) use of systemic chemotherapy to decrease the risk of metastatic disease. To optimize outcomes, it is critical to be able to appropriately risk stratify patients. Specifically, it is important to identify patients with a high risk for locoregional recurrence and for whom de-escalation would be contraindicated. In addition, identification of patients at risk for metastatic disease would allow use of induction chemotherapy to limit metastatic disease. The results from this report confirm earlier reports that the rate of distant control is equivalent between HPV-positive and HPV-negative patients. Furthermore, they show that patients with HPV-positive cancers who have T4 primary tumors or N3 nodal disease at are at substantial increased risks for distant metastasis. In addition, patients with N2c neck disease had reduced distant control if they were treated with radiation alone. Although clinical decisions should not be based on retrospective data analysis, the data can be used to inform future clinical trials.

B. A. Murphy, MD

Induction Chemotherapy Followed by Either Chemoradiotherapy or Bioradiotherapy for Larynx Preservation: the TREMPLIN Randomized Phase II Study

Lefebvre JL, Pointreau Y, Rolland F, et al (Centre Oscar Lambret, Lille, France; Centre Hospitalier Universitaire Pierre Bretonneau, Tours, France; Institut de Cancerologie de l'Ouest Rene Gauducheau, France; et al)
J Clin Oncol 31:853-859, 2013

Purpose.—To compare the efficacy and safety of induction chemotherapy (ICT) followed by chemoradiotherapy (CRT) or bioradiotherapy (BRT) for larynx preservation (LP).

Patients and Methods.—Previously untreated patients with stage III to IV larynx/hypopharynx squamous cell carcinoma received three cycles of ICT—docetaxel and cisplatin 75 mg/m^2 each on day 1 and fluorouracil 750 mg/m^2 per day on days 1 through 5. Poor responders (<50% response) underwent salvage surgery. Responders (≥50% response) were randomly assigned to conventional radiotherapy (RT; 70 Gy) with concurrent cisplatin 100 mg/m^2 per day on days 1, 22, and 43 of RT (arm A) or concurrent cetuximab 400 mg/m^2 loading dose and 250 mg/m^2 per week during RT (arm B). Primary end point was LP at 3 months. Secondary end points were larynx function preservation (LFP) and overall survival (OS) at 18 months.

Results.—Of the 153 enrolled patients, 116 were randomly assigned after ICT (60, arm A; 56, arm B). Overall toxicity of both CRT and BRT was substantial following ICT. However, treatment compliance was higher in the BRT arm. In an intent-to-treat analysis, there was no significant difference in LP at 3 months between arms A and B (95% and 93%, respectively), LFP (87% and 82%, respectively), and OS at 18 months (92% and 89%, respectively). There were fewer local treatment failures in arm A than in arm B; salvage surgery was feasible in arm B only.

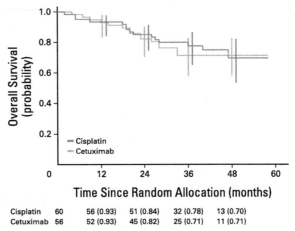

FIGURE 2.—Overall survival (intent to treat) for the subgroup of patients who were responding to induction chemotherapy. (Reprinted from Lefebvre JL, Pointreau Y, Rolland F, et al. Induction chemotherapy followed by either chemoradiotherapy or bioradiotherapy for larynx preservation: the TREMPLIN randomized phase II Study. *J Clin Oncol.* 2013;31:853-859, Reprinted with permission. © 2013, American Society of Clinical Oncology. All rights reserved.)

Conclusion.—There is no evidence that one treatment was superior to the other or could improve the outcome reported with ICT followed by RT alone (French Groupe Oncologie Radiothérapie Tête et Cou [GORTEC] 2000-01 trial [Induction CT by Cisplatin, 5FU With or Without Docetaxel in Patients With T3 and T4 Larynx and Hypopharynx Carcinoma]). The protocol that can best compare with RT alone after ICT is still to be determined (Fig 2).

▶ There are 2 approaches for radiation-based function preservation in patients with locally advanced squamous carcinoma of the larynx: induction chemotherapy followed by radiation in responders (surgical salvage for nonresponders) vs concurrent chemoradiotherapy (CCR). In general, CCR has been favored by clinicians in the United States, whereas an induction approach has been favored by many clinicians in Europe. In a large, randomized trial conducted mainly in Europe, the use of docetaxel (T), cisplatin (P), and 5-flurouracil (F) (TPF) as induction therapy was found to enhance treatment larynx preservation when compared with cisplatin-fluorouracil.[1] It was felt that this regimen should be the standard induction regimen on which further treatment should be based. Investigators report the results of a randomized, phase II trial evaluating induction therapy with TPF followed by 1 of 2 concurrent treatment regimens: high-dose cisplatin or single-agent cetuximab. Of note, there was no significant difference in the incidence of grade 3 or 4 mucositis. There was an increase in grade 4 dermatologic toxicity in patients treated with cetuximab. The incidence of toxicities during CCR was high. Dose modification during CCR caused by toxicity was required in 57% and 34% of patients treated with cisplatin and cetuximab, respectively. The decreased rate of dose delivery of cetuximab after induction therapy with TPF may be secondary to residual treatment-related effects. Overall survival and local control were equal between arms. When compared with results from therapy with TPF followed by radiation alone, there was no evidence of benefit to either chemoradiotherapy with cisplatin or cetuximab after TPF induction.

B. A. Murphy, MD

Reference

1. Pointreau Y, Garaud P, Chpaet S, et al. Randomized trial of induction chemotherapy with cisplatin and 5-fluorouracil with or without docetaxel for larynx preservation. *J Natl Cancer Inst.* 2009;101:498-506.

Long-Term Results of RTOG 91-11: A Comparison of Three Nonsurgical Treatment Strategies to Preserve the Larynx in Patients With Locally Advanced Larynx Cancer

Forastiere AA, Zhang Q, Weber RS, et al (Sydney Kimmel Comprehensive Cancer Ctr at Johns Hopkins, Baltimore, MD; Radiation Therapy Oncology Group Statistical Ctr, Philadelphia, PA; The Univ of Texas MD Anderson Cancer Ctr, Houston; et al)
J Clin Oncol 31:845-852, 2013

Purpose.—To report the long-term results of the Intergroup Radiation Therapy Oncology Group 91-11 study evaluating the contribution of chemotherapy added to radiation therapy (RT) for larynx preservation.

Patients and Methods.—Patients with stage III or IV glottic or supraglottic squamous cell cancer were randomly assigned to induction cisplatin/fluorouracil (PF) followed by RT (control arm), concomitant cisplatin/RT, or RT alone. The composite end point of laryngectomy-free survival (LFS) was the primary end point.

Results.—Five hundred twenty patients were analyzed. Median follow-up for surviving patients is 10.8 years. Both chemotherapy regimens significantly improved LFS compared with RT alone (induction chemotherapy v RT alone: hazard ratio [HR], 0.75; 95% CI, 0.59 to 0.95; $P = .02$; concomitant chemotherapy v RT alone: HR, 0.78; 95% CI, 0.78 to 0.98; $P = .03$). Overall survival did not differ significantly, although there was a possibility of worse outcome with concomitant relative to induction chemotherapy (HR, 1.25; 95% CI, 0.98 to 1.61; $P = .08$). Concomitant cisplatin/RT significantly improved the larynx preservation rate over induction PF followed by RT (HR, 0.58; 95% CI, 0.37 to 0.89; $P = .0050$) and over RT alone ($P < .001$), whereas induction PF followed by RT was not better than treatment with RT alone (HR, 1.26; 95% CI, 0.88 to 1.82; $P = .35$). No difference in late effects was detected, but deaths not attributed to larynx cancer or treatment were higher with concomitant chemotherapy (30.8% v 20.8% with induction chemotherapy and 16.9% with RT alone).

Conclusion.—These 10-year results show that induction PF followed by RT and concomitant cisplatin/RT show similar efficacy for the composite end point of LFS. Locoregional control and larynx preservation were significantly improved with concomitant cisplatin/RT compared with the induction arm or RT alone. New strategies that improve organ preservation and function with less morbidity are needed.

▶ RTOG 91-11 is a randomized, 3-arm trial comparing radiation alone, induction chemotherapy using 3 cycles of cisplatin/5-flurouracil followed by radiation, and concurrent chemoradiation using high-dose cisplatin every 21 days for 3 cycles in patients with locally advanced laryngeal cancer. The initial results were published in 2003. In this report, the investigators provide long-term data regarding toxicity and treatment outcomes. There was no significant difference in late effects in any of the 3 treatments arms. It should be noted, however, that toxicity data were obtained from a review of chart information that documented patient reports. In all likelihood, this dramatically underreports the effects of late tissue damage. Despite these limitations, 30% to 38% of patients experienced at least one grade 3 or greater toxicity. The incidence rate of toxicity was highest among patients treated with chemoradiation. More aggressive late toxicity assessment and reporting is needed to understand the true incidence and its impact on symptom burden, functionality, and quality of life. Patients treated with chemoradiation had a better rate of larynx preservation. Long-term survival data indicate that there is a nonsignificant improvement in overall survival favoring induction therapy (39% induction therapy vs 28% chemoradiation vs 32% radiation only). The reason for this observation is unknown. It may be postulated that chemoradiation results in unrecognized long-term health effects that adversely impact survival.

B. A. Murphy, MD

Randomized Phase III Trial of Induction Chemotherapy With Docetaxel, Cisplatin, and Fluorouracil Followed by Surgery Versus Up-Front Surgery in Locally Advanced Resectable Oral Squamous Cell Carcinoma
Zhong L-P, Zhang C-P, Ren G-X, et al (Shanghai Jiao Tong Univ School of Medicine, China; et al)
J Clin Oncol 31:744-751, 2013

Purpose.—To evaluate induction chemotherapy with docetaxel, cisplatin, and fluorouracil (TPF) followed by surgery and postoperative radiotherapy versus up-front surgery and postoperative radiotherapy in patients with locally advanced resectable oral squamous cell carcinoma (OSCC).

Patients and Methods.—A prospective open-label phase III trial was conducted. Eligibility criteria included untreated stage III or IVA locally advanced resectable OSCC. Patients received two cycles of TPF induction chemotherapy (docetaxel 75 mg/m^2 on day 1, cisplatin 75 mg/m^2 on day 1, and fluorouracil 750 mg/m^2 on days 1 to 5) followed by radical surgery and postoperative radiotherapy (54 to 66 Gy) versus up-front radical surgery and postoperative radiotherapy. The primary end point was overall survival (OS). Secondary end points included local control and safety.

Results.—Of the 256 patients enrolled onto this trial, 222 completed the full treatment protocol. There were no unexpected toxicities, and induction chemotherapy did not increase perioperative morbidity. The clinical response rate to induction chemotherapy was 80.6%. After a median follow-up of 30 months, there was no significant difference in OS (hazard ratio [HR], 0.977; 95% CI, 0.634 to 1.507; $P = .918$) or disease-free survival (HR, 0.974; 95% CI, 0.654 to 1.45; $P = .897$) between patients treated with and without TPF induction. Patients in the induction chemotherapy arm with a clinical response or favorable pathologic response ($\leq 10\%$ viable tumor cells) had superior OS and locoregional and distant control.

Conclusion.—Our study failed to demonstrate that TPF induction chemotherapy improves survival compared with up-front surgery in patients with resectable stage III or IVA OSCC.

▶ Trials conducted in the 1980s failed to show an advantage to induction therapy before surgery. Furthermore, it is generally agreed that oral cavity cancers are best treated with primary resection followed by adjunctive radiation-based therapy if indicated by pathologic risk factors. Induction therapy has been investigated as a method for identification of good-risk patients for whom definitive radiation therapy is a therapeutic alternative to surgery; however, because of mixed results from clinical trials, this approach has not been adopted widely. The authors of this study investigate the role of a triple drug induction chemotherapy (docetaxel, cisplatin, and 5-fluorouracil) before surgical resection in patients with oral cavity tumors to determine whether there is an improvement in survival. The authors report a high rate of clinical complete response (72.9%) and a modest rate of pathological complete response (27.7%). Unfortunately, this did not result in improved survival.

B. A. Murphy, MD

Cisplatin and Radiotherapy With or Without Erlotinib in Locally Advanced Squamous Cell Carcinoma of the Head and Neck: A Randomized Phase II Trial

Martins RG, Parvathaneni U, Bauman JE, et al (Univ of Washington, Seattle; Univ of New Mexico, Albuquerque; et al)
J Clin Oncol 31:1415-1421, 2013

Purpose.—The combination of cisplatin and radiotherapy is a standard treatment for patients with locally advanced squamous cell carcinoma of the head and neck (SCCHN). Cetuximab-radiotherapy is superior to radiotherapy alone in this population, validating epidermal growth factor receptor (EGFR) as a target. Erlotinib is a small-molecule inhibitor of EGFR. Adding EGFR inhibition to standard cisplatin-radiotherapy may improve efficacy.

Patients and Methods.—Patients with locally advanced SCCHN were randomly assigned to receive cisplatin 100 mg/m^2 on days 1, 22, and 43

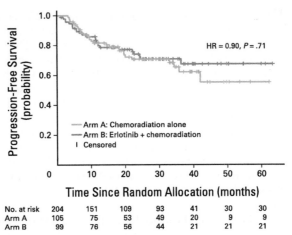

FIGURE 2.—Progression-free survival by treatment arm. HR, hazard ratio. (Reprinted from Martins RG, Parvathaneni U, Bauman JE, et al. Cisplatin and radiotherapy with or without erlotinib in locally advanced squamous cell carcinoma of the head and neck: a randomized phase II trial. *J Clin Oncol.* 2013;31:1415-1421, Reprinted with permission. © 2013, American Society of Clinical Oncology. All rights reserved.)

combined with 70 Gy of radiotherapy (arm A) or the same chemoradiotherapy with erlotinib 150 mg per day, starting 1 week before radiotherapy and continued to its completion (arm B). The primary end point was complete response rate (CRR), evaluated by central review. The secondary end point was progression-free survival (PFS). Available tumors were tested for p16 and EGFR by fluorescent in situ hybridization.

Results.—Between December 2006 and October 2011, 204 patients were randomly assigned. Arms were well balanced for all patient characteristics including p16, with the exception of more women on arm A. Patients on arm B had more rash, but treatment arms did not differ regarding rates of other grade 3 or 4 toxicities. Arm A had a CRR of 40% and arm B had a CRR of 52% ($P = .08$) when evaluated by central review. With a median follow-up time of 26 months and 54 progression events, there was no difference in PFS (hazard ratio, 0.9; $P = .71$).

Conclusion.—Erlotinib did not increase the toxicity of cisplatin and radiotherapy in patients with locally advanced HNSCC but failed to significantly increase CRR or PFS (Fig 2).

▶ Concurrent chemoradiation (CCR) is an integral part of therapy for either primary or adjuvant therapy for head and neck cancer patients with locally advanced disease. Depending on the setting, trials comparing CCR with radiation have only shown improved outcomes, including larynx preservation, disease-specific survival (DFS), and overall survival (OS). Improved outcomes, however, come at the expense of increased toxicity. Unfortunately, even aggressive CCR fails to cure a subset of high-risk patients. Thus, identification of effective, less-toxic radiation-sensitizing regimens is needed. The investigators conducted a large, randomized, phase II trial to determine whether the addition of erlotinib to chemoradiation with standard-dose cisplatin resulted in improved complete response rates or progression-free survival. Results failed to show any benefit from the addition of erlotinib to CCR with cisplatin. The results are similar to those reported for RTOG 0522, a randomized, phase III trial of concurrent accelerated radiation plus cisplatin with or without cetuximab for stage III to IV head and neck cancer. The RTOG trial, which randomly selected 895 patients, failed to show any improvement in OS or DFS. Thus, outside of a clinical trial, the combined use of an epidermal growth factor receptor (EGFR) inhibitor with chemoradiation should not be used. The question still remains as to whether replacing chemotherapy with an EGFR inhibitor in low-risk patients provides equivalent treatment outcomes with improved acute and late symptom burden.

B. A. Murphy, MD

Associations among speech, eating, and body image concerns for surgical patients with head and neck cancer
Fingeret MC, Hutcheson KA, Jensen K, et al (The Univ of Texas MD Anderson Cancer Ctr, Houston)
Head Neck 35:354-360, 2013

Background.—Body image can be affected by bodily experiences extending beyond physical appearance. This study evaluated associations among speech, eating, and body image concerns for surgically treated patients with oral cavity, midface, and cutaneous cancers of the head and neck.

Methods.—Using a cross-sectional design, 280 participants completed the Body Image Scale, a survey evaluating disease-specific body image issues, and the Functional Assessment of Cancer Therapy Scale—General.

Results.—Participants with speech and eating concerns reported the highest levels of body image/appearance dissatisfaction compared with those without such concerns. This group also reported greater cognitive and behavioral difficulties associated with body image concerns and significantly higher levels of interest in psychosocial interventions to address appearance-related difficulties compared with all other participants.

Conclusions.—Findings point to the need for more comprehensive psychosocial care for patients with head and neck malignancies reporting speech and eating difficulties, which extend beyond functional rehabilitation.

▶ Alterations in body image are known to accompany diseases that cause disfigurement. In the field of oncology, body image has been studied most extensively in patients with breast cancer. Data pertaining to alterations in body image are scant in other tumor types. That being said, head and neck cancers have the potential to dramatically impact body image because they can leave highly visible scars, alterations in tissue symmetry, and changes in skin or soft tissue texture. In addition to impacting appearance, head and neck cancers have the potential to affect function: organs critical to sight, speech, swallowing, hearing, taste, and smell may be impaired by either cancer or its treatment. The relationship between function and body image has not been previously explored in the head and neck population. Fingeret conducted a cross-sectional analysis of 280 patients with head and neck or skin cancer to assess body image (using the Body Image Scale), its relationship with general function (measured using the FACT-G), and a study-specific survey that queried head and neck—specific physical, functional, and social issues. Results showed that body image disturbance was highest among patients with functional impairment (speech and eating). The results of this study are important because they highlight the need to study the impact of both disfigurement and dysfunction on body image in head and neck cancer patients.

B. A. Murphy, MD

Cisplatin and fluorouracil with or without panitumumab in patients with recurrent or metastatic squamous-cell carcinoma of the head and neck (SPECTRUM): an open-label phase 3 randomised trial
Vermorken JB, on behalf of the SPECTRUM investigators (Antwerp Univ Hosp, Edegem, Belgium; et al)
Lancet Oncol 14:697-710, 2013

Background.—Previous trials have shown that anti-EGFR monoclonal antibodies can improve clinical outcomes of patients with recurrent or metastatic squamous-cell carcinoma of the head and neck (SCCHN). We assessed the efficacy and safety of panitumumab combined with cisplatin and fluorouracil as first-line treatment for these patients.

Methods.—This open-label phase 3 randomised trial was done at 126 sites in 26 countries. Eligible patients were aged at least 18 years; had histologically or cytologically confirmed SCCHN; had distant metastatic or locoregionally recurrent disease, or both, that was deemed to be incurable by surgery or radiotherapy; had an Eastern Cooperative Oncology Group performance status of 1 or less; and had adequate haematological, renal, hepatic, and cardiac function. Patients were randomly assigned according to a computer-generated randomisation sequence (1:1; stratified by previous treatment, primary tumour site, and performance status) to one of two groups. Patients in both groups received up to six 3-week cycles of intravenous cisplatin (100 mg/m^2 on day 1 of each cycle) and fluorouracil (1000 mg/m^2 on days 1—4 of each cycle); those in the experimental group also received intravenous panitumumab (9 mg/kg on day 1 of each cycle). Patients in the experimental group could choose to continue maintenance panitumumab every 3 weeks. The primary endpoint was overall survival and was analysed by intention to treat. In a prospectively defined retrospective analysis, we assessed tumour human papillomavirus (HPV) status as a potential predictive biomarker of outcomes with a validated p16-INK4A (henceforth, p16) immunohistochemical assay. Patients and investigators were aware of group assignment; study statisticians were masked until primary analysis; and the central laboratory assessing p16 status was masked to identification of patients and treatment. This trial is registered with ClinicalTrials.gov, number NCT00460265.

Findings.—Between May 15, 2007, and March 10, 2009, we randomly assigned 657 patients: 327 to the panitumumab group and 330 to the control group. Median overall survival was 11·1 months (95% CI 9·8-12·2) in the panitumumab group and 9·0 months (8·1-11·2) in the control group (hazard ratio [HR] 0·873, 95% CI 0·729-1·046; p=0·1403). Median progression-free survival was 5·8 months (95% CI 5·6-6·6) in the panitumumab group and 4·6 months (4·1-5·4) in the control group (HR 0·780, 95% CI 0·659-0·922; p=0·0036). Several grade 3 or 4 adverse events were more frequent in the panitumumab group than in the control group: skin or eye toxicity (62 [19%] of 325 included in safety analyses vs six [2%] of 325), diarrhoea (15 [5%] vs four [1%]), hypomagnesaemia (40 [12%] vs 12 [4%]), hypokalaemia (33 [10%] vs 23 [7%]), and dehydration (16 [5%] vs seven [2%]). Treatment-related deaths occurred in 14 patients (4%) in the panitumumab group and eight (2%) in the control group. Five (2%) of the fatal adverse events in the panitumumab group were attributed to the experimental agent. We had appropriate samples to assess p16 status for 443 (67%) patients, of whom 99 (22%) were p16 positive. Median overall survival in patients with p16-negative tumours was longer in the panitumumab group than in the control group (11·7 months [95% CI 9·7-13·7] vs 8·6 months [6·9-11·1]; HR 0·73

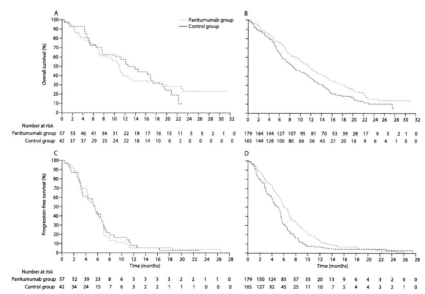

FIGURE 5.—Overall and progression-free survival by p16 status. Overall survival in p16-positive (A) and p16-negative (B) patients. Progression-free survival in p16-positive (C) and p16-negative (D) patients. p16=p16-INK4A. (Reprinted from The Lancet Oncology. Vermorken JB, on behalf of the SPECTRUM investigators. Cisplatin and fluorouracil with or without panitumumab in patients with recurrent or metastatic squamous-cell carcinoma of the head and neck (SPECTRUM): an open-label phase 3 randomised trial. *Lancet Oncol.* 2013;14:697-710, Copyright 2013, with permission from Elsevier.)

[95% CI 0·58-0·93]; $p=0·0115$), but this difference was not shown for p16-positive patients (11·0 months [7·3-12·9] vs 12·6 months [7·7-17·4]; 1·00 [0·62-1·61]; $p=0·998$). In the control group, p16-positive patients had numerically, but not statistically, longer overall survival than did p16-negative patients (HR 0·70 [95% CI 0·47-1·04]).

Interpretation.—Although the addition of panitumumab to chemotherapy did not improve overall survival in an unselected population of patients with recurrent or metastatic SCCHN, it improved progression-free survival and had an acceptable toxicity profile. p16 status could be a prognostic and predictive marker in patients treated with panitumumab and chemotherapy. Prospective assessment will be necessary to validate our biomarker findings (Fig 5).

▶ Cetuximab, an anti—epidermal growth factor receptor (EGFR) monoclonal antibody, in combination with platinum-based chemotherapy, improved overall survival in patients with metastatic/recurrent head and neck cancer when compared with chemotherapy alone.[1] Panitumumab, a fully human anti-EGFR monoclonal antibody, is associated with a decreased risk of anaphylactic reactions. In this study, investigators wanted to determine whether panitumumab improved survival when combined with systemic chemotherapy in patients with metastatic/recurrent head and neck cancer. No survival advantage was noted in the unselected study population; however, in the subset of patients with p16-negative tumors, results showed an increase in median survival from 8.6 to 11.7 months when panitumumab was added to chemotherapy. This study is the first to underscore the potential difference in response to systemic chemotherapy for patients with metastatic/recurrent head and neck cancer based on human papillomavirus status. Previously, when designing treatment trials directed at this population, investigators would consider the following important prognostic indicators: performance status, time since completion of prior therapy, and whether patients had received prior therapy directed at metastatic or recurrent disease. Future studies will need to be stratified based on HPV status, or they will need to design clinical trials specifically for HPV+ and HPV-patients.

B. A. Murphy, MD

Reference

1. Vermorken JB, Mesia R, Rivera F, et al. Platinum-based chemotherapy plus cetuximab in head and neck cancer. *N Engl J Med*. 2008;359:1116-1127.

A systematic review of head and neck cancer quality of life assessment instruments

Ojo B, Genden EM, Teng MS, et al (Mount Sinai School of Medicine, NY; et al)
Oral Oncol 48:923-937, 2012

Although quality of life (QOL) is an important treatment outcome in head and neck cancer (HNC), cross-study comparisons have been hampered by the heterogeneity of measures used and the fact that reviews of HNC QOL instruments have not been comprehensive to date. We performed a systematic review of the published literature on HNC QOL instruments from 1990 to 2010, categorized, and reviewed the properties of the instruments using international guidelines as reference. Of the 2766 articles retrieved, 710 met the inclusion criteria and used 57 different head and neck-specific instruments to assess QOL. A review of the properties of these utilized measures and identification of areas in need of further research is presented. Given the volume and heterogeneity of QOL measures, there is no gold standard questionnaire. Therefore, when selecting instruments, researchers should consider not only psychometric properties but also research objectives, study design, and the pitfalls and benefits of combining different measures. Although great strides have been made in the assessment of QOL in HNC and researchers now have a plethora of quality instruments to choose from, more work is needed to improve the clinical utility of these measures in order to link QOL research to clinical practice. This review provides a platform for head and neck-specific instrument comparisons, with suggestions of important factors to consider in the systematic selection of QOL instruments, and is a first step towards translation of QOL assessment into the clinical scene.

▶ "Quality of life" is a term that has become synonymous with "symptom burden" and "functional outcomes." However, strictly speaking, "quality of life" refers to a global construct that describes a patient's general sense of well-being. Health-related quality of life confines itself to factors related to disease and treatment that impact well-being. Most health-related quality-of-life tools will address several specific domains, including functional, physical, emotional, and social well-being. In addition to general quality-of-life tools, symptom-specific and tumor site—specific measurement tools have been developed.

Head and neck cancer and its treatment results in tremendous symptom burden and impaired functionality, which can, in turn, decrease quality of life. With increasingly aggressive multimodality therapy, there has been a dramatic escalation in the acute and late toxicities of therapy. We are only now beginning to recognize the myriad problems head and neck cancer patients face and the profound impact on their day-to-day existence. To better understand adverse treatment-related effects, there has been a proliferation of patient-reported outcome measures. Some of these tools are designed to asses overall symptom burden, whereas others assess specific problems, such as swallowing, in a more in-depth manner. For the average reader, keeping up with the available tools is a daunting task. Ojo et al have made this task simpler by conducting an extensive review of tools directed at assessing quality of life, symptom burden, and functional impairment. The content, validity, and reliability are summarized in easy-to-read tables. This is a must-read article for anyone who treats head and neck cancer.

B. A. Murphy, MD

Evaluation of Human Papillomavirus Antibodies and Risk of Subsequent Head and Neck Cancer

Kreimer AR, Johansson M, Waterboer T, et al (Natl Insts of Health, Rockville, MD; International Agency for Res on Cancer, Lyon, France; German Inst of Human Nutrition Potsdam Rehbruecke, Nuthetal, Germany; et al)
J Clin Oncol 31:2708-2715, 2013

Purpose.—Human papillomavirus type 16 (HPV16) infection is causing an increasing number of oropharyngeal cancers in the United States and Europe. The aim of our study was to investigate whether HPV antibodies are associated with head and neck cancer risk when measured in prediagnostic sera.

Methods.—We identified 638 participants with incident head and neck cancers (patients; 180 oral cancers, 135 oropharynx cancers, and 247 hypopharynx/larynx cancers) and 300 patients with esophageal cancers as well as 1,599 comparable controls from within the European Prospective Investigation Into Cancer and Nutrition cohort. Prediagnostic plasma samples from patients (collected, on average, 6 years before diagnosis) and control participants were analyzed for antibodies against multiple proteins of HPV16 as well as HPV6, HPV11, HPV18, HPV31, HPV33, HPV45, and HPV52. Odds ratios (ORs) of cancer and 95% CIs were calculated, adjusting for potential confounders. All-cause mortality was evaluated among patients using Cox proportional hazards regression.

Results.—HPV16 E6 seropositivity was present in prediagnostic samples for 34.8% of patients with oropharyngeal cancer and 0.6% of controls (OR, 274; 95% CI, 110 to 681) but was not associated with other cancer sites. The increased risk of oropharyngeal cancer among HPV16 E6 seropositive participants was independent of time between blood collection and diagnosis and was observed more than 10 years before diagnosis. The all-cause mortality ratio among patients with oropharyngeal cancer was 0.30 (95% CI, 0.13 to 0.67), for patients who were HPV16 E6 seropositive compared with seronegative.

Conclusion.—HPV16 E6 seropositivity was present more than 10 years before diagnosis of oropharyngeal cancers (Table 2).

▶ Human papillomavirus (HPV) is a known cause of oropharyngeal carcinomas. One question that researchers have been interested in answering is the temporal relationship between HPV exposure and the development of oropharyngeal cancers. To answer this question, investigators in 10 European countries linked clinical databases with a serum repository of almost 400 000 patients who

TABLE 2.—ORs by HPV16 Serology Status for Cancer of the Oral Cavity, Oropharynx, Larynx, and Esophagus

Serology Status	Controls (n = 1,599)		Oral Cavity Cancer (n = 180)				Oropharynx Cancer (n = 135)				Larynx Cancer (n = 247)*				Esophageal Cancer (n = 300)			
	No. of Participants	%	No. of Patients	%	OR	95% CI	No. of Patients	%	OR	95% CI	No. of Patients	%	OR	95% CI	No. of Patients	%	OR	95% CI
HPV16 oncoproteins																		
E6																		
Seronegative	1,590	99.4	178	98.9	1		88	65.2	1		244	98.8	1		299	99.7	1	
Seropositive	9	0.6	2	1.1	1.3	0.3 to 6.9	47	34.8	274	110 to 681	3	1.2	3.8	0.8 to 17.6	1	0.3	0.6	.1 to 5.2
E7																		
Seronegative	1,421	88.9	155	86.1	1		108	80.0	1		217	87.9	1		272	90.7	1	
Seropositive	178	11.1	25	13.9	1.2	0.7 to 1.9	27	20.0	2.4	1.5 to 3.9	30	12.1	0.9	0.5 to 1.4	28	9.3	0.7	0.5 to 1.2
HPV16 other early proteins																		
E1																		
Seronegative	1,536	96.1	165	91.7	1		113	83.7	1		226	91.5	1		283	94.3	1	
Seropositive	63	3.9	15	8.3	2.1	1.1 to 3.9	22	16.3	5.7	3.2 to 10.0	21	8.5	2.2	1.2 to 3.9	17	5.7	1.7	0.9 to 3.0
E2																		
Seronegative	1,527	95.5	170	94.4	1		102	75.6	1		234	94.7	1		286	95.3	1	
Seropositive	72	4.5	10	5.6	1.0	0.5 to 2.1	33	24.4	9.5	5.7 to 15.8	13	5.3	1.0	0.5 to 1.9	14	4.7	0.9	0.5 to 1.7
E4																		
Seronegative	1,437	89.9	165	91.7	1		120	88.9	1		218	88.3	1		276	92.0	1	
Seropositive	162	10.1	15	8.3	0.8	0.5 to 1.5	15	11.1	1.3	0.7 to 2.4	29	11.7	1.2	0.7 to 1.9	24	8.0	0.8	0.5 to 1.2
HPV16 late protein																		
L1																		
Seronegative	1,270	79.4	138	76.7	1		79	58.5	1		187	75.7	1		231	77.0	1	
Seropositive	329	20.6	42	23.3	1.2	0.8 to 1.7	56	41.5	3.1	2.1 to 4.5	60	24.3	1.3	0.9 to 1.8	69	23.0	1.1	0.8 to 1.6

NOTE. All ORs were adjusted for sex, age at enrollment (in 5-year age categories), country, tobacco (never, former, current), and alcohol use (never/ever and continuous values in gm/day at recruitment).

Abbreviations: HPV, human papillomavirus; OR, odds ratio.

*The larynx cancer category includes 31 participants with hypopharyngeal cancer.

donated samples between 1992 and 2000. The development and maintenance of large databases of this type are a herculean effort on the part of investigators and reflect substantial monetary investment. That being said, the potential gain of knowledge is well worth the effort. In this analysis, serum samples were tested for antibodies to L1 (a major capsid protein), early oncoproteins E6 and E7, and other early proteins associated with selected carcinogenic and noncarcinogenic HPV serotypes. Thirty-five percent of patients with oropharyngeal cancer were HPV16 E6 seropositive compared with 1% for controls. Because the HPV status of the tumors was not reported and the ability of HVP E6 antibody to identify HPV-associated tumors has yet to be established, the true incidence of HPV-associated tumors in this study is unknown. Given the patient characteristics and excellent survival of the antibody-positive cohort, it is highly likely that the oropharyngeal cancers associated with HPV E6 antibody were indeed caused by HPV. The most striking results from the study indicate that antibodies to HPV16 were present an average of 6 years before the documentation of oropharyngeal cancer with a latency of greater than 10 years in a significant subset of patients. It is unknown whether the antibodies are produced in response to persistent HPV infection, preinvasive cancer, or slowly developing invasive cancer that is asymptomatic or clinically undetectable. For never-smoking patients with HPV E6 antibodies, the 10-year risk of oropharyngeal cancer development is 7% for women and 23% for men. Of note, specimens collected from oral cavity and laryngeal and esophageal cancers have low rates of HPV E6 seropositivity, confirming the unique role of HPV in the pathogenesis of oropharyngeal cancers.

B. A. Murphy, MD

Management of Human Papillomavirus–Positive and Human Papillomavirus–Negative Head and Neck Cancer
Mehra R, Ang KK, Burtness B (Fox Chase Cancer Ctr, Philadelphia, PA; MD Anderson Cancer Ctr, Houston, TX)
Semin Radiat Oncol 22:194-197, 2012

A subset of squamous cell carcinomas of the head and neck is now known to be caused by oncogenic human papillomavirus (HPV) infection. Viral-associated malignancies arise predominantly from the oropharynx and are generally more responsive to treatment compared with non-HPV squamous cell head and neck carcinomas. Although many patients with HPV-positive disease lack the traditional risk factors of tobacco and alcohol use, retrospective recursive partitioning analysis indicates that patients with a >10 pack-year smoking history and HPV-positive disease may be at intermediate risk for survival. This warrants further study in a prospective clinical trial. Thus, current clinical trials that are being designed to study curative treatment regimens, such as transoral surgery or combinations of radiation with systemic therapy, are being developed separately for HPV-positive and HPV-negative disease with attention to tobacco history. This review will discuss some of the ongoing research efforts for HPV-positive and HPV-negative head and neck carcinomas.

▶ Squamous cell carcinoma of the head and neck region is notoriously caused by smoking and, in some cases, by smoking and excessive alcohol intake. A subset of head and neck cancers was identified several years ago in patients without a smoking history plus or minus alcohol use but found to be associated with human papillomavirus (HPV) infections. The good news about the HPV-positive tumors is that they have been found to have a more favorable outcome and often require less aggressive therapy to attain that good outcome.

This article is an excellent review of the current strategies of treating head and neck cancers with or without associated HPV infections. The authors have nicely included a perspective on smoking history with patients who have HPV-positive tumors. If the smoking history is significant (ie, > 10 years) then these HPV-positive tumors may not be as favorable as those without the smoking history. Thus, this smoking and HPV group needs special attention, especially about trials to assess outcomes and the possible need for more aggressive therapies compared with the nonsmoking HPV-positive tumors.

C. Lawton, MD

history. This review will discuss some of the ongoing research efforts for HPV-positive and HPV-negative head and neck carcinoma.

C. Lawton, MD

12 Pediatric Cancer

Hematologic Disorders

Association Between Radiotherapy vs No Radiotherapy Based on Early Response to VAMP Chemotherapy and Survival Among Children With Favorable-Risk Hodgkin Lymphoma

Metzger ML, Weinstein HJ, Hudson MM, et al (Univ of Tennessee, Memphis; Massachusetts General Hosp, Boston; et al)
JAMA 307:2609-2616, 2012

Context.—More than 90% of children with favorable-risk Hodgkin lymphoma can achieve long-term survival, yet many will experience toxic effects from radiation therapy. Pediatric oncologists strive for maintaining excellent cure rates while minimizing toxic effects.

Objective.—To evaluate the efficacy of 4 cycles of vinblastine, Adriamycin (doxorubicin), methotrexate, and prednisone (VAMP) in patients with favorable–risk Hodgkin lymphoma who achieve a complete response after 2 cycles and do not receive radiotherapy.

Design, Setting, and Patients.—Multi-institutional, unblinded, non-randomized single group phase 2 clinical trial to assess the need for radiotherapy based on early response to chemotherapy. Eighty-eight eligible patients with Hodgkin lymphoma stage I and II (<3 nodal sites, no B symptoms, mediastinal bulk, or extranodal extension) enrolled between March 3, 2000, and December 9, 2008. Follow-up data are current to March 12, 2012.

Interventions.—The 47 patients who achieved a complete response after 2 cycles received no radiotherapy, and the 41 with less than a complete response were given 25.5 Gy-involved-field radiotherapy.

Main Outcome Measures.—Two-year event-free survival was the primary outcome measure. A 2-year event-free survival of greater than 90% was desired, and 80% was considered to be unacceptably low.

Results.—Two-year event-free survival was 90.8% (95% CI, 84.7%-96.9%). For patients who did not require radiotherapy, it was 89.4% (95% CI, 80.8%-98.0%) compared with 92.5% (95% CI, 84.5%-100%) for those who did (*P* = .61). Most common acute adverse effects were neuropathic pain (2% of patients), nausea or vomiting (3% of patients), neutropenia (32% of cycles), and febrile neutropenia (2% of patients). Nine patients (10%) were hospitalized 11 times (3% of cycles) for febrile neutropenia or nonneutropenic infection. Long-term adverse effects after radiotherapy were asymptomatic compensated hypothyroidism in 9 patients (10%), osteonecrosis and moderate osteopenia in 2 patients each (2%), subclinical pulmonary dysfunction in 12 patients (14%), and asymptomatic left ventricular dysfunction in 4 patients (5%). No second malignant neoplasms were observed.

Conclusions.—Among patients with favorable–risk Hodgkin lymphoma and a complete early response to chemotherapy, the use of limited radiotherapy resulted in a high rate of 2-year event-free survival.

Trial Registration.—clinicaltrials.gov Identifier: NCT00145600.

▶ Treatment of any of the pediatric malignancies is always a double-edged sword. On the one side, it is imperative to give enough treatment, including surgery with or without chemotherapy or radiation, to eliminate the disease, and on the other side, physicians really do not want to overtreat so as to mitigate toxicity, both acute and late. Thus, studies like this are critical to achieve the best outcomes for the pediatric patients.

Pediatric Hodgkin lymphoma is a very curable malignancy, especially for the favorable-risk subgroup. With cure rates in the 90% range, there are questions as to how to help decrease the risk of subsequent treatment toxicities. The addition of radiation for these patients is known to be associated with an increased risk of secondary malignancies and other nonmalignant complications (pending the site of radiation). Therefore, the data in this study that show an equivalency between children who achieved an early complete response without radiation and children who received radiation and chemotherapy because of a lesser response are very significant. The patients who did not need the radiation benefited from a decrease in harmful effects on the lungs, thyroid, bones, and heart and likely with longer follow-up will benefit in terms of a decrease in secondary malignancies.

C. Lawton, MD

Therapy prolongation improves outcome in multisystem Langerhans cell histiocytosis
Gadner H, for the Histiocyte Society (Children's Cancer Res Inst and St. Anna Children's Hosp, Vienna, Austria; et al)
Blood 121:5006-5014, 2013

Langerhans cell histiocytosis (LCH)-III tested risk-adjusted, intensified, longer treatment of multisystem LCH (MS-LCH), for which optimal therapy has been elusive. Stratified by risk organ involvement (high [RO+] or low [RO−] risk groups), >400 patients were randomized. RO+ patients received 1 to 2 six-week courses of vinblastine+prednisone (Arm A) or vinblastine+prednisone+methotrexate (Arm B). Response triggered milder continuation therapy with the same combinations, plus 6-mercaptopurine, for 12 months total treatment. 6/12-week response rates (mean,

71%) and 5-year survival (84%) and reactivation rates (27%) were similar in both arms. Notably, historical comparisons revealed survival superior to that of identically stratified RO+ patients treated for 6 months in predecessor trials LCH-I (62%) or LCH-II (69%, $P < .001$), and lower 5-year reactivation rates than in LCH-I (55%) or LCH-II (44%, $P < .001$). RO− patients received vinblastine+prednisone throughout. Response by 6 weeks triggered randomization to 6 or 12 months total treatment. Significantly lower 5-year reactivation rates characterized the 12-month Arm D (37%) compared with 6-month Arm C (54%, $P = .03$) or to 6-month schedules in LCH-I (52%) and LCH-II (48%, $P < .001$). Thus, prolonging treatment decreased RO− patient reactivations in LCH-III, and although methotrexate added no benefit, RO+ patient survival and reactivation rates have substantially improved in the 3 sequential trials. (Trial No NCT00276757 www.ClinicalTrials.gov).

▶ The discussion of whether Langerhans cell histiocytosis (LCH) is an inflammatory, immune-mediated disorder or a neoplasm has been going on for decades. The documentation favoring the latter explanation, however, has increased, including the demonstration of clonality, alterations in p53 regulation, the presence of shortened telomeres, and, most critically, the recent findings of *BRAF1* mutations in 50% to 60% of cells along with nearly uniform activation of the ERK pathway. Thus, LCH properly belongs in this YEAR BOOK OF ONCOLOGY, and the report by Gadner et al possibly represents the debut of such reviews. This study describes the results of the LCH III International Trial. Building on the results of the LCH I and II trials, this trial randomized 2 important questions. Patients with risk of organ involvement and multisystem disease were randomly assigned to receive standard therapy with or without methotrexate. The results were negative, but definitive, in that methotrexate did not improve overall responses, survival, or recurrence rates. However, those who received methotrexate had a significantly increased risk of development of grade 3 and 4 toxicities. Patients without risk of organ involvement and multisystem disease were randomly assigned to receive either 6 months or 12 months of maintenance therapy. The results showed a significant reduction in the recurrence rate for those who received 12 months of maintenance therapy. Of note, there was no change in the incidence of diabetes insipidus among any of the randomized cohorts. When overall survival was compared with the results from LCH I and II trials (a dangerous statistical leap), there appeared to be a significantly improved overall survival with the LCH III trial. Because initial response rates did not differ, one can hypothesize that, if such historical comparisons are true, then possibly supportive care or improved treatment for those with up-front refractory disease might be responsible. These results show how real progress in a rare disease can be made through international cooperation. They also show that significant improvements in overall response rates are still needed in this enigmatic disease.

R. J. Arceci, MD, PhD

Leukemia

The role of matched sibling donor allogeneic stem cell transplantation in pediatric high-risk acute myeloid leukemia: results from the AML-BFM 98 study

Klusmann J-H, Reinhardt D, Zimmermann M, et al (Med School Hannover, Germany; et al)
Haematologica 97:21-29, 2012

Background.—The role of allogeneic stem cell transplantation in post-remission management of children with high-risk acute myeloid leukemia remains controversial. In the multi-center AML-BFM 98 study we prospectively evaluated the impact of allogeneic stem cell transplantation in children with high-risk acute myeloid leukemia in first complete remission.

Design and Methods.—HLA-typed patients with high-risk acute myeloid leukemia, who achieved first complete remission (n = 247), were included in this analysis. All patients received double induction and consolidation. Based on the availability of a matched-sibling donor, patients were allocated by genetic chance to allogeneic stem cell transplantation (n = 61) or chemotherapy-only (i.e. intensification and maintenance therapy; n = 186). The main analysis was done on an intention-to-treat basis according to this allocation.

Results.—Intention-to-treat analysis did not show a significantly different 5-year disease-free survival (49 ± 6% *versus* 45 ± 4%, $P_{\text{log rank}} = 0.44$) or overall survival (68 ± 6% *versus* 57 ± 4%, $P_{\text{log rank}} = 0.17$) between the matched-sibling donor and no-matched-sibling donor groups, whereas late adverse effects occurred more frequently after allogeneic stem cell transplantation (72.5% *versus* 31.8%, $P_{\text{Fischer}} < 0.01$). These results were confirmed by as-treated analysis corrected for the time until transplantation (5-year overall survival: 72 ± 8% *versus* 60 ± 4%, $P_{\text{Mantel-Byar}}$ 0.21). Subgroup analysis demonstrated improved survival rates for patients with 11q23 aberrations allocated to allogeneic stem cell transplantation (5-year overall survival: 94 ± 6% *versus* 52 ± 7%, $P_{\text{log rank}} = 0.01$; n = 18 *versus* 49) in contrast to patients without 11q23 aberrations (5-year overall survival: 58 ± 8% *versus* 55 ± 5%, $P_{\text{log rank}} = 0.66$).

Conclusions.—Our analyses defined a genetic subgroup of children with high-risk acute myeloid leukemia who benefited from allogeneic stem cell transplantation in the prospective multi-center AML-BFM 98 study. For the remainder of the pediatric high-risk acute myeloid leukemia patients the prognosis was not improved by allogeneic stem cell transplantation, which was, however, associated with a higher rate of late sequelae. (ClinicalTrials.gov Identifier: #NCT00111345).

▶ Although the role of bone marrow transplantation in pediatric acute myeloid leukemia (AML) has decreased as chemotherapeutic regimens have improved overall outcome, there are still a group of patients with quite poor prognosis for whom transplantation continues to be used without a great deal of data to definitively demonstrate its role. Klusmann et al have provided some hints to indicate that a subgroup of patients with high-risk AML may indeed benefit from transplantation. Although they observed no difference in outcome for the overall AML-BFM (Berlin-Frankfurt-Muenster) 98 study for those who received vs those who did not receive a transplant, a subgroup of patients with AML characterized by chromosome 11q23 alternations showed significant benefit in overall survival if they underwent a transplant. Not surprisingly, the effect seemed to emanate from those with t(4;11), t(6;11), and t(10;11) translocations and not t(9;11) or t(11;19) translocations, which have been shown in previous studies not to be particularly poor prognostic markers. Although the numbers and the age of this trial do not provide definitive data for emphatically directed treatment choices, the study points out the continued need to rigorously investigate the role, if any, of transplantation in patients with high-risk AML.

R. J. Arceci, MD, PhD

Nonadherence to Oral Mercaptopurine and Risk of Relapse in Hispanic and Non-Hispanic White Children With Acute Lymphoblastic Leukemia: A Report From the Children's Oncology Group

Bhatia S, Landier W, Shangguan M, et al (City of Hope, Duarte, CA; et al)
J Clin Oncol 30:2094-2101, 2012

Purpose.—Systemic exposure to mercaptopurine (MP) is critical for durable remissions in children with acute lymphoblastic leukemia (ALL). Nonadherence to oral MP could increase relapse risk and also contribute to inferior outcome in Hispanics. This study identified determinants of adherence and described impact of adherence on relapse, both overall and by ethnicity.

Patients and Methods.—A total of 327 children with ALL (169 Hispanic; 158 non-Hispanic white) participated. Medication event-monitoring system caps recorded date and time of MP bottle openings. Adherence rate, calculated monthly, was defined as ratio of days of MP bottle opening to days when MP was prescribed.

Results.—After 53,394 person-days of monitoring, adherence declined from 94.7% (month 1) to 90.2% (month 6; $P < .001$). Mean adherence over 6 months was significantly lower among Hispanics (88.4% v 94.8%; $P < .001$), patients age ≥ 12 years (85.7% v 93.1%; $P < .001$), and patients from single-mother households (80.6% v 93.1%; $P = .001$). A progressive increase in relapse was observed with decreasing adherence (reference: adherence $\geq 95\%$; 94.9% to 90%: hazard ratio [HR], 4.1; 95% CI, 1.2 to 13.5; $P = .02$; 89.9% to 85%: HR, 4.0; 95% CI, 1.0 to 15.5; $P = .04$; <85%: HR. 5.7; 95% CI, 1.9 to 16.8; $P = .002$). Cumulative incidence of relapse ($\pm$ standard deviation) was higher among Hispanics (16.5% $\pm$ 4.0% v 6.3% $\pm$ 2.2%; $P = .02$). Association between Hispanic ethnicity and relapse (HR, 2.6; 95% CI, 1.1 to 6.1; $P = .02$) became nonsignificant (HR, 1.8; 95% CI, 0.6 to 5.2; $P = .26$) after adjusting for adherence and socioeconomic status. At adherence rates $\geq 90\%$, Hispanics continued to demonstrate higher relapse, whereas at rates <90%, relapse risk was comparable to that of non-Hispanic whites.

Conclusion.—Lower adherence to oral MP increases relapse risk. Ethnic difference in relapse risk differs by level of adherence—an observation currently under investigation.

▶ Although dozens of publications on molecular biomarkers are published detailing how a distinct ribonucleic acid expression pattern or set of gene mutations impacts the prognosis of various cancers, a relatively understudied area is medication compliance. The study by Bhatia et al examines compliance to taking oral 6-mercaptopurine in a cohort of children with acute lymphoblastic leukemia (ALL). Several potentially important findings emerged from the results. First was that 44% of children with ALL may be taking ≤95% of the recommended doses of 6-mercaptopurine and may be at risk for higher frequency of leukemia relapse. Second, Hispanic patients, particularly those older than 12 years of age, are in a single-mother household, or are of lower socioeconomic status, have a significantly lower compliance and a concomitant increased incidence of leukemia relapse. Of further interest, Hispanic ethnicity and relapse were nonsignificant when adjusted for medication adherence and socioeconomic status. Although one could certainly question whether electronically recording that a bottle of medication was opened proves that a patient took the medication (eg, one could open the bottle and remove several days of pills and take them but this would be recorded as noncompliance), the likelihood is that the measure reflected the reality of compliance. Clearly, increased efforts need to be made to assure medication compliance, as the cost of 6-mercaptopurine during maintenance therapy is a great deal less life threatening and costly than dealing with recurrent leukemia.

R. J. Arceci, MD, PhD

Second Malignant Neoplasms After Treatment of Childhood Acute Lymphoblastic Leukemia
Schmiegelow K, Levinsen MF, Attarbaschi A, et al (Rigshospitalet, Copenhagen, Denmark; St Anna Children's Hosp, Vienna, Austria; et al)
J Clin Oncol 31:2469-2476, 2013

Purpose.—Second malignant neoplasms (SMNs) after diagnosis of childhood acute lymphoblastic leukemia (ALL) are rare events.

Patients and Methods.—We analyzed data on risk factors and outcomes of 642 children with SMNs occurring after treatment for ALL from 18 collaborative study groups between 1980 and 2007.

Results.—Acute myeloid leukemia (AML; n = 186), myelodysplastic syndrome (MDS; n = 69), and nonmeningioma brain tumor (n = 116) were the most common types of SMNs and had the poorest outcome (5-year survival rate, 18.1% ± 2.9%, 31.1% ± 6.2%, and 18.3% ± 3.8%, respectively). Five-year survival estimates for AML were 11.2% ± 2.9% for 125 patients diagnosed before 2000 and 34.1% ± 6.3% for 61 patients diagnosed after 2000 ($P < .001$); 5-year survival estimates for MDS were 17.1% ± 6.4% (n = 36) and 48.2% ± 10.6% (n = 33; $P = .005$). Allogeneic stem-cell transplantation failed to improve outcome of secondary myeloid malignancies after adjusting for waiting time to transplantation. Five-year survival rates were above 90% for patients with meningioma, Hodgkin lymphoma, thyroid carcinoma, basal cell carcinoma, and parotid gland tumor, and 68.5% ± 6.4% for those with non-Hodgkin lymphoma. Eighty-nine percent of patients with brain tumors had received cranial irradiation. Solid tumors were associated with cyclophosphamide exposure, and myeloid malignancy was associated with topoisomerase II inhibitors and starting doses of methotrexate of at least 25 mg/m^2 per week and mercaptopurine of at least 75 mg/m^2 per day. Myeloid malignancies with monosomy 7/5q- were associated with high hyperdiploid ALL karyotypes, whereas 11q23/*MLL*-rearranged AML or MDS was associated with ALL harboring translocations of t(9;22), t(4;11), t(1;19), and t(12;21) ($P = .03$).

Conclusion.—SMNs, except for brain tumors, AML, and MDS, have outcomes similar to their primary counterparts.

▶ One of the ironic tragedies of the successful treatment of childhood acute lymphoblastic leukemia is the occurrence of treatment-related secondary malignancies. The incidence of these treatment-related cancers has been documented in several publications. Schmiegelow et al now take such analyses a bit further and examine the survival after the occurrence of second malignancies. Their results are important in that they show an extremely poor outcome for survivors who develop secondary acute myeloid leukemia and myelodysplastic syndrome but not meningiomas, Hodgkin lymphoma, thyroid carcinoma, basal cell carcinoma, or parotid gland tumors. The development of secondary myeloid malignancies was associated with the usual suspects of topoisomerase II inhibitors but also higher doses and exposures of methotrexate and 6-mercaptopurine. Also of considerable interest was that 89% of patients who develop brain tumors had received cranial radiation, suggesting either increased germ line predisposition or alternative explanations of brain tumor development. Although the incidence of these secondary malignancies, especially myeloid disorders and brain tumors, might be expected to decrease over time because of the decreased exposure to topoisomerase II inhibitors and cranial radiation, it will be important to carefully monitor survivors, as we have been wrong on such issues before.

R. J. Arceci, MD, PhD

Results of the AIEOP AML 2002/01 multicenter prospective trial for the treatment of children with acute myeloid leukemia
Pession A, for the AIEOP AML Study Group (Università di Bologna, Italy; et al)
Blood 122:170-178, 2013

We evaluated the outcome of 482 children with acute myeloid leukemia (AML) other than promyelocytic leukemia enrolled in the AIEOP-AML-2002/01 trial. Treatment was stratified according to risk group; hematopoietic stem cell transplantation (HSCT) was broadly used in high-risk (HR) children. Patients with core-binding-factor leukemia achieving complete remission (CR) after the first induction course were considered standard risk (SR, 99 patients), whereas the others (n = 383) were assigned to the HR group. Allogeneic (ALLO) or autologous (AUTO)-HSCT was employed, respectively, in 141 and 102 HR patients in CR1 after consolidation therapy. CR, early death, and induction failure rates were 87%, 3%, and 10%, respectively. Relapse occurred in 24% of patients achieving CR. The 8-year overall (OS), event-free (EFS), and disease-free survival (DFS) were 68%, 55%, and 63%, respectively. OS, EFS, and DFS for SR and HR patients were 83%, 63%, and 66% and 64%, 53%, and 62% respectively. DFS was 63% and 73% for HR patients given AUTO-HSCT and ALLO-HSCT, respectively. In multivariate analysis for EFS, risk group, WBC >100 × 10^9/L at diagnosis and monosomal karyotype predicted poorer outcome. These findings indicate that risk-oriented treatment and broad use of HSCT result in a long-term EFS comparing favorably with previously published studies on childhood AML.

▶ An increasing number of oncologists are calling for a decrease in the long and large randomized phase III trial, in part because they are slow in initiating, slow in being completed, and take prolonged periods of time to report. They have also not been strongly biologically driven in terms of the questions being asked. The report by Pession et al on the AIEOP AML 2002/01 multicenter, prospective trial fits comfortably within those criticisms. The study defined patients by risk groups that have been changed in the interim (the question of autologous transplantation has been previously reported in other studies), no analysis of minimal residual disease was reported, and the usually good and bad prognostic factors were identified. Thus, although such data are clearly important to publish, one might consider a nonjournal publication approach to report such information as part of a global database of treatment and outcomes for particular diseases. The balance between resource utilization and scientific advancement remains a difficult field to navigate.

R. J. Arceci, MD, PhD

Clonal selection in xenografted TAM recapitulates the evolutionary process of myeloid leukemia in Down syndrome
Saida S, Watanabe K, Sato-Otsubo A, et al (Kyoto Univ, Japan; The Univ of Tokyo, Japan; et al)
Blood 121:4377-4387, 2013

Transient abnormal myelopoiesis (TAM) is a clonal pre-leukemic disorder that progresses to myeloid leukemia of Down syndrome (ML-DS) through the accumulation of genetic alterations. To investigate the mechanism of leukemogenesis in this disorder, a xenograft model of TAM was established using NOD/Shi-*scid*, IL-2Rγ^{null} mice. Serial engraftment after transplantation of cells from a TAM patient who developed ML-DS a year later demonstrated their self-renewal capacity. A *GATA1* mutation and no copy number alterations (CNA) were detected in the primary patient sample by conventional genomic sequencing and CNA profiling. However, in serial transplantations, engrafted TAM-derived cells showed the emergence of divergent subclones with another *GATA1* mutation and various CNAs, including a 16q deletion and 1q gain, which are clinically associated with ML-DS. Detailed genomic analysis identified minor subclones with 16q deletion or this distinct *GATA1* mutation in the primary patient sample. These results suggest that genetically heterogeneous subclones with varying leukemia-initiating potential already exist in the neonatal TAM phase, and ML-DS may develop from a pool of such minor clones through clonal selection. Our xenograft model of TAM may provide unique insight into the evolutionary process of leukemia.

▶ The biology to explain the extremely high incidence of leukemia in children with Down syndrome or trisomy 21 has remained a mystery. One clue has been thought to reside in the enigmatic disorder of neonates with trisomy 21 called transient abnormal myelopoiesis (TAM) or transient myeloproliferative disorder, which usually regresses over the course of a few weeks to a few months but in roughly 20% to 30% of cases evolves into true acute myeloid leukemias (AML). The identification of *GATA1* mutations as a uniform marker of TAM, along with the presence of the background trisomy 21, has suggested these are early genetic hits with potential to evolve into AML. Saida et al report on the use of a novel immunodeficient mouse system for exploiting xenografts from children with TAM, a previously very low yield approach. The observed definitive clonal evolution in the xenograft model was also, in some instances, similar to that observed in patients who develop AML. The results provide a potentially important model for studying the clonal evolution of AML in a xenograft setting, and this model might be able to be applied to other myelodysplastic syndromes and other myeloproliferative syndromes, including transition from chronic to acute phase chronic myelogenous leukemia. Such a xenograft model would allow the potential to study approaches to intervene in the process as well. The work presents a nice example as to how a rare disease in children can potentially light the way to understanding more common disorders in adults.

R. J. Arceci, MD, PhD

Dasatinib in Children and Adolescents With Relapsed or Refractory Leukemia: Results of the CA180-018 Phase I Dose-Escalation Study of the Innovative Therapies for Children With Cancer Consortium

Zwaan CM, Rizzari C, Mechinaud F, et al (Erasmus Med Ctr (MC)/Sophia Children's Hosp, Rotterdam, the Netherlands; Univ of Milano-Bicocca, Italy; Royal Children's Hosp, Melbourne, Victoria, Australia; et al)
J Clin Oncol 31:2460-2468, 2013

Purpose.—Dasatinib is a potent BCR-ABL inhibitor with proven efficacy in adults with newly diagnosed chronic myeloid leukemia (CML) in chronic phase (CP) and in imatinib-resistant/intolerant disease. This phase I study of the Innovative Therapies for Children with Cancer Consortium assessed dasatinib safety and efficacy in pediatric patients.

Patients and Methods.—Escalating once-daily dasatinib doses (60 to 120 mg/m^2) were administered to children (n = 58) with (i) imatinib-pretreated CML or Philadelphia chromosome (Ph)—positive acute lymhoblastic leukemia (ALL) and (ii) treatment-refractory Ph-negative ALL or acute myeloid leukemia (AML).

Results.—Dasatinib safety and efficacy profiles compared favorably with those in adults. The most common drug-related nonhematologic adverse events were nausea (31%, all grades; 2%, grade 3 to 4), headache (22%, 3%), diarrhea (21%, 0%), and vomiting (17%, 2%). Of 17 patients with CML-CP, 14 (82%) achieved complete cytogenetic response (CCyR) and eight (47%) achieved major molecular response. After ≥24 months of follow-up, median complete hematologic response (CHR) and major cytogenetic response (MCyR) durations were not reached. Of 17 patients with advanced-phase CML or Ph-positive ALL, six (35%) achieved confirmed CHR and 11 (65%) achieved CCyR. Median MCyR duration was 4.6 months (95% CI, 2.1 to 17.4 months). No patient with Ph-negative ALL or AML responded. Dasatinib pediatric pharmacokinetic parameters were comparable with those in adult studies, showing rapid absorption (time to reach maximum concentration, 0.5 to 6.0 hours) and elimination (mean half-life, 3.0 to 4.4 hours).

Conclusion.—Dasatinib 60 mg/m^2 and 80 mg/m^2 once-daily dosing were selected for phase II studies in children with Ph-positive leukemias.

▶ The introduction of novel targeted therapies for children with cancer has usually lagged behind that in adults. The study by Zwaan et al is no exception but, nevertheless, presents some important results testing dasatinib in children who have relapsed or refractory leukemia. The results in patients with chronic myeloid leukemia in chronic phase are similar to those observed in adults, including pharmacokinetic parameters. Somewhat surprisingly, no patients with Ph-negative acute lymphoblastic leukemia (ALL) or acute myeloid leukemia (AML) responded to dasatinib. Although the number of these patients was low (9 for ALL and 15 for AML), the clear lack of response for such a tyrosine kinase inhibitor is disappointing. It is possible that less-specific kinase inhibitors may prove more useful. However, the overall similarities with results compared with those observed in adults, especially the toxicity profiles and pharmacokinetics, re-emphasized the need to accelerate the testing of new agents sooner in children than is currently being done. The chance of such children dying from their cancers is clearly much greater than them dying from such targeted therapies.

R. J. Arceci, MD, PhD

Development and validation of a single-cell network profiling assay-based classifier to predict response to induction therapy in paediatric patients with *de novo* acute myeloid leukaemia: a report from the Children's Oncology Group
Lacayo NJ, Alonzo TA, Gayko U, et al (Children's Oncology Group, Arcadia, CA; Nodality Inc., South San Francisco, CA)
Br J Haematol 162:250-262, 2013

Single cell network profiling (SCNP) is a multi-parameter flow cytometry technique for simultaneous interrogation of intracellular signalling pathways. Diagnostic paediatric acute myeloid leukaemia (AML) bone marrow samples were used to develop a classifier for response to induction therapy in 53 samples and validated in an independent set of 68 samples. The area under the curve of a receiver operating characteristic curve (AUC_{ROC}) was calculated to be $0 \cdot 85$ in the training set and after exclusion of induction deaths, the AUC_{ROC} of the classifier was $0 \cdot 70$ ($P = 0 \cdot 02$) and $0 \cdot 67$ ($P = 0 \cdot 04$) in the validation set when induction deaths (intent to treat) were included. The highest predictive accuracy was noted in the cytogenetic intermediate risk patients (AUC_{ROC} $0 \cdot 88$, $P = 0 \cdot 002$), a subgroup that lacks prognostic/predictive biomarkers for induction response. Only white blood cell count and cytogenetic risk were associated with response to induction therapy in the validation set. After controlling for these variables, the SCNP classifier score was associated with complete remission ($P = 0 \cdot 017$), indicating that the classifier provides information independent of other clinical variables that were jointly associated with response. This is the first validation of an SCNP classifier to predict response to induction chemotherapy. Herein we demonstrate the usefulness of quantitative SCNP under modulated conditions to provide independent information on AML disease biology and induction response.

▶ Predicting the initial response of a cancer to the prescribed, conventional therapy has been an elusive goal of oncologists. This is especially important in that although often a percentage of patients will respond to such treatment, a significant number will not respond but, nevertheless, still experience the toxicities of chemotherapy. This approach is costly to patients and to health care systems. The potential for rapid analysis of diagnosis specimens that could predict the response to treatment would be extremely useful. Lacayo et al show that single-cell network profiling evaluation of newly diagnosed acute myeloid leukemia (AML) samples is able to provide a significantly high (the area under the curve of a receiver operating characteristic curve 0.88) predictive accuracy for determining whether patients will achieve an initial first remission. Of interest, this approach was most useful in patients with intermediate-risk AML and not for good-risk or high-risk AML. Does this suggest that the test, by virtue of how it is performed, represents a subset of cellular signaling responses only relevant to the intermediate-risk AML? Whether such an approach will be relevant to the responses to more targeted therapies will be a future challenge.

R. J. Arceci, MD, PhD

Randomized trial comparing liposomal daunorubicin with idarubicin in induction for pediatric acute myeloid leukemia – Results from Study AMLBFM 2004

Creutzig U, Zimmermann M, Bourquin J-P, et al (Hannover Med School, Germany; Univ of Zurich, Switzerland; et al)
Blood 122:37-43, 2013

Outcomes of patients with acute myeloid leukemia (AML) improve significantly by intensification of induction. To further intensify anthracycline dosage without increasing cardiotoxicity, we compared potentially less cardiotoxic liposomal daunorubicin (L-DNR) to idarubicin at a higher-than-equivalent dose (80 vs 12 mg/m^2 per day for 3 days) during induction. In the multicenter therapy-optimization trial AML-BFM 2004, 521 of 611 pediatric patients (85%) were randomly assigned to L-DNR or idarubicin induction. Five-year results in both treatment arms were similar (overall survival 76% ± 3% [L-DNR] vs 75% ± 3% [idarubicin], $P_{logrank} = .65$; event-free survival [EFS] 59% ± 3% vs 53% ± 3%, $P_{logrank} = .25$; cumulative incidence of relapse 29% ± 3% vs 31% ± 3%, $P_{(Gray)} = .75$), as were EFS results for standard (72% ± 5% vs 68% ± 5%, $P_{logrank} = .47$) and high-risk (51% ± 4% vs 46% ± 4%, $P_{logrank} = .45$) patients. L-DNR resulted in significantly better probability of EFS in patients with t(8;21). Overall, treatment-related mortality was lower with L-DNR than idarubicin (2/257 vs 10/264 patients, $P = .04$). Grade 3/4 cardiotoxicity was rare after induction (4 L-DNR vs 5 idarubicin). Only 1 L-DNR and 3 idarubicin patients presented with subclinical or mild cardiomyopathy during follow-up. In conclusion, at the given dose, L-DNR has overall antileukemic activity comparable to idarubicin, promises to be more active in subgroups, and causes less treatment-related mortality. This trial was registered at www.clinicaltrials.gov as #NCT00111345.

▶ Success in the treatment of patients with acute myeloid leukemia (AML) has come at the expense of dose intensification and accompanying toxicity. Attempts to introduce new agents with high levels of antileukemia activity but with low cross-resistant toxicity have been largely unsuccessful. In addition, as anthracyclines are one of the 2 mainstay active drugs in AML treatment, their cardiotoxicity in children has been particularly concerning. To this end, the AML-BFM 2004 clinical trial attempted to test the introduction of a liposomal anthracycline (daunorubicin), which had potentially less cardiotoxicity. The study randomly assigned 85% of patients to either receive the liposomal daunorubicin or conventional idarubicin. The study unfortunately gave the liposomal daunorubicin at a 1.33-fold higher anthracycline dose, thus, tempering conclusions that might have resulted from using equivalent doses. Nevertheless, the results show that the liposomal daunorubicin cohort experiences a lower treatment-related mortality, although the numbers were low (1 patient in the liposomal cohort vs 6 in the idarubicin group). No differences in overall survival or event-free survival (EFS) were observed except in patients with AML characterized by t(8;21); in this group the liposomal daunorubicin had an improved EFS. The conclusions are early, and late cardiotoxicity showed no difference as well, although the authors try to put a positive spin on this as indicating that more anthracycline can be given without increasing cardiotoxicity. Whether this holds up in longer follow-up is unclear. It would have been of interest to examine MDR1-like transporters and drug efflux in this patient population, as liposomal anthracyclines are known to partially circumvent this drug efflux transporter and drug resistance mechanism. Regardless of the caveats, the introduction of this new agent in pediatric AML is important, and time will be the judge as to its cardiac toxicity—sparing characteristics.

R. J. Arceci, MD, PhD

Treatment reduction for children and young adults with low-risk acute lymphoblastic leukaemia defined by minimal residual disease (UKALL 2003): a randomised controlled trial
Vora A, Goulden N, Wade R, et al (Sheffield Children's Hosp, UK; Great Ormond Street Hosp, London, UK; Univ of Oxford, UK)
Lancet Oncol 14:199-209, 2013

Background.—Minimal residual disease (MRD) is the most sensitive and specific predictor of relapse risk in children with acute lymphoblastic leukaemia (ALL) during remission. We assessed whether treatment intensity could be adjusted for children and young adults according to MRD risk stratification.

Methods.—Between Oct 1, 2003 and June 30, 2011, consecutive children and young adults (aged 1–25 years) with ALL from the UK and Ireland were recruited. Eligible patients were categorised into clinical standard, intermediate, and high risk groups on the basis of a combination of National Cancer Institute (NCI) criteria, cytogenetics, and early response to induction therapy, which was assessed by bone marrow blast counts taken at days 8 (NCI high-risk patients) and 15 (NCI standard-risk patients) after induction began. Clinical standard-risk and intermediate-risk patients were assessed for MRD. Those classified as MRD low risk (undetectable MRD at the end of induction [day 29] or detectable MRD at day 29 that became undetectable by week 11) were randomly assigned

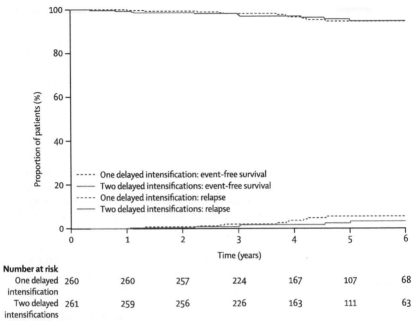

Number at risk

	0	1	2	3	4	5	6
One delayed intensification	260	260	257	224	167	107	68
Two delayed intensifications	261	259	256	226	163	111	63

FIGURE 4.—Event-free survival and relapse in MRD low-risk patients MRD=minimal residual disease. (Reprinted from The Lancet Oncology. Vora A, Goulden N, Wade R, et al. Treatment reduction for children and young adults with low-risk acute lymphoblastic leukaemia defined by minimal residual disease (UKALL 2003): a randomised controlled trial. *Lancet Oncol.* 2013;14:199-209, Copyright 2013, with permission from Elsevier.)

to receive one or two delayed intensification courses. Patients had received induction, consolidation, and interim maintenance therapy before they began delayed intensification. Delayed intensification consisted of pegylated asparaginase on day 4; vincristine, dexamethasone (alternate weeks), and doxorubicin for 3 weeks; and 4 weeks of cyclophosphamide and cytarabine. Computer randomisation was done with stratification by MRD result and balancing for sex, age, and white blood cell count at diagnosis by method of minimisation. Patients, clinicians, and data analysts were not masked to treatment allocation. The primary outcome was event-free survival (EFS), which was defined as time to relapse, secondary tumour, or death. Our aim was to rule out a 7% reduction in EFS in the group given one delayed intensification course relative to that given two delayed intensification courses. Analyses were by intention to treat. This trial is registered, number ISRCTN07355119.

Findings.—Of 3207 patients registered in the trial overall, 521 MRD low-risk patients were randomly assigned to receive one (n=260) or two (n=261) delayed intensification courses. Median follow-up of these patients was 57 months (IQR 42–72). We recorded no significant difference in EFS between the group given one delayed intensification (94·4% at 5 years, 95% CI 91·1–97·7) and that given two delayed intensifications (95·5%, 92·8–98·2; unadjusted odds ratio 1·00, 95% CI

$0 \cdot 43 - 2 \cdot 31$; two-sided p=$0 \cdot 99$). The difference in 5-year EFS between the two groups was $1 \cdot 1\%$ (95% CI $-5 \cdot 6$ to $2 \cdot 5$). 11 patients (actuarial relapse at 5 years $5 \cdot 6\%$, 95% CI $2 \cdot 3$-$8 \cdot 9$) given one delayed intensification and six ($2 \cdot 4\%$, $0 \cdot 2 - 4 \cdot 6$) given two delayed intensifications relapsed (p=$0 \cdot 23$). Three patients ($1 \cdot 2\%$, $0 - 2 \cdot 6$) given two delayed intensifications died of treatment-related causes compared with none in the group given one delayed intensification (p=$0 \cdot 08$). We recorded no significant difference between groups for serious adverse events and grade 3 or 4 toxic effects; however, the second delayed intensification course was associated with one (<1%) treatment-related death, and 74 episodes of grade 3 or 4 toxic effects in 45 patients (17%).

Interpretation.—Treatment reduction is feasible for children and young adults with ALL who are predicted to have a low risk of relapse on the basis of rapid clearance of MRD by the end of induction therapy (Fig 4).

▶ It is not common in oncology to be in a position to consider backing off on treatment because the cure rate is sufficiently high enough that there is the possibility that some patients are being overtreated with resultant adverse side effects. This is indeed the case for a subset of children with low-risk acute lymphoblastic leukemia (ALL), and Vora et al directly, although modestly, address this question based on what is considered a strong prognostic biomarker, that is, minimal residual disease at the end of induction therapy. The study randomly assigned 521 patients with low-risk disease defined by having a minimal residual disease-negative bone marrow (nondetectable leukemia cells at the 0.001% detection level) to receive either 1 or 2 courses of delayed intensification. No difference in event-free survival was observed, thus, showing the noninferiority of the reduced treatment approach. An additional issue is that although one might argue that the reduction of therapy was not very significant, the facts regarding toxicity would argue otherwise in that the second course of delayed intensification was associated with significant morbidity and possibly mortality. This is an important study not only because of the successful reduction in therapy in a subgroup of children with ALL, but also because of the fact that the decision tree was based on a key prognostic biomarker.

R. J. Arceci, MD, PhD

Neuro-Oncology

High Frequency of Germline *SUFU* Mutations in Children With Desmoplastic/Nodular Medulloblastoma Younger Than 3 Years of Age

Brugières L, Remenieras A, Pierron G, et al (Institut Gustave Roussy, Villejuif, France; Institut Curie, Paris, France; et al)
J Clin Oncol 30:2087-2093, 2012

Purpose.—Germline mutations of the *SUFU* gene have been shown to be associated with genetic predisposition to medulloblastoma, mainly in families with multiple cases of medulloblastoma and/or in patients with symptoms similar to those of Gorlin syndrome. To evaluate the contribution of these mutations to the genesis of sporadic medulloblastomas, we screened a series of unselected patients with medulloblastoma for germline *SUFU* mutations.

Patients and Methods.—A complete mutational analysis of the *SUFU* gene was performed on genomic DNA in all 131 consecutive patients treated for medulloblastoma in the pediatrics department of the Institut Gustave Roussy between 1972 and 2009 and for whom a blood sample was available.

Results.—We identified eight germline mutations of the *SUFU* gene: one large genomic duplication and seven point mutations. Mutations were identified in three of three individuals with medulloblastoma with extensive nodularity, four of 20 with desmoplastic/nodular medulloblastomas, and one of 108 with other subtypes. All eight patients were younger than 3 years of age at diagnosis. The mutations were inherited from the healthy father in four of six patient cases in which the parents accepted genetic testing; de novo mutations accounted for the other two patient cases. Associated events were macrocrania in six patients, hypertelorism in three patients, and multiple basal cell carcinomas in the radiation field after age 18 years in one patient.

Conclusion.—These data indicate that germline *SUFU* mutations were responsible for a high proportion of desmoplastic medulloblastoma in children younger than 3 years of age. Genetic testing should be offered to all children diagnosed with sonic hedgehog—driven medulloblastoma at a young age.

▶ Inherited predisposition of cancer has been a key area of investigation in pediatric oncology, leading to the Knudson "2-hit" hypothesis based on children with retinoblastoma, *p53* mutations leading to Li-Fraumeni syndrome, adenomatous polyposis coli, and Lynch syndrome, among many others. Germline mutations of the *SUFU* gene have been identified in several publications to be a strong predisposition to the development of desmoplastic/nodular medulloblastomas in young children. Brugières et al investigated the incidence of *SUFU* mutations in a series of 131 consecutive patients who seemingly had sporadic medulloblastomas. Only 8 mutations were noted, but 6 of these turned out to be germline, in children younger than 3 years of age, and of the desmoplastic/nodular subtype known to be driven by the sonic hedgehog pathway. Although the numbers are not terribly impressive in overall frequency of the *SUFU* mutations, the fact that most of the mutations found were germline raises the important need to carefully screen all young children with the desmoplastic/nodular subtype of medulloblastoma.

R. J. Arceci, MD, PhD

Solid Tumors

G-CSF Receptor Positive Neuroblastoma Subpopulations Are Enriched in Chemotherapy-Resistant or Relapsed Tumors and Are Highly Tumorigenic

Hsu DM, Agarwal S, Benham A, et al (Texas Children's Cancer Ctr, Houston; Baylor College of Medicine, Houston, TX)

Cancer Res 73:4134-4146, 2013

Neuroblastoma is a neural crest-derived embryonal malignancy, which accounts for 13% of all pediatric cancer mortality, primarily due to tumor recurrence. Therapy-resistant cancer stem cells are implicated in tumor relapse, but definitive phenotypic evidence of the existence of these cells has been lacking. In this study, we define a highly tumorigenic subpopulation in neuroblastoma with stem cell characteristics, based on the expression of CSF3R, which encodes the receptor for granulocyte colony-stimulating factor (G-CSF). G-CSF receptor positive (aka G-CSFr⁺ or CD114⁺) cells isolated from a primary tumor and the NGP cell line by flow cytometry were highly tumorigenic and capable of both self-renewal and differentiation to progeny cells. CD114⁺ cells closely resembled embryonic and induced pluripotent stem cells with respect to their profiles of cell cycle, miRNA, and gene expression. In addition, they reflect a primitive undifferentiated neuroectodermal/neural crest phenotype revealing a developmental hierarchy within neuroblastoma tumors. We detected this dedifferentiated neural crest subpopulation in all established neuroblastoma cell lines, xenograft tumors, and primary tumor specimens analyzed. Ligand activation of CD114 by the addition of exogenous G-CSF to CD114⁺ cells confirmed intact STAT3 upregulation, characteristic of G-CSF receptor signaling. Together, our data describe a novel distinct subpopulation within neuroblastoma with enhanced tumorigenicity and a stem cell-like phenotype, further elucidating the complex heterogeneity of solid tumors such as neuroblastoma. We propose that this subpopulation may represent an additional target for novel therapeutic approaches to this aggressive pediatric malignancy.

▶ There have probably been more review articles written regarding cancer stem cells than definitive research papers. Immunophenotypic or functional definitions vary and are limited by the models being used. Nevertheless, the existence and behavior of cancer stem or initiating cells is a fundamentally important one. Hsu et al report on a novel marker, the granulocyte colony-stimulating factor receptor (CD114), for a putative subset of cells with features of neuroblastoma stem cells. Although CD114 has been mostly associated with granulocytic differentiation, there are considerable data to support its role through STAT3 activation in the neural lineage. Although the CD114 expressing population of cells in neuroblastoma does not represent a discretely staining population, but more of a continuum of expression, they usually account for less than 1% of the total population, depending on where one places the flow cytometer gates. The CD114-positive population does have the capacity to form neuroblastoma after xenografting and, interestingly, has a higher percentage of cells in the S phase of the cell cycle than the CD14-negative/low population. This is an unusual observation, as many other cancer stem cells are considered more mitotically quiescent. Nevertheless, the observations of this report are potentially important. It would have been of considerable interest to see functional drug responses of this population of cells and their percentage differences with different clinical stages of neuroblastoma.

R. J. Arceci, MD, PhD

Outcome After Surgery Alone or With Restricted Use of Chemotherapy for Patients With Low-Risk Neuroblastoma: Results of Children's Oncology Group Study P9641
Strother DR, London WB, Schmidt ML, et al (Univ of Calgary and Alberta Children's Hosp, Canada; Children's Hosp Boston and Dana-Farber Cancer Inst, MA; Univ of Illinois at Chicago College of Medicine; et al)
J Clin Oncol 30:1842-1848, 2012

Purpose.—The primary objective of Children's Oncology Group study P9641 was to demonstrate that surgery alone would achieve 3-year overall survival (OS) ≥95% for patients with asymptomatic International Neuroblastoma Staging System stages 2a and 2b neuroblastoma (NBL). Secondary objectives focused on other low-risk patients with NBL and on those who required chemotherapy according to protocol-defined criteria.

Patients and Methods.—Patients underwent maximally safe resection of tumor. Chemotherapy was reserved for patients with, or at risk for, symptomatic disease, with less than 50% tumor resection at diagnosis, or with unresectable progressive disease after surgery alone.

Results.—For all 915 eligible patients, 5-year event-free survival (EFS) and OS were 89% ± 1% and 97% ± 1%, respectively. For patients with asymptomatic stage 2a or 2b disease, 5-year EFS and OS were 87% ± 2% and 96% ± 1%, respectively. Among patients with stage 2b disease, EFS and OS were significantly lower for those with unfavorable histology or diploid tumors, and OS was significantly lower for those ≥18 months old. For patients with stage 1 and 4s NBL, 5-year OS rates were 99% ± 1% and 91% ± 1%, respectively. Patients who required chemotherapy at diagnosis achieved 5-year OS of 98% ± 1%. Of all patients observed after surgery, 11.1% experienced recurrence or progression of disease.

Conclusion.—Excellent survival rates can be achieved in asymptomatic low-risk patients with stages 2a and 2b NBL after surgery alone. Immediate use of chemotherapy may be restricted to a minority of patients with low-risk NBL. Patients with stage 2b disease who are older or have diploid or unfavorable histology tumors fare less well. Future studies will seek to refine risk classification.

▶ Neuroblastoma represents a rare and heterogeneous childhood cancer that has been extensively studied both clinically and molecularly. Even with the extensive amount of analyses, the prognostic factors of age, histology, stage, and *MYCN* amplification remain the key elements in risk definition and treatment stratification. One subgroup of patients that has remained an important challenge is those with low-stage disease. The major question in this group has been how much therapy such patients should receive. Strother et al report on the Children's Oncology Group P9641 experience and show that patients with asymptomatic stage 2a or 2b disease with favorable histology who are less than 18 months of age have excellent outcomes after surgery alone. Importantly, the outcome was significantly worse for patients ≥18 months of age and with tumor histology; comparison with previous studies would suggest that such a group might benefit from treatment more directed toward intermediate-risk patients. These results are important and consistent with the experience from European trials. The results suggest that a subgroup of patients with low-risk disease do not need to experience the short- or long-term consequences of chemotherapy. Why even an incomplete resection of the neuroblastoma in patients with such low-risk disease should be curative remains an important and unexplained mystery.

R. J. Arceci, MD, PhD

The Use of Computed Tomography in Pediatrics and the Associated Radiation Exposure and Estimated Cancer Risk
Miglioretti DL, Johnson E, Williams A, et al (Univ of Washington, Seattle; Kaiser Permanente Hawaii, Honolulu; et al)
JAMA Pediatr 167:1-8, 2013

Importance.—Increased use of computed tomography (CT) in pediatrics raises concerns about cancer risk from exposure to ionizing radiation.

Objectives.—To quantify trends in the use of CT in pediatrics and the associated radiation exposure and cancer risk.

Design.—Retrospective observational study.

Setting.—Seven US health care systems.

Participants.—The use of CT was evaluated for children younger than 15 years of age from 1996 to 2010, including 4 857 736 child-years of observation. Radiation doses were calculated for 744 CT scans performed between 2001 and 2011.

Main Outcomes and Measures.—Rates of CT use, organ and effective doses, and projected lifetime attributable risks of cancer.

Results.—The use of CT doubled for children younger than 5 years of age and tripled for children 5 to 14 years of age between 1996 and 2005, remained stable between 2006 and 2007, and then began to decline. Effective doses varied from 0.03 to 69.2 mSv per scan. An effective dose of 20 mSv or higher was delivered by 14% to 25% of abdomen/pelvis scans, 6% to 14% of spine scans, and 3% to 8% of chest scans. Projected lifetime attributable risks of solid cancer were higher for younger patients and girls than for older patients and boys, and they were also higher for patients who underwent CT scans of the abdomen/pelvis or spine than for patients who underwent other types of CT scans. For girls, a radiation-induced solid cancer is projected to result from every 300 to 390 abdomen/pelvis scans, 330 to 480 chest scans, and 270 to 800 spine scans, depending on age. The risk of leukemia was highest from head scans for children younger than 5 years of age at a rate of 1.9 cases per 10 000 CT scans. Nationally, 4 million pediatric CT scans of the head, abdomen/pelvis, chest, or spine performed each year are projected to cause 4870 future cancers. Reducing the highest 25% of doses to the median might prevent 43% of these cancers.

Conclusions and Relevance.—The increased use of CT in pediatrics, combined with the wide variability in radiation doses, has resulted in many children receiving a high-dose examination. Dose-reduction strategies targeted to the highest quartile of doses could dramatically reduce the number of radiation-induced cancers.

▶ The exposure of patients to potentially cancer-inducing doses (there probably is no safe dose) of radiation through diagnostic imaging has been examined for many years without definitive conclusions. The concern has been of particular interest to those who care for children in part because of their potential increased susceptibility to radiation-induced cancer. Ironically, one group of individuals who are exposed to multiple imaging modalities is children who have cancer. Because secondary malignancies are a major long-term concern for such children, who are often cured of their original cancer, the risk of diagnostic imaging is particularly important. Miglioretti et al show a significantly increased incidence of solid tumors in children who have experienced one or more computed tomography (CT) scans. Of interest, young girls were at highest risk as well as those children undergoing CT scanning of the abdomen, pelvis, or spine. The authors note that the data suggest that the roughly 4 million pediatric CT scans done each year may result in about 4900 future cancers. In pediatric oncology, we have had a growing concern about the utility of follow-up CT scans for patients as well as the often intense imaging of patients admitted for fever and neutropenia. Miglioretti et al provide important data that should alert all of us to image only when necessary and then with a modality that minimizes exposure to ionizing radiation.

R. J. Arceci, MD, PhD

Miscellaneous

High Risk of Symptomatic Cardiac Events in Childhood Cancer Survivors
van der Pal HJ, van Dalen EC, van Delden E, et al (Emma Children's Hosp/Academic Med Centre, Amsterdam, the Netherlands; et al)
J Clin Oncol 30:1429-1437, 2012

Purpose.—To evaluate the long-term risk for validated symptomatic cardiac events (CEs) and associated risk factors in childhood cancer survivors (CCSs).

Patients and Methods.—We determined CEs grade 3 or higher: congestive heart failure (CHF), cardiac ischemia, valvular disease, arrhythmia and/or pericarditis (according to Common Terminology Criteria for Adverse Events [CTCAE], version 3.0) in a hospital-based cohort of 1,362 5-year CCSs diagnosed between 1966 and 1996. We calculated both marginal and cause-specific cumulative incidence of CEs and cause-specific cumulative incidence of separate events. We analyzed different risk factors in multivariable Cox regression models.

Results.—Overall, 50 CEs, including 27 cases of CHF, were observed in 42 survivors (at a median attained age of 27.1 years). The 30-year cause-specific cumulative incidence of CEs was significantly increased after treatment with both anthracyclines and cardiac irradiation (12.6%; 95% CI, 4.3% to 20.3%), after anthracyclines (7.3%; 95% CI, 3.8% to 10.7%), and after cardiac irradiation (4.0%; 95% CI, 0.5% to 7.4%) compared with other treatments. In the proportional hazards analyses, anthracycline (dose), cardiac irradiation (dose), combination of these treatments, and congenital heart disease were significantly associated with developing a CE. We demonstrated an exponential relationship between the cumulative anthracycline dose, cardiac irradiation dose, and risk of CE.

Conclusion.—CCSs have a high risk of developing symptomatic CEs at an early age. The most common CE was CHF. Survivors treated with both anthracyclines and radiotherapy have the highest risk; after 30 years, one in eight will develop severe heart disease. The use of potentially cardiotoxic treatments should be reconsidered for high-risk groups, and frequent follow-up for high-risk survivors is needed.

▶ The development of adverse late sequelae of treatment of disease in children with cancer has come under increasingly intense scrutiny after success with treating such patients over the last several decades. One of most studied areas is late cardiac events. The study by van der Pal et al is noteworthy for several important reasons. They studied 1 362 5-year survivors of childhood cancer for the 30-year cause-specific incidence of cardiac problems. The incidence was significantly increased in those patients who received both anthracyclines and radiation to the heart (approximately 13% cumulative incidence) with significant congestive heart failure being the most common complication. After 30 years, a staggering figure of 1 in 8 survivors with the combination of anthracycline and cardiac radiation exposure were shown to have developed severe heart disease. The current hope is that with more modern treatments, such high cardiac event rates will be significantly reduced. However, it is doubtful such events will be eliminated in the near future. And although identification of predisposing risk factors that would predict that certain children were at higher risk than others because of genetic factors, several reports have shown that such predisposing polymorphisms are likely to exist. However, the different reports have not come to any consensus on which polymorphisms are relevant. In the meantime, we need to take these sobering results seriously enough to work toward avoiding or reducing anthracycline and cardiac radiation exposures in this most vulnerable population.

R. J. Arceci, MD, PhD

13 Sarcoma

Efficacy and safety of regorafenib for advanced gastrointestinal stromal tumours after failure of imatinib and sunitinib (GRID): an international, multicentre, randomised, placebo-controlled, phase 3 trial
Demetri GD, on behalf of all GRID study investigators (Ludwig Ctr at Dana-Farber Cancer Inst and Harvard Med School, Boston, MA; et al)
Lancet 381:295-302, 2013

Background.—Until now, only imatinib and sunitinib have proven clinical benefit in patients with gastrointestinal stromal tumours (GIST), but almost all metastatic GIST eventually develop resistance to these agents, resulting in fatal disease progression. We aimed to assess efficacy and safety of regorafenib in patients with metastatic or unresectable GIST progressing after failure of at least imatinib and sunitinib.

Methods.—We did this phase 3 trial at 57 hospitals in 17 countries. Patients with histologically confirmed, metastatic or unresectable GIST, with failure of at least previous imatinib and sunitinib were randomised in a 2:1 ratio (by computer-generated randomisation list and interactive voice response system; preallocated block design (block size 12); stratified by treatment line and geographical region) to receive either oral regorafenib 160 mg daily or placebo, plus best supportive care in both groups, for the first 3 weeks of each 4 week cycle. The study sponsor, participants, and investigators were masked to treatment assignment. The primary endpoint was progression-free survival (PFS). At disease progression, patients assigned placebo could crossover to open-label regorafenib. Analyses were by intention to treat. This trial is registered with ClinicalTrials.gov, number NCT01271712.

Results.—From Jan 4, to Aug 18, 2011, 240 patients were screened and 199 were randomised to receive regorafenib (n = 133) or matching placebo (n = 66). Data cutoff was Jan 26, 2012. Median PFS per independent blinded central review was $4 \cdot 8$ months (IQR $1 \cdot 4 - 9 \cdot 2$) for regorafenib and 0.9 months ($0 \cdot 9 - 1 \cdot 8$) for placebo (hazard ratio [HR] $0 \cdot 27$, 95% CI $0 \cdot 19 - 0 \cdot 39$; $p < 0 \cdot 0001$). After progression, 56 patients (85%) assigned placebo crossed over to regorafenib. Drug-related adverse events were reported in 130 (98%) patients assigned regorafenib and 45 (68%) patients assigned placebo. The most common regorafenib-related adverse events of grade 3 or higher were hypertension (31 of 132, 23%), hand-foot skin reaction (26 of 132, 20%), and diarrhoea (seven of 132, 5%).

Interpretation.—The results of this study show that oral regorafenib can provide a significant improvement in progression-free survival compared with placebo in patients with metastatic GIST after progression on standard treatments. As far as we are aware, this is the first clinical trial to show benefit from a kinase inhibitor in this highly refractory population of patients.

▶ Gastrointestinal stromal tumors (GIST) are the most common sarcomas of the gastrointestinal tract. Unlike certain other sarcomas of the GI tract, GIST are not very responsive to chemotherapy. The introduction of the first tyrosine kinase inhibitor (TKI) tested in GIST, imatinib, provided the first effective therapy for GIST. Studies since then have identified a second TKI, sunitinib, as having activity in patients whose tumors are resistant to imatinib. This study evaluates a third agent, regorafenib, which is a multikinase inhibitor that targets several protein kinases, including those involved in the regulation of tumor angiogenesis (VEGFR1-3, TEK), oncogenesis (KIT, RET, RAF1, BRAF, and BRAF^{V600E}), and the tumor microenvironment (PDGFR and FGFR). The study population was a group of patients who had shown clinical resistance to both imatinib and sunitinib; hence, this was a very refractory patient population. The phase III trial was placebo controlled and included 199 patients. Regorafenib therapy achieved a superior progression-free survival with a striking hazard ratio of 0.27 with the most common side effects being hypertension, hand-foot syndrome, and diarrhea. These data provide a basis for considering regorafenib as the third-line treatment of choice for GIST refractory to imatinib and sunitinib.

J. T. Thigpen, MD

Results of an International Randomized Phase III Trial of the Mammalian Target of Rapamycin Inhibitor Ridaforolimus Versus Placebo to Control Metastatic Sarcomas in Patients After Benefit From Prior Chemotherapy
Demetri GD, Chawla SP, Ray-Coquard I, et al (Dana-Farber Cancer Inst and Harvard Med School, Boston, MA; International Inst of Clinical Studies, Santa Monica, CA; Centre LéonBérard Cancer Ctr, Lyon, France; et al)
J Clin Oncol 31:2485-2492, 2013

Purpose.—Aberrant mammalian target of rapamycin (mTOR) signaling is common in sarcomas and other malignancies. Drug resistance and toxicities often limit benefits of systemic chemotherapy used to treat metastatic sarcomas. This large randomized placebo-controlled phase III trial evaluated the mTOR inhibitor ridaforolimus to assess maintenance of disease control in advanced sarcomas.

Patients and Methods.—Patients with metastatic soft tissue or bone sarcomas who achieved objective response or stable disease with prior chemotherapy were randomly assigned to receive ridaforolimus 40 mg or placebo once per day for 5 days every week. Primary end point was progression-free survival (PFS); secondary end points included overall survival (OS), best target lesion response, safety, and tolerability.

Results.—A total of 711 patients were enrolled, and 702 received blinded study drug. Ridaforolimus treatment led to a modest, although significant, improvement in PFS per independent review compared with placebo (hazard ratio [HR], 0.72; 95% CI, 0.61 to 0.85; $P = .001$; median PFS, 17.7 v 14.6 weeks). Ridaforolimus induced a mean 1.3% decrease in target lesion size versus a 10.3% increase with placebo ($P < .001$). Median OS with ridaforolimus was 90.6 weeks versus 85.3 weeks with placebo (HR, 0.93; 95% CI, 0.78 to 1.12; $P = .46$). Adverse events (AEs) more common with ridaforolimus included stomatitis, infections, fatigue, thrombocytopenia, noninfectious pneumonitis, hyperglycemia, and rash. Grade ≥ 3 AEs were more common with ridaforolimus than placebo (64.1% v 25.6%).

Conclusion.—Ridaforolimus delayed tumor progression to a small statistically significant degree in patients with metastatic sarcoma who experienced benefit with prior chemotherapy. Toxicities were observed with ridaforolimus, as expected with mTOR inhibition. These data provide a foundation on which to further improve control of sarcomas.

▶ Advanced soft-tissue sarcomas remain incredibly difficult to effectively treat and remain in great need of effective, new treatment approaches. Inhibition of the mammalian target of rapamycin (mTOR) pathway has been one of those possible new approaches that have shown encouraging preclinical and early-phase clinical trial work. Demetri et al report on a randomized, blinded study of more than 700 patients with metastatic sarcoma who had experienced some benefit from prior chemotherapy. The results lead one to the analogy of whether you believe a glass is half full or half empty. The facts show that the addition of ridaforolimus extended progression-free survival by 3 weeks, decreased tumor size significantly, and extended overall survival by about 5 weeks. However, the group of patients who received ridaforolimus experienced more adverse effects than the control group. Also, no attempts to measure target inhibition were used, and no quality of life was studied. So we are left with another, to quote the authors, treatment demonstrating "a small, statistically significant" effect while compromising a patient's quality of life, if one assumes adverse effects. A major question is what to do with such results. Should we declare partial victory and move on to combination therapy with other inhibitors? Or should we conclude that mTOR inhibition may be only modestly interesting and minimally useful, leading to the further conclusion that maybe we are barking up the wrong tree.

R. J. Arceci, MD, PhD

14 Supportive Care

A combined pain consultation and pain education program decreases average and current pain and decreases interference in daily life by pain in oncology outpatients: A randomized controlled trial
Oldenmenger WH, Sillevis Smitt PAE, van Montfort CAGM, et al (Erasmus MC, Rotterdam, The Netherlands)
Pain 152:2632-2639, 2011

Pain education programs (PEP) and pain consultations (PC) have been studied to overcome patient-related and professional-related barriers in cancer pain management. These interventions were studied separately, not in combination, and half of the studies reported a significant improvement in pain. Moreover, most PEP studies did not mention the adequacy of pain treatment. We studied the effect of PC combined with PEP on pain and interference by pain with daily functioning in comparison to standard care (SC). Patients were randomly assigned to SC (n = 37) or PC-PEP (n = 35). PEP consisted of patient-tailored pain education and weekly monitoring of pain and side effects. We measured overall reduction in pain intensity and daily interference over an 8-week period as well as adequacy of pain treatment and adherence. The overall reduction in pain intensity and daily interference was significantly greater after randomization to PC-PEP than to SC (average pain 31% vs 20%, $P = .03$; current pain 30% vs 16%, $P = .016$; interference 20% vs 2.5%, $P = .01$). Adequacy of pain management did not differ between the groups. Patients were more adherent to analgesics after randomization to PC-PEP than to SC ($P = .03$). In conclusion, PC-PEP improves pain, daily interference, and patient adherence in oncology outpatients (Fig 2).

▶ Pain is a common problem in cancer patients; unfortunately, pain control is often inadequate. Most patients are candidates for both pharmacologic and non-pharmacologic therapies. Unfortunately, physicians often rely heavily on pharmacologic treatment and fail to use other techniques to optimize outcome. Studies of patient education as a method to improve pain outcomes by enhancing knowledge, addressing biases, and improving communication skills have shown mixed results; however, multiple meta-analyses demonstrate moderate effect size with sociobehavioral interventions including education. This study adds to the growing literature supporting the use of sociobehavior techniques to improve pain control in the cancer population. In this study, an educational intervention was paired with a pain consultation and weekly nursing contact with the patient to ensure adequate attention to pain control issues. The

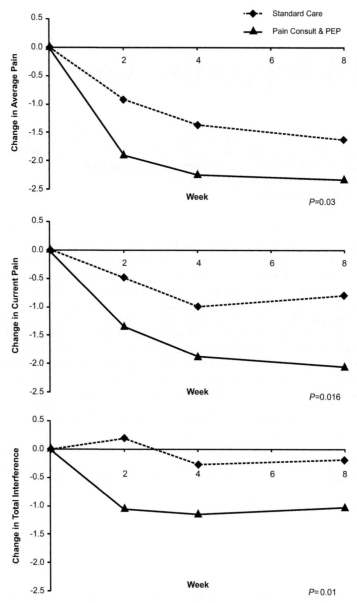

FIGURE 2.—Mean changes in pain scores and daily interference, compared with baseline, over time in the standard care (N = 37) and pain consultation and pain education program (N = 35) groups. (Reprinted from Oldenmenger WH, Sillevis Smitt PAE, van Montfort CAGM, et al. A combined pain consultation and pain education program decreases average and current pain and decreases interference in daily life by pain in oncology outpatients: a randomized controlled trial. *Pain*. 2011;152:2632-2639, with permission from IASP.)

intervention was compared with standard care. Results demonstrated an improvement in pain intensity for patients in the intervention arm. More importantly, patients in the intervention arm had a decreased interference in daily activity secondary to pain.

B. A. Murphy, MD

Cytokine use and survival in the first-line treatment of ovarian cancer: A Gynecologic Oncology Group Study
Stehman FB, Brady MF, Thigpen JT, et al (Indiana Univ School of Medicine, Indianapolis; Roswell Park Cancer Inst, Buffalo, NY; Univ of Mississippi Med Ctr, Jackson; et al)
Gynecol Oncol 127:495-501, 2012

Background.—Granulocyte colony stimulating factor (G-CSF) and erythropoietin stimulating agents (ESA) may be used to support patients during chemotherapy. We assessed whether G-CSF or ESA were associated with progression or death in patients with ovarian cancer.

Methods.—Patients with ovarian cancer following surgery, were on a protocol to evaluate bevacizumab with chemotherapy. Guidelines for administering G-CSF and ESA were specified in the protocol. Overall survival (OS) was analyzed with landmark procedures and multivariate, time-dependent hazard models.

Results.—Eighteen-hundred-seventy-three women were enrolled, with no differences in clinical and pathologic variables among treatment group. Performance status, hemoglobin, and white cell counts were associated with G-CSF and/or ESA usage during treatment. Nine patients received no protocol directed therapy, leaving 1864 patients for this review. One-thousand-one-hundred-twenty-five patients received neither ESA nor G-CSF; 311 received G-CSF but no ESA; 241 received ESA but no G-CSF; and 187 received both. Median survival following a five month landmark from the start of treatment was 34 versus 38 months for those who did versus did not receive ESA (multivariate hazard ratio: 0.989; 95% confidence interval: 0.849–1.15) and 40 versus 37 months for those who did versus did not receive G-CSF (multivariate hazard ratio: 0.932; 95% confidence interval: 0.800–1.08).

Conclusions.—Neither ESA nor G-CSF had a negative impact on survival after adjustment of prognostic factors among patients with ovarian cancer receiving chemotherapy. ESA may appear to be associated with shorter survival in univariate analyses because factors prognostic for ESA use are also prognostic for progression-free survival.

▶ Based on 3 phase III trials and 3 large community-based studies in the late 1990s, erythropoietin was approved for use in cancer patients to maintain a hemoglobin level of greater than 12 g/dL. The observation that led to approval was the significant improvement in quality of life of patients whose hemoglobins were brought up to 12 g/dL. Strikingly, the greatest improvement occurred during the last increment from 11 to 12 g/dL. Retrospective studies subsequently suggested that, at least in cervical cancer, there might be as much as a 25% reduction in mortality associated with erythropoietin use. The resultant widespread use of erythropoietin was brought to sudden and dramatic halt when 3 studies seeking to raise hemoglobin to an even higher level of as much as 15 g/dL suggested that there was a decrement in survival associated with the use of erythropoietin. The US Food and Drug Administration authored a black box warning for the package insert that stated that there was a decrement in survival in several cancers, including cervix cancer. The warning incorrectly cited a report from Gynecologic Oncology Group (GOG) 191, which randomly assigned patients to chemotherapy with erythropoietin, as showing a reduction in survival time. The actual report from GOG 191[1] concluded as follows: "Thromboembolic events (TE) are common in cervical cancer patients receiving [chemotherapy and radiotherapy]. Difference in TE rate between the two treatments was not statistically significant. The impact of maintaining Hgb level > 12.0 g/dl on [progression-free survival], [overall survival], and local control remains undetermined." From the same publication, "...the observed differences with respect to recurrence status between treatment regimens are not statistically significant ($P = .6471$)." Because of these discrepancies, investigators from the GOG undertook to examine the use of cytokines and the relationship to survival in a large ovarian cancer study, GOG 218, which evaluated the impact of bevacizumab on ovarian cancer outcome. As the abstract above shows, there was no negative impact of the use of either granulocyte colony-stimulating factor or erythropoietin on survival after adjustment for known prognostic factors associated with ovarian cancer. To quote the investigators, "Erythropoietin stimulating agents (ESA) may appear to be associated with shorter survival in univariate analyses because factors prognostic for ESA use are also prognostic for progression-free survival."

J. T. Thigpen, MD

Reference

1. Thomas G, Ali S, Hoebers FJ, et al. Phase III trial to evaluate the efficacy of maintaining hemoglobin levels above 12.0 g/dL with erythropoietin vs above 10.0 g/dL without erythropoietin in anemic patients receiving concurrent radiation and cisplatin for cervical cancer. *Gynecol Oncol.* 2008;108:317-325.

15 Miscellaneous

Suicide and Cardiovascular Death after a Cancer Diagnosis
Fang F, Fall K, Mittleman MA, et al (Karolinska Institutet, Stockholm, Sweden; Örebro Univ and Örebro Univ Hosp, Sweden; Beth Israel Deaconess Med Ctr and Harvard Med School; et al)
N Engl J Med 366:1310-1318, 2012

Background.—Receiving a diagnosis of cancer is a traumatic experience that may trigger immediate adverse health consequences beyond the effects of the disease or treatment.

Methods.—Using Poisson and negative binomial regression models, we conducted a historical cohort study involving 6,073,240 Swedes to examine the associations between a cancer diagnosis and the immediate risk of suicide or death from cardiovascular causes from 1991 through 2006. To adjust for unmeasured confounders, we also performed a nested, self-matched case-crossover analysis among all patients with cancer who died from suicide or cardiovascular diseases in the cohort.

Results.—As compared with cancer-free persons, the relative risk of suicide among patients receiving a cancer diagnosis was 12.6 (95% confidence interval [CI], 8.6 to 17.8) during the first week (29 patients; incidence rate, 2.50 per 1000 person-years) and 3.1 (95% CI, 2.7 to 3.5) during the first year (260 patients; incidence rate, 0.60 per 1000 person-years). The relative risk of cardiovascular death after diagnosis was 5.6 (95% CI, 5.2 to 5.9) during the first week (1318 patients; incidence rate, 116.80 per 1000 person-years) and 3.3 (95% CI, 3.1 to 3.4) during the first 4 weeks (2641 patients; incidence rate, 65.81 per 1000 person-years). The risk elevations decreased rapidly during the first year after diagnosis. Increased risk was particularly prominent for cancers with a poor prognosis. The case-crossover analysis largely confirmed results from the main analysis.

Conclusions.—In this large cohort study, patients who had recently received a cancer diagnosis had increased risks of both suicide and death from cardiovascular causes, as compared with cancer-free persons. (Funded by the Swedish Council for Working Life and Social Research and others.)

▶ Receiving a diagnosis of cancer of any form can be a traumatic event. Often the public perception of a cancer diagnosis is equivalent to a death sentence. Thus, many patients who receive a diagnosis of cancer may feel overwhelmed and hopeless. This feeling could lead to cardiovascular events, such as a heart attack, stroke, or, potentially, clinical depression with suicidal thoughts or actions.

As much as one assumes that the above is true, quantitating the risk of these events is critical to understand the magnitude of them and the potential interventions.

These data from Sweden represent the kind of data that are needed to quantitate these risks. The relative risk of suicide in the first week after a cancer diagnosis is 12.6, a staggering number. The relative risk of a cardiovascular event resulting in death was 5.6 during the first week after diagnosis, which is also frightening.

These data suggest a significant need for psychosocial support in patients receiving a cancer diagnosis. It also calls for careful study of such an intervention to avoid these often needless fatal outcomes.

C. Lawton, MD

Article Index

Chapter 1: Cancer Biology

Earlier Age of Onset of *BRCA* Mutation-Related Cancers in Subsequent Generations   1

Punctuated Evolution of Prostate Cancer Genomes   2

Cytokine release syndrome after blinatumomab treatment related to abnormal macrophage activation and ameliorated with cytokine-directed therapy   3

Genomic and Epigenomic Landscapes of Adult De Novo Acute Myeloid Leukemia   4

Development of a Prognostic Model for Breast Cancer Survival in an Open Challenge Environment   5

Chapter 2: Cancer Prevention

Multivitamins in the prevention of cancer in men: the Physicians' Health Study II randomized controlled trial   7

Chapter 3: Cancer Therapies

Statin use and reduced cancer-related mortality   9

Predictive Gene Signature in MAGE-A3 Antigen-Specific Cancer Immunotherapy   10

Chapter 4: Chemotherapy: Mechanisms and Side Effects

Patients' Expectations about Effects of Chemotherapy for Advanced Cancer   13

Chapter 5: Breast Cancer

Assessing the Impact of a Cooperative Group Trial on Breast Cancer Care in the Medicare Population   15

Association Between Age at Diagnosis and Disease-Specific Mortality Among Postmenopausal Women With Hormone Receptor–Positive Breast Cancer   17

Pain Outcomes in Patients With Advanced Breast Cancer and Bone Metastases: Results From a Randomized, Double-Blind Study of Denosumab and Zoledronic Acid   18

Active Smoking and Breast Cancer Risk: Original Cohort Data and Meta-Analysis   19

Effect of Three Decades of Screening Mammography on Breast-Cancer Incidence   20

The benefits and harms of breast cancer screening: an independent review   22

Effect of three decades of screening mammography on breast-cancer incidence   23

Estrogen Plus Progestin and Breast Cancer Incidence and Mortality in the Women's Health Initiative Observational Study   25

Exemestane Versus Anastrozole in Postmenopausal Women With Early Breast Cancer: NCIC CTG MA.27—A Randomized Controlled Phase III Trial   26

Long-term effects of continuing adjuvant tamoxifen to 10 years versus stopping at 5 years after diagnosis of oestrogen receptor-positive breast cancer: ATLAS, a randomised trial 27

Evaluation of breast amorphous calcifications by a computer-aided detection system in full-field digital mammography 29

Locally Advanced Breast Cancer: MR Imaging for Prediction of Response to Neoadjuvant Chemotherapy—Results from ACRIN 6657/I-SPY TRIAL 31

Preoperative Breast MRI Can Reduce the Rate of Tumor-Positive Resection Margins and Reoperations in Patients Undergoing Breast-Conserving Surgery 35

Computer-aided Detection of Masses at Mammography: Interactive Decision Support Versus Prompts 40

Breast Cancer: Assessing Response to Neoadjuvant Chemotherapy by Using US-guided Near-Infrared Tomography 43

High risk of non-sentinel node metastases in a group of breast cancer patients with micrometastases in the sentinel node 47

An Updated Meta-Analysis on the Effectiveness of Preoperative Prophylactic Antibiotics in Patients Undergoing Breast Surgical Procedures 50

Axillary Dissection Versus No Axillary Dissection in Older Patients With T1N0 Breast Cancer: 15-Year Results of a Randomized Controlled Trial 52

Reduced Incidence of Breast Cancer–Related Lymphedema following Mastectomy and Breast Reconstruction versus Mastectomy Alone 55

Clinically Used Breast Cancer Markers Such As Estrogen Receptor, Progesterone Receptor, and Human Epidermal Growth Factor Receptor 2 Are Unstable Throughout Tumor Progression 57

CHEK2*1100delC Heterozygosity in Women With Breast Cancer Associated With Early Death, Breast Cancer–Specific Death, and Increased Risk of a Second Breast Cancer 59

Variability in Reexcision Following Breast Conservation Surgery 62

Everolimus in Postmenopausal Hormone-Receptor–Positive Advanced Breast Cancer 63

A Prospective Surveillance Model for Physical Rehabilitation of Women With Breast Cancer: Chemotherapy-Induced Peripheral Neuropathy 67

Efficacy of Cognitive Behavioral Therapy and Physical Exercise in Alleviating Treatment-Induced Menopausal Symptoms in Patients With Breast Cancer: Results of a Randomized, Controlled, Multicenter Trial 68

Prognostic Impact of Pregnancy After Breast Cancer According to Estrogen Receptor Status: A Multicenter Retrospective Study 69

Cost Effectiveness of Fracture Prevention in Postmenopausal Women Who Receive Aromatase Inhibitors for Early Breast Cancer 71

Chapter 6: Genitourinary

Radiotherapy with or without Chemotherapy in Muscle-Invasive Bladder Cancer 75

Diagnostic Performance of PCA3 to Detect Prostate Cancer in Men with Increased Prostate Specific Antigen: A Prospective Study of 1,962 Cases 76

Cost-effectiveness analysis of SBRT versus IMRT: an emerging initial radiation treatment option for organ-confined prostate cancer — 77

Radical Prostatectomy in Austria From 1992 to 2009: An Updated Nationwide Analysis of 33,580 Cases — 79

Interval to Biochemical Failure as a Biomarker for Cause-Specific and Overall Survival After Dose-Escalated External Beam Radiation Therapy for Prostate Cancer — 80

Conventional versus hypofractionated high-dose intensity-modulated radiotherapy for prostate cancer: preliminary safety results from the CHHiP randomised controlled trial — 81

Management of Older Men With Clinically Localized Prostate Cancer: The Significance of Advanced Age and Comorbidity — 83

Quality-of-Life Effects of Prostate-Specific Antigen Screening — 83

Intermittent Androgen Suppression for Rising PSA Level after Radiotherapy — 85

Radical Prostatectomy versus Observation for Localized Prostate Cancer — 86

Variation in Use of Androgen Suppression With External-Beam Radiotherapy for Nonmetastatic Prostate Cancer — 87

Long-Term Results of an RTOG Phase II Trial (00-19) of External-Beam Radiation Therapy Combined With Permanent Source Brachytherapy for Intermediate-Risk Clinically Localized Adenocarcinoma of the Prostate — 88

Intensity-Modulated Radiation Therapy, Proton Therapy, or Conformal Radiation Therapy and Morbidity and Disease Control in Localized Prostate Cancer — 90

Germline Mutations in *HOXB13* and Prostate-Cancer Risk — 91

Prostate-Cancer Mortality at 11 Years of Follow-up — 92

Racial Differences in Bone Mineral Density and Fractures in Men Receiving Androgen Deprivation Therapy for Prostate Cancer — 93

Long-term quality of life outcome after proton beam monotherapy for localized prostate cancer — 94

Long-term outcomes from a prospective trial of stereotactic body radiotherapy for low-risk prostate cancer — 96

Adverse Effects of Robotic-Assisted Laparoscopic Versus Open Retropubic Radical Prostatectomy Among a Nationwide Random Sample of Medicare-Age Men — 97

Increased Survival with Enzalutamide in Prostate Cancer after Chemotherapy — 98

Chapter 7: Gynecology

ACR Appropriateness Criteria® Pretreatment Planning of Invasive Cancer of the Cervix — 101

Incorporation of bevacizumab in the treatment of recurrent and metastatic cervical cancer: a phase III randomized trial of the Gynecologic Oncology Group — 102

Phase II trial of nab-paclitaxel in the treatment of recurrent or persistent advanced cervix cancer: A gynecologic oncology group study — 103

A systematic review of randomized trials assessing human papillomavirus testing in cervical cancer screening — 105

Chemotherapy for advanced and recurrent cervical carcinoma: Results from cooperative group trials — 106

Phase II trial of combination bevacizumab and temsirolimus in the treatment of recurrent or persistent endometrial carcinoma: A Gynecologic Oncology Group study — 107

Did GOG99 and PORTEC1 change clinical practice in the United States? — 108

Adjuvant Radiotherapy for Stage I Endometrial Cancer: An Updated Cochrane Systematic Review and Meta-analysis — 110

Adjuvant Therapy for High-Grade, Uterus-Limited Leiomyosarcoma: Results of a Phase 2 Trial (SARC 005) — 111

Recurrence and Survival After Random Assignment to Laparoscopy Versus Laparotomy for Comprehensive Surgical Staging of Uterine Cancer: Gynecologic Oncology Group LAP2 Study — 112

Long-Term Ovarian Cancer Survival Associated With Mutation in BRCA1 or BRCA2 — 113

Patient reported outcomes of a randomized, placebo-controlled trial of bevacizumab in the front-line treatment of ovarian cancer: A Gynecologic Oncology Group Study — 114

Results of Annual Screening in Phase I of the United Kingdom Familial Ovarian Cancer Screening Study Highlight the Need for Strict Adherence to Screening Schedule — 116

Randomized, Open-Label, Phase III Study Comparing Patupilone (EPO906) With Pegylated Liposomal Doxorubicin in Platinum-Refractory or -Resistant Patients With Recurrent Epithelial Ovarian, Primary Fallopian Tube, or Primary Peritoneal Cancer — 117

Abagovomab As Maintenance Therapy in Patients With Epithelial Ovarian Cancer: A Phase III Trial of the AGO OVAR, COGI, GINECO, and GEICO—The MIMOSA Study — 118

A phase II trial of docetaxel and bevacizumab in recurrent ovarian cancer within 12 months of prior platinum-based chemotherapy — 120

Declining Second Primary Ovarian Cancer After First Primary Breast Cancer — 121

Chapter 8: Gastrointestinal

Effect of Oxaliplatin, Fluorouracil, and Leucovorin With or Without Cetuximab on Survival Among Patients With Resected Stage III Colon Cancer: A Randomized Trial — 123

Randomized trial of short-course radiotherapy versus long-course chemoradiation comparing rates of local recurrence in patients with T3 rectal cancer: Trans-Tasman Radiation Oncology Group trial 01.04 — 124

Preoperative versus postoperative chemoradiotherapy for locally advanced rectal cancer: results of the German CAO/ARO/AIO-94 randomized phase III trial after a median follow-up of 11 years — 126

Colorectal-Cancer Incidence and Mortality with Screening Flexible Sigmoidoscopy — 127

Colonoscopic Polypectomy and Long-Term Prevention of Colorectal-Cancer Deaths — 128

Association of *KRAS* G13D Tumor Mutations With Outcome in Patients With Metastatic Colorectal Cancer Treated With First-Line Chemotherapy With or Without Cetuximab   129

Regorafenib monotherapy for previously treated metastatic colorectal cancer (CORRECT): an international, multicentre, randomised, placebo-controlled, phase 3 trial   131

Estrogen Plus Progestin and Colorectal Cancer Incidence and Mortality   132

Aspirin Use, Tumor *PIK3CA* Mutation, and Colorectal-Cancer Survival   133

Open-Label, Multicenter, Randomized Phase III Trial of Adjuvant Chemoradiation Plus Interferon Alfa-2b Versus Fluorouracil and Folinic Acid for Patients With Resected Pancreatic Adenocarcinoma   135

Carbohydrate Antigen 19-9 is a Prognostic and Predictive Biomarker in Patients With Advanced Pancreatic Cancer Who Receive Gemcitabine-Containing Chemotherapy: A Pooled Analysis of 6 Prospective Trials   137

EGFR pathway biomarkers in erlotinib-treated patients with advanced pancreatic cancer: translational results from the randomised, crossover phase 3 trial AIO-PK0104   138

Re-resection for Isolated Local Recurrence of Pancreatic Cancer is Feasible, Safe, and Associated with Encouraging Survival   140

Long-Term Update of US GI Intergroup RTOG 98-11 Phase III Trial for Anal Carcinoma: Survival, Relapse, and Colostomy Failure With Concurrent Chemoradiation Involving Fluorouracil/Mitomycin Versus Fluorouracil/Cisplatin   143

Chapter 9: Hematologic Malignancies

Secondary genetic lesions in acute myeloid leukemia with inv(16) or t(16;16): a study of the German-Austrian AML Study Group (AMLSG)   145

Sequential gain of mutations in severe congenital neutropenia progressing to acute myeloid leukemia   146

DNA methylation changes are a late event in acute promyelocytic leukemia and coincide with loss of transcription factor binding   147

Dexamethasone exposure and asparaginase antibodies affect relapse risk in acute lymphoblastic leukemia   148

The genetic basis of early T-cell precursor acute lymphoblastic leukaemia   149

inv(16)/t(16;16) acute myeloid leukemia with non–type A *CBFB-MYH11* fusions associate with distinct clinical and genetic features and lack *KIT* mutations   150

Prognostic Relevance of Integrated Genetic Profiling in Acute Myeloid Leukemia   151

Retinoic Acid and Arsenic Trioxide for Acute Promyelocytic Leukemia   152

The level of residual disease based on mutant *NPM1* is an independent prognostic factor for relapse and survival in AML   153

Clonal evolution in relapsed *NPM1*-mutated acute myeloid leukemia   155

Epigenetic silencing of *microRNA-193a* contributes to leukemogenesis in t(8;21) acute myeloid leukemia by activating the *PTEN*/PI3K signal pathway   156

A phase 3 study of gemtuzumab ozogamicin during induction and postconsolidation therapy in younger patients with acute myeloid leukemia   157

Chapter 10: Thoracic Cancer

Lung Cancer That Harbors a *HER2* Mutation: Epidemiologic Characteristics and
Therapeutic Perspectives 159

Effect of crizotinib on overall survival in patients with advanced non-small-cell
lung cancer harbouring *ALK* gene rearrangement: a retrospective analysis 160

Natural History and Molecular Characteristics of Lung Cancers Harboring *EGFR*
Exon 20 Insertions 162

Mechanisms of Acquired Crizotinib Resistance in ALK-Rearranged Lung Cancers 163

Genotypic and Histological Evolution of Lung Cancers Acquiring Resistance to
EGFR Inhibitors 164

Fibroblast Growth Factor Receptor 1 Gene Amplification Is Associated With Poor
Survival and Cigarette Smoking Dosage in Patients With Resected Squamous Cell
Lung Cancer 165

Randomized Phase II Study of Ixabepilone or Paclitaxel Plus Carboplatin in
Patients With Non–Small-Cell Lung Cancer Prospectively Stratified by Beta-3
Tubulin Status 167

Erlotinib versus standard chemotherapy as first-line treatment for European
patients with advanced EGFR mutation-positive non-small-cell lung cancer
(EURTAC): a multicentre, open-label, randomised phase 3 trial 168

Randomized Phase II Study of Dacomitinib (PF-00299804), an Irreversible
Pan–Human Epidermal Growth Factor Receptor Inhibitor, Versus Erlotinib in
Patients With Advanced Non–Small-Cell Lung Cancer 170

Aflibercept and Docetaxel Versus Docetaxel Alone After Platinum Failure in
Patients With Advanced or Metastatic Non–Small-Cell Lung Cancer:
A Randomized, Controlled Phase III Trial 172

Pemetrexed Versus Pemetrexed and Carboplatin As Second-Line Chemotherapy in
Advanced Non–Small-Cell Lung Cancer: Results of the GOIRC 02-2006
Randomized Phase II Study and Pooled Analysis With the NVALT7 Trial 173

Incorporating Bevacizumab and Erlotinib in the Combined-Modality Treatment of
Stage III Non–Small-Cell Lung Cancer: Results of a Phase I/II Trial 174

Phase II Trial of Erlotinib Plus Concurrent Whole-Brain Radiation Therapy for
Patients With Brain Metastases From Non–Small-Cell Lung Cancer 176

Chapter 11: Head and Neck

Induction chemotherapy followed by concurrent chemoradiotherapy (sequential
chemoradiotherapy) versus concurrent chemoradiotherapy alone in locally
advanced head and neck cancer (PARADIGM): a randomized phase 3 trial 179

Phase III Randomized, Placebo-Controlled Trial of Docetaxel With or Without
Gefitinib in Recurrent or Metastatic Head and Neck Cancer: An Eastern
Cooperative Oncology Group Trial 180

Deintensification Candidate Subgroups in Human Papillomavirus–Related
Oropharyngeal Cancer According to Minimal Risk of Distant Metastasis 182

Induction Chemotherapy Followed by Either Chemoradiotherapy or
Bioradiotherapy for Larynx Preservation: the TREMPLIN Randomized Phase II
Study 183

Long-Term Results of RTOG 91-11: A Comparison of Three Nonsurgical Treatment Strategies to Preserve the Larynx in Patients With Locally Advanced Larynx Cancer   185

Randomized Phase III Trial of Induction Chemotherapy With Docetaxel, Cisplatin, and Fluorouracil Followed by Surgery Versus Up-Front Surgery in Locally Advanced Resectable Oral Squamous Cell Carcinoma   186

Cisplatin and Radiotherapy With or Without Erlotinib in Locally Advanced Squamous Cell Carcinoma of the Head and Neck: A Randomized Phase II Trial   187

Associations among speech, eating, and body image concerns for surgical patients with head and neck cancer   189

Cisplatin and fluorouracil with or without panitumumab in patients with recurrent or metastatic squamous-cell carcinoma of the head and neck (SPECTRUM): an open-label phase 3 randomised trial   190

A systematic review of head and neck cancer quality of life assessment instruments   193

Evaluation of Human Papillomavirus Antibodies and Risk of Subsequent Head and Neck Cancer   194

Management of Human Papillomavirus—Positive and Human Papillomavirus—Negative Head and Neck Cancer   196

Chapter 12: Pediatric Cancer

Association Between Radiotherapy vs No Radiotherapy Based on Early Response to VAMP Chemotherapy and Survival Among Children With Favorable-Risk Hodgkin Lymphoma   199

Therapy prolongation improves outcome in multisystem Langerhans cell histiocytosis   200

The role of matched sibling donor allogeneic stem cell transplantation in pediatric high-risk acute myeloid leukemia: results from the AML-BFM 98 study   202

Nonadherence to Oral Mercaptopurine and Risk of Relapse in Hispanic and Non-Hispanic White Children With Acute Lymphoblastic Leukemia: A Report From the Children's Oncology Group   203

Second Malignant Neoplasms After Treatment of Childhood Acute Lymphoblastic Leukemia   204

Results of the AIEOP AML 2002/01 multicenter prospective trial for the treatment of children with acute myeloid leukemia   205

Clonal selection in xenografted TAM recapitulates the evolutionary process of myeloid leukemia in Down syndrome   206

Dasatinib in Children and Adolescents With Relapsed or Refractory Leukemia: Results of the CA180-018 Phase I Dose-Escalation Study of the Innovative Therapies for Children With Cancer Consortium   208

Development and validation of a single-cell network profiling assay-based classifier to predict response to induction therapy in paediatric patients with *de novo* acute myeloid leukaemia: a report from the Children's Oncology Group   209

Randomized trial comparing liposomal daunorubicin with idarubicin in induction for pediatric acute myeloid leukemia — Results from Study AMLBFM 2004   210

Treatment reduction for children and young adults with low-risk acute
lymphoblastic leukaemia defined by minimal residual disease (UKALL 2003): a
randomised controlled trial   211

High Frequency of Germline *SUFU* Mutations in Children With Desmoplastic/
Nodular Medulloblastoma Younger Than 3 Years of Age   213

G-CSF Receptor Positive Neuroblastoma Subpopulations Are Enriched in
Chemotherapy-Resistant or Relapsed Tumors and Are Highly Tumorigenic   215

Outcome After Surgery Alone or With Restricted Use of Chemotherapy for Patients
With Low-Risk Neuroblastoma: Results of Children's Oncology Group Study
P9641   216

The Use of Computed Tomography in Pediatrics and the Associated Radiation
Exposure and Estimated Cancer Risk   217

High Risk of Symptomatic Cardiac Events in Childhood Cancer Survivors   218

Chapter 13: Sarcoma

Efficacy and safety of regorafenib for advanced gastrointestinal stromal tumours
after failure of imatinib and sunitinib (GRID): an international, multicentre,
randomised, placebo-controlled, phase 3 trial   221

Results of an International Randomized Phase III Trial of the Mammalian Target of
Rapamycin Inhibitor Ridaforolimus Versus Placebo to Control Metastatic
Sarcomas in Patients After Benefit From Prior Chemotherapy   222

Chapter 14: Supportive Care

A combined pain consultation and pain education program decreases average and
current pain and decreases interference in daily life by pain in oncology
outpatients: A randomized controlled trial   225

Cytokine use and survival in the first-line treatment of ovarian cancer:
A Gynecologic Oncology Group Study   227

Chapter 15: Miscellaneous

Suicide and Cardiovascular Death after a Cancer Diagnosis   229

Author Index

A

Abel U, 135
Agarwal S, 215
Aiello Bowles EJ, 62
Ajani JA, 143
Akhter N, 50
Alberts DS, 103
Alberts SR, 123
Alfano CM, 67
Alonzo TA, 209
Alvarez EA, 107
Amini A, 176
Anastassiou D, 5
Anderson GL, 25
Andreotti RF, 101
Ang KK, 196
Ardizzoni A, 173
Ardoino I, 52
Argiris A, 180
Attarbaschi A, 204
Auvinen A, 83
Azim HA Jr, 69

B

Baca SC, 2
Barnette KG, 93
Barry MJ, 97
Baselga J, 63
Bauer HM, 105
Bauer TM, 137
Bauman JE, 187
Beekman R, 146
Benham A, 215
Berger I, 79
Bhatia S, 203
Blackhall F, 170
Blessing JA, 103
Bleyer A, 20, 23
Blinder VS, 71
Body J-J, 18
Boeck S, 138
Boike TP, 77
Bojesen SE, 9
Boni L, 173
Boracchi P, 52
Bourquin J-P, 210
Brady MF, 227
Brady WE, 107
Brooks JD, 96
Brugières L, 213
Bukhanov K, 29

Bullinger L, 155
Burger RA, 114
Burmeister B, 124
Burtness B, 196

C

Campone M, 63
Card A, 55
Cardenes HR, 101
Catalano PJ, 13
Celik I, 129
Chawla SP, 222
Chen H, 1
Cheng WY, 5
Chlebowski RT, 25, 132
Christen WG, 7
Christodouleas JP, 87
Ciuleanu TE, 172
Clark LH, 108
Cleeland CS, 18
Coen JJ, 94
Colombo N, 117
Crawford ED, 76
Creutzig U, 210
Cronin A, 13
Crook JM, 85
Crosby MA, 55

D

Davies C, 27
de Gonzalez AB, 121
Dearnaley D, 81
Debus J, 135
DeFusco PA, 43
Demetri GD, 221, 222
Dias-Santagata D, 164
Dimopoulos M, 117
Ding L, 149
Dizier B, 10
Du J, 145
Duijts SFA, 68
Duncan G, 85

E

Edelman MJ, 167
Eiada R, 29
El-Rayes BF, 137

Elkin EB, 71
Ewing CM, 91

F

Fall K, 229
Fang F, 229
Figueroa ME, 151
Fingeret MC, 189
Fisher RJ, 124
Forastiere AA, 185
Fraser L, 116
Funk MJ, 108

G

Gadner H, 200
Gallagher PM, 97
Gao L, 156
Gapstur SM, 19
Gaudet MM, 19
Gayko U, 209
Gaziano JM, 7
Genden EM, 193
Ghebremichael M, 180
Gilbert J, 180
Gill H, 96
Goldin GH, 90
Gönen M, 151
Gorbunova V, 172
Goss PE, 26
Goulden N, 211
Grothey A, 131
Gunderson LL, 143

H

Hackert T, 140
Haddad R, 179
Hancock ML, 93
Harter P, 118
Hartwig W, 140
Hebestreit K, 147
Heijnsdijk EA, 83
Hensley ML, 111
Hodges JC, 77
Hoffman KE, 83
Holmfeldt L, 149
Hsu DM, 71
Huang HQ, 114
Huang SH, 182
Hudson MM, 199

Hupse R, 40
Hutcheson KA, 189
Hutson K, 50
Hylton NM, 31

I

Ingle JN, 26
Ito K, 71

J

James ND, 75
Jensen K, 189
Jensen M-B, 47
Johansson M, 194
Johnson E, 217
Johnson N, 110
Jung A, 138

K

Kang DR, 165
Kapadia NS, 80
Karlsson E, 57
Katayama R, 163
Kawedia JD, 148
Khan TM, 163
Kim DJ, 165
Kim HR, 165
King CR, 96
Kitchener HC, 110
Klusmann J-H, 202
Ko EM, 108
Komaki R, 176
Kong A, 110
Kopecky KJ, 157
Kreimer AR, 194
Kroman N, 69
Krönke J, 155
Krzakowski M, 170
Kutarska E, 117

L

Lacayo NJ, 209
Landier W, 203
Landrum LM, 103
Lange EM, 91
Lapolla J, 120
Laubender RP, 138
Lawrence MS, 2
Lawton CA, 88
Leath CA III, 106

Lee WR, 88
Lefebvre JL, 183
Lepage B, 159
Levinsen MF, 204
Li X, 137
Li Y, 156
Liao X, 133
Liersch T, 126
Lin H-Y, 120
Lindström LS, 57
Lisse IM, 47
Litton JK, 1
Liu C, 148
Liu J, 55
Lo PC, 162
Lo-Coco F, 152
Lobbes MB, 40
Lochhead P, 133
London WB, 216
Long HJ, 102
Lotan Y, 77
Louahed J, 10
Luo X, 156

M

Maki RG, 111
Manchanda R, 116
Manson JE, 25
Markopoulos C, 17
Martelli G, 52
Martins RG, 187
Maude SL, 3
Mazières J, 159
McCahill LE, 62
McLaughlin JR, 113
McNeely ML, 67
Mechinaud F, 208
Mehra R, 196
Merkel S, 126
Metzger ML, 199
Meyer AM, 90
Miglioretti DL, 217
Mittleman MA, 229
Miyamoto J, 105
Monk BJ, 114
Moody J, 113
Moore DT, 174
Morgans AK, 93

N

Nair S, 123
Ngan SY, 124

Nielsen SF, 9
Niemierko A, 94
Nishihara R, 133
Nishino M, 162
Nordestgaard BG, 9, 59

O

Obdeijn I-M, 35
O'Brien MJ, 128
O'Callaghan CJ, 85
Ojo B, 193
Oldenburg HSA, 68
Oldenmenger WH, 225
Olson K, 80
O'Neill A, 179
O'Sullivan B, 182
Ou Yang TH, 5
Oxnard GR, 162

P

Paesmans M, 69
Paly JJ, 94
Parvathaneni U, 187
Paschka P, 145
Patanwala IY, 105
Patel JP, 151
Pei D, 148
Pession A, 205
Peters S, 159
Petersdorf SH, 157
Pharoah P, 59
Piccart M, 63
Piedmonte MR, 112
Pierron G, 213
Pointreau Y, 183
Pollack CE, 87
Prandi D, 2
Pritchard KI, 26

R

Rabinowits G, 179
Ramalingam SS, 170
Ramlau R, 172
Ray AM, 91
Ray-Coquard I, 222
Ready K, 1
Reinhardt D, 202
Remenieras A, 213
Ren G-X, 186

Rheingold SR, 3
Ricci A Jr, 43
Rizzari C, 208
Roberts KB, 15
Rohde C, 147
Rolland F, 183
Rosell R, 168
Rosen B, 113
Rosenthal AN, 116
Rove KO, 76

S

Sabbatini P, 118
Saida S, 206
Sajid MS, 50
Samulski M, 40
Sanders MA, 146
Sandler HM, 80
Sargent DJ, 123
Sato-Otsubo A, 206
Sauer R, 126
Scambia G, 118
Scaranelo AM, 29
Scher HI, 98
Schlenk RF, 145
Schlichting M, 129
Schmidt J, 135
Schmidt ML, 216
Schmiegelow K, 204
Schneider C-P, 167
Schoen RE, 127
Schonfeld SJ, 121
Schoofs T, 147
Schröder FH, 92
Schwind S, 150
Sequist LV, 164
Sesso HD, 7
Shangguan M, 203
Shaw AT, 160, 163
Shayegi N, 153
Sheets NC, 90
Siegel CL, 101
Sill M, 102
Sillevis Smitt PAE, 225
Simon MS, 132
Single RM, 62
Siu LL, 182
Skinner JS, 97

Slovak M, 157
Socinski MA, 174
Solomon BJ, 160
Soulos PR, 15
Spirtos NM, 112
Spronk S, 35
Stehman FB, 227
Stinchcombe TE, 174
Stopeck A, 18
Straughn JM Jr, 106
Strobel O, 140
Strother DR, 216
Stubblefield MD, 67
Sumo G, 81
Sun J, 19
Swisher-McClure S, 87
Syndikus I, 81

T

Teachey DT, 3
Tejpar S, 129
Teleanu V, 155
Teng MS, 193
Tewari KS, 102
Thigpen JT, 227
Tilanus-Linthorst MMA, 35
Tiseo M, 173
Trabulsi EJ, 76
Tsai C-M, 167
Tvedskov TF, 47

U

Ulloa-Montoya F, 10

V

Valkhof MG, 146
van Beurden M, 68
van Dalen EC, 218
van de Velde CJH, 17
van de Water W, 17
van Delden E, 218
van der Pal HJ, 218
van Montfort CAGM, 225

Vermorken JB, 190
Visvanathan K, 121
Vora A, 211

W

Wactawski-Wende J, 132
Wade R, 211
Walker JL, 107, 112
Waltman BA, 164
Watanabe K, 206
Waterboer T, 194
Wathen JK, 111
Weber RS, 185
Weeks JC, 13
Wehrberger C, 79
Weinstein HJ, 199
Weischer M, 59
Welch HG, 20, 23
Welsh JW, 176
Wenham RM, 120
Wever EM, 83
Wilking UM, 57
Williams A, 217
Willinger M, 79
Wilt TJ, 86
Winawer SJ, 128
Winter KA, 143

Y

Yan Y, 88
Yeap BY, 160
Yu JB, 15

Z

Zauber AG, 128
Zhang C-P, 186
Zhang J, 149
Zhang Q, 185
Zhong L-P, 186
Zhu Q, 43
Zimmermann M, 202, 210
Zwaan CM, 208

Printed and bound by CPI Group (UK) Ltd, Croydon, CR0 4YY

08/05/2025

01864755-0002